AF616672

Combating CANCER

Diagnosis, Therapy and Nanomedicine

Combating CANCER

Diagnosis, Therapy and Nanomedicine

HD Kumar, PhD
Varanasi, India

Swati Kumar, MD
Milwaukee, Wisconsin, USA

Vitasta Publishing Pvt. Ltd.
New Delhi

Published by
Vitasta Publishing Pvt. Ltd.
2/15, Ansari Road, Daryaganj,
New Delhi – 110 002

ISBN 81-89766-44-9

Disclaimer

The information contained in this book is for general educational purposes and for use by biologists, biotechnologists and the medical fraternity. Neither the authors nor the publisher give any warranty on accuracy, completeness, functionality, usefulness or other assurances as to such information. They disclaim all responsibility for any loss, damage to property or personal injury suffered directly or indirectly from reliance on such information. Individuals who wish to adopt or use any of the methods, techniques, prescriptions, or suggestions contained in the book must first consult qualified medical practitioners and oncologists and seek their expert advice.

Typeset and cover design by Vitasta Publishing Pvt. Ltd., New Delhi
Printed at Saurabh Printers Pvt. Ltd., New Delhi

Contents

Contents

Preface

Cancer is a dreaded disease all over the world. Its incidence has been rising at an alarming rate in rapidly developing countries such as China and India where life expectancy is increasing substantially. The incidence shows global variations, suggesting that different risk factors operate in different parts of the world. These risks are mostly related to lifestyle and diet but viruses and parasites may also be causative agents in some cases.

Everywhere, prevention is advocated as the best strategy. Anti-smoking campaigns and healthful diets rich in nutraceuticals and antioxidants can prove highly effective preventatives. Recent researches have suggested that the wonder vitamin (vitamin D) protects against several internal cancers.

To look for natural plant, animal and microbial products and exploit their properties has been the mainstay of the biotechnology industries. In drug discovery, for instance, novel natural products with interesting structures and biological attributes are being increasingly reported. Without such discoveries, a significant therapeutic deficit can take place in several important clinical areas including cancer, especially solid tumours and immune-inflammatory diseases.

Molecular genetics, robotics, miniaturization, massively parallel preparation and detection systems, and automatic data analysis drive the search for drug-discovery leads, while modern 'omics' technologies and use of suitable biomarkers have materially assisted medical researchers and physicians in effective diagnosis of various cancers.

Exciting developments and explosive progress in nanoscience, nanotechnology, nanobiotechnology and nanomedicine are now impacting research in all aspects of cancer. Various kinds of nanoparticles are being explored for use in biomedical applications, including diagnosis and therapy of cancers.

Nanoengineering of particle surfaces to carry payloads, ligands or drugs to identified targets is attracting keen interest of oncologists. Monolayer protected nanoparticles, magnetic nanoparticles, plasmonically heated gold nanoparticles, nanoshell-enabled photonics-based imaging and therapy of cancer, and nanosized medicines based on polymer conjugates exemplify some hot areas in cancer nanotechnology today.

Cancer stem cells, structure and selection of viral carbohydrates and their possible use for drug and vaccine design, cancer epigenetics, and companion diagnostics for mutation-targeted cancer therapies are also emerging as prospective strategies for combating cancer. Several of these and other emerging techniques are futuristic or in the pipeline. Many of them may well mature in the coming few years and, following clinical trials, could potentially reach the clinic when they could change the way how cancer is identified and treated.

We have attempted to summarize briefly the current status of research in the fast-moving areas listed above as also in some allied and associated aspects of cancer diagnostics and biomedicine. Rather than covering older and historical aspects, we have focused on issues of current interest and emerging possibilities hovering on the near-term biomedical horizon, for informing students, teachers and researchers in medicine (allopathy and ayurveda), oncology, immunology, pathology (diagnostics), nanobiotechnology and the practising physicians.

HD Kumar
Swati Kumar

Preface

Cancer is a dreaded disease all over the world. Its incidence has been rising at an alarming rate in rapidly developing countries such as China and India where life expectancy is increasing substantially. The incidence shows wide variations, suggesting that different risk factors operate in different [illegible]. These risk factors are mostly related to lifestyle and diet but viruses and parasites may also be causative agents in some cases.

Everywhere, prevention is advocated as the best strategy. Avoiding smoking, and engaging in healthful diets rich in nutraceuticals and antioxidants, have proved highly effective preventatives. Recent researches have suggested that the sunshine vitamin (vitamin D) protects against several internal cancers.

To look for natural plant, animal and microbial products and to exploit their properties has been the mainstay of the biotechnology industries. In drug discovery, for instance, novel natural products with interesting structures and biological attributes are being increasingly [illegible]. Without such discoveries, a significant therapeutic deficit can take place in several important clinical areas including cancer, especially solid tumours and [illegible] inflammatory diseases.

[illegible] parallel preparation and [illegible] systems [illegible] which modern [illegible] medical research and [illegible] that hosts of [illegible].

Exciting developments and explosive progress in nanoscience, nanotechnology, nanobiotechnology and nanomedicine are now impacting research in all aspects of cancer. Various kinds of nanoparticles are being explored for use in biomedical applications, including diagnosis and therapy of cancers.

Newer approaches [illegible] to identi- [illegible]

Cancer stem [illegible] use [illegible] and [illegible] design, cancer [illegible] and [illegible] targeted cancer therapies are also [illegible] combating cancer. Several of these and other emerging techniques are [illegible] the pipeline. Many of them may well mature in the coming few years and, following clinical trials, could potentially [illegible] how they could change the way [illegible] identified and treated.

We have attempted to summarize briefly the current status of research in the fast moving areas listed above as also in some allied and associated aspects of cancer diagnosis and biomedicine. Rather than covering old and historic aspects, we have focused on topics of current interest and emerging possibilities, [illegible] on the near-term biomedical horizon, for informing students, teachers and researchers in medicine (allopathy and ayurveda), oncology, immunology, pathology, diagnostics, nanobiotechnology and the practising physicians.

HD Kumar
Swati Kumar

Acknowledgements

For writing this monograph, we have depended inter alia, on the literature supplied by the Indian National Science Academy, New Delhi.

We thank all those who very kindly provided reprints, newsletters, monographs and other gray literature from time to time.

We also thank several leading experts and active researchers who very kindly granted permission to reproduce some of their published illustrations (figures or tables).

HD Kumar is indebted to his friends ON Srivastava, Ashok Kumar, SP Vyas, Vinay Sharma and TS Misra for help from time to time. He also thanks the members and Chairman of the UNEP Panel on Environmental Effects of Ozone Depletion for their suggestions and support since 1989.

The bulk of the material in this monograph has been written by HD Kumar. Swati Kumar contributed significantly through several discussions and correspondence and by making available many reviews and research papers published in journals not otherwise easily accessible in Varanasi.

The senior author HD Kumar alone is, however, responsible for any errors of commission or omission, or for any other flaws in the book. We would welcome any criticism or suggestions for improvement.

We thank our publisher Renu Kaul Verma, Managing Director, Vitasta Publishing Pvt. Ltd., KK Raman, Editor–Science and Production Manager, and other staff of Vitasta Publishing Pvt. Ltd., for their keen interest, critical editing and high quality production of the book.

Several drafts of the monograph were patiently typed and composed by Rang Nath Singh, whose ardent support and diligence has helped making this a reality.

Abbreviations

[25(OH)D]	25-hydroxyvitamin D
Abl	Abelson leukaemia
ADCC	Antibody-dependent cell-mediated cytotoxicity
Ag:Ab	Antigen:antibody
AKs	Actinic keratoses
ALL	Acute lymphoblastic leukaemia
AMPK	AMP-activating protein kinase
APC	Adenomatous polyposis coli
APCs	Antigen-presenting cells
APML	Acute promyelocytic leukaemia
AR	Androgen receptor
BC	Breast cancer
BCBLs	Body cavity based lymphomas
BCC	Basal cell carcinoma
BCG	Bacillus Calmette–Guerin
BCR/Ig	B receptor
BCR-ABL	Breakpoint cluster region–Abelson
BCS	BC-specific survival
BDNF	Brain-derived neutrotrophic factor
bFGF	Basic fibroblast growth factor
BFP	Blue fluorescent protein
BioMEMS	Biological microelectronic mechanical systems
BKV	BK virus
BL	Burkitt's lymphoma
BRMs	Biological response modifiers
CAFs	Carcinoma-associated fibroblasts

CALI	Chromophore-assisted laser inactivation
CAM	Cell-adhesion molecule
CAST	Cardiac arrhythmic suppression trial
CCAT	Cancer complementary and alternative therapies
CDC	Complement dependent cytotoxicity
CDGE	Common disease genetic and epigenetic hypothesis
CE	Capillary electrophoresis
CEA	Carcinoembryonic antigen
CFTR	Cystic fibrosis transmembrane conductance regulator
CGA	Cancer genome atlas
ChAT	Choline acetyltransferase
CHHFBC	Collaborative group on hormonal factors in breast cancer
CM	Cutaneous melanoma
CML	Chronic myeloid leukaemia
CMV	Cytomegalovirus
CNS	Central nervous system
CNT	Carbon nanotube
COX2	Cyclooxygenase 2
CPDs	Cyclobutane pyrimidine dimers
CRC	Colorectal cancer
CT	Computed tomography
CTCs	Circulating tumour cells
CTLs	Cytotoxic T-lymphocytes
CTVT	Canine transmissible venereal tumour
DACH	Diaminocyclohexane
DCs	Dendritic cells
DDFS	Distant disease-free survival
DEN	Diethylnitrosamine
DIGE	Differential in-gel electrophoresis
Dll4	Notch ligand Delta-like 4
DLA	Dog leukocyte antigen
DMR	Differentially methylated region

DSBs	Double strand breaks
dsDNA	Double-stranded DNA
DTPA	Diethylenetriaminepentaacetic
EBV	Epstein–Barr virus
ECG	Electrocardiogram
EGF	Epidermal growth factor
EGFR	Epidermal growth factor receptor
EMT	Epithelial-mesenchymal transition
EPCs	Endothelial precursor cells
EPR	Enhanced permeability and retention
EPXs	Endoperoxides
ER	Estrogen receptor
ERBB2	E-rb-b2 erythroblastic leukaemia viral oncogene homolog 2
ERK	Extracellular signal-regulated kinase
ESCs	Embryonic stem cells
ESL	Evidence suggesting lack of carcinogenicity
ESTs	Expressed sequence tags
EXAFS	Extended X-ray absorption fine structure
f-CNT	Functionalized CNT
FDA	Federal Drug Administration
FDCs	Follicular dendritic cells
FETs	Field effect transistors
FGF	Fibroblast growth factor
FGFR	Fibroblast growth factor receptors
FGFs	Fibroblast growth factors
FISH	Fluorescent in situ hybridization
FITC	Fluorescein isothiocyanate
f-MWNT	Functionalized MWNT
FRET	Fluorescence resonance energy transfer
FRs	Folate receptors
f-SWNT	Functionalized SWNT
GalNAc	N-acetyl-galactosamine core

GARBAN	Genome analysis and rapid biological annotation
GCC	Guanylyl cyclase C
G-CSF	Granulocyte colony-stimulating factor
GFP	Green fluorescent protein
GIST	Gastrointestinal stromal tumours
HGF	Hepatocyte growth factor
HIF	Hypoxia-inducible factor
HIV	Human immunodeficiency virus
HLA	Human leukocyte antigen
HNPCC	Hereditary non-polyposis colon carcinoma
hnRNP-K	Heterogenous nuclear ribonucleoprotein K
HPMA	N-(2-hydroxypropyl) methacrylamide
HPV	Human papilloma virus
HPVs	Human papillomaviruses
HRTEM	High-resolution transmission electron microscope
HSC	Hematopoietic stem cell
HSV	Herpes simplex virus
iAb-lib	Intracellular antibody library
IBDs	Inflammatory bowel diseases
ICA	Independent component analysis
IFN-α	Interferon-α
IGFs	Insulin-like growth factors
IHC	Immunohistochemistry
IL-13α	Interleukin 13 receptor-α
IL-6	Interleukin-6
IMAC-LC-MS/MS	Immobilized metal-affinity chromatography combined with liquid chromatography-tandem mass spectrometry
iPSCs	Induced pluripotent stem cells
JCV	JC virus
KLH	Keyhole limpet haemocyanin
KS	Kaposi's sarcoma
KSHV	Kaposi's sarcoma-associated herpesvirus

LAB	Lactic acid bacteria
LC-MS/MS	Liquid chromatography-tandem mass spectrometry
LHRH	Luteinising hormone-releasing hormone
LOC	Laboratory-on-a-chip
LOH	Loss of heterozygosity
LOI	Loss of imprinting
LPS	Lipopolysaccharide
MAbs	Monoclonal antibodies
MAC	Membrane attack complex
MAPK	Mitogen-activated protein kinase
MAQC	Micro-array quality control
MC1R	Melanocortin 1 receptor
MCD	Multicentric Castelman's disease
MDC1	Mediator of DNA damage checkpoint 1
MEFs	Mouse embryonic fibroblasts
MHC	Major histocompatibility complex
MITF	Micro-ophthalmia-associated transcription factor
MLL	Mixed lineage leukaemia gene
MMPs	Matrix metalloproteases
MMTV	Mouse mammary tumour virus
MPCs	Monolayer-protected clusters
MpNPs	Monolayer-protected nanoparticles
MRI	Magnetic resonance imaging
MSP	Macrophage-stimulating protein
MST1R	Macrophage-stimulating 1 receptor
mtDNA	Mitochondrial DNA
MT-SP1	Membrane-type serine protease 1
Mw	Molecular weight
MWNT	Multiwalled CNT
NCAM	Neural CAM
NDV	Newcastle disease virus
NIR	Near infrared

NIRF	Near-infrared fluorescence imaging
NK	Natural killer
NMSC	Non-melanoma skin cancer
NPC	Nasopharyngeal carcinoma
NPs	Nanoparticles
NrCAM	Neuronal CAM
NSCLC	Non-small cell lung carcinoma
NWs	Nanowires
ONC	Oncogene
Osbpy	Tris(2'2-bipyridyl) dichloroosmium (II)
PAR1	Protease-activated receptor 1
PARP	Poly(ADP-ribose) polymerase
PCA	Principal component analysis
PDEPT	Polymer-directed enzyme pro-drug therapy
PDFs	Pair distribution functions
PDGFR	Platelet-derived growth factor receptor
PDMS	Polydimethylsiloxane
PDT	Photodynamic therapy
PEG	Poly(ethylene) glycol
pEGFP	Plasmid encoding EGFP
PELs	Primary effusion lymphomas
PET	Positron emission tomography
PGA	Poly(glutamic) acid
PGCs	Primordial germ cells
PI3K	Phosphoinositide 3-kinase
PIP_2	Phosphatidylinositol 4,5-bisphosphate
PIP_3	Phosphatidylinositol 3,4,5-triphosphate
PML	Progressive multifocal leukoencephalopathy
PSA	Prostate-specific antigen
PSK	Polysaccharide-K
PSMA	Prostate-specific membrane antibody
PSP	Polysaccharide-P

PSVs	Pseudoviruses
PTEN	Phosphatase and tensin homologue
PTES	Phenyltriethoxysilane
PyMT	Polyomavirus middle T antigen
QDs (q.ds)	Quantum dots
qRT-PCR	Quantitative reverse transcription polymerase chain reaction
R6G	Rhodamine 6G
RA	Rheumatoid arthritis
RAP80	Receptor-associated protein 80
RES	Reticuloendothelial system
ROS	Reactive oxygen species
RTD	Resistive temperature detector
RTK	Receptor tyrosine kinase
Rubpy	Tris(2'2-bipyridyl)dichlororuthenium(II)
SAGE	Serial analysis of gene expression
SARMs	Selective androgen-receptor modulators
SAXS	Small-angle X-ray scattering
SBT	Streptovidin-binding protein
SCC	Squamous cell carcinoma
scFv	Single chain Fv
SCLC	Small cell lung carcinoma
SELDI-MS	Surface-enhanced laser desorption ionization mass spectrometry
SEREX	Serological analysis of recombinant cDNA expression libraries
SERMs	Selective oestrogen-receptor modulators
shRNA	Short-hairpin RNA
siRNA	Short-interfering RNA
SMANCS	Poly(styrene-co-maleic anhydride)-neocarzinostatin
SNPs	Single nucleotide polymorphisms
SPECT	Single-photon emission CT
SPIO	Superparamagnetic iron oxides
ssDNA	Single-stranded DNA

SWNT	Single-walled CNT
TAAs	Tumour-associated antigens
TAMs	Tumour-associated macrophages
TEM	Transmission electron microscope
TEOS	Tetraethyl orthosilicate
TGF-β1	Transforming growth factor-β1
TGF-β	Transforming growth factor
TILS	Tumour-infiltrating T lymphocytes
TLR	Toll-like receptors
TMA	Tissue micro-array
TMZ	Temozolomide
TNF-α	Tumour necrosis factor-α
TOR	Target of rapamycin
TPs	Tumour touch preps
TRAFs	Tumour necrosis factor receptor associated factors
TRAP	Tartrate-resistant acid phosphatase
TSG	Tumour-suppressor gene
uPA	Urokinase plasminogen activator
USPIO	Ultrasmall superparamagnetic iron oxides
VCAM1	Vascular cell-adhesion molecule 1
VEGF	Vascular endothelial growth factor
VEGFR	Vascular endothelial growth factor receptor
vGPCR	Viral G-protein-coupled receptor
VLPs	Virus-like particles
VPCs	Vector producer cells
VSV	Vesicular stomatitis virus
VTES	Triethoxyvinylsilane
Xp	Xeroderma pigmentosum
YFP	Yellow fluorescent protein

1 Understanding Cancer

Introduction

Cancer is not only a most tragic disease but also most enigmatic. A cancerous tumour is very well adapted for survival in its own horrible way—its cells go on dividing long after normal cells stop dividing. Tumour cells destroy adjoining tissues to make room for themselves. They somehow induce the body to supply them with energy which they need for their growth. The tumours that afflict us are no alien parasites resorting to elegant strategies for attacking our bodies. Rather, they are made of our own cells that have turned against us. Nor does cancer exemplify some bizarre rarity. While a woman in the US has a 39 per cent chance of being diagnosed with some type of cancer in her lifetime, a man has 45 per cent chances (Zimmer, 2007).

Essentially, cancer is a disease of multicellularity. The complex, multicellular bodies of vertebrate animals evolved by the emergence of new genes that could control how cells divided—such as by stopping the cells' reproduction once an organ attained its adult size. But bodies also present a great risk. Whenever a body-cell divides, its DNA has a small chance of acquiring a cancer-causing mutation. Whenever a cell divides, it is at some risk of developing into cancer. Rare mutations can sometimes cause a cell to lose restraint and to continue to multiply uncontrollably. Other mutations can aggravate the problem by allowing deranged cells to invade surrounding tissues and spread through the body. Or they may allow tumour cells to evade the immune system or attract blood vessels that can supply fresh oxygen (Zimmer, 2007).

Cancer-causing changes to DNA allow some cells to reproduce more effectively than non-cancerous cells. But although our bodies are vulnerable to cancer, they also carry some potential to obstruct it by adopting various strategies. One of the most effective defensive strategies is tumour suppressor proteins. Some of these proteins prevent cancer by monitoring how a cell reproduces. If the cell multiplies abnormally, the proteins either induce it to die or to become senescent. The cell can then survive but can no longer divide. Though tumour suppressor proteins play a crucial role in our survival, it has also recently emerged that in some respects, we would be better off without them (see Crespi and Summers, 2005, 2006; Zimmer, 2007).

The word cancer does not refer to just one disease. It encompasses about a hundred different entities. It is a class of diseases or disorders characterized by uncontrolled division of cells and their ability to invade other tissues, either by direct growth into adjacent tissue through 'invasion' or by implantation into distant sites by 'metastasis'. Cancer exemplifies a remarkably complex disease that affects nearly every tissue lineage in our bodies. It arises from normal cells as a consequence of various mutations affecting many genes. It is widespread and often lethal. Basic cancer research, including molecular biology, biochemistry, cancer genomics and proteomics, attempts to sort out the similarities and differences amongst all these entities. The unregulated growth usually results from some damage to DNA or mutations in genes that code for proteins controlling cell division. These mutations may be induced by:

- Chemical or physical agents called 'carcinogens';
- Exposure to radioactive materials;
- Heredity or genetic factors;
- Viruses that insert their DNA into the human genome;
- Environmental factors such as pollution and alcohol.

Based on this basic research, clinical trials are carried out and usually entail testing new treatments, such as a new drug on patients with a certain cancer. New drugs (sunitinib, sorafenib) have been developed to prolong the lives of patients suffering from kidney cancer that has spread widely in the body. These drugs differ from cisplatinum and vinorelbine used to cure patients who have undergone surgery for early lung cancer.

The conventional treatment of cancer includes surgery, chemotherapy, immunotherapy, radiation therapy or hormonal suppression. Unfortunately, these therapies have significant side effects, including leucopenia, thrombocytopenia, hair loss, nausea and vomiting, diarrhoea, reverse acidity, poor appetite, anaemia and other related immunocompromised disorders. Even after treatment, the chances of a relapse are quite high.

While for many subsets of cancer, cure is possible, for some others, lives can be prolonged. Over half a century ago, breast cancer used to be treated by surgery alone. Usually, women were not given any additional treatment (adjuvants) after the surgery. At least 75 per cent of the patients relapsed and eventually died of advanced metastatic disease.

Forty-five years ago, the first chemotherapy trials were started with CMF (three-drug combination of cyclophosphamide, methotrexate and 5-fluorouracil). Tamoxifen, an anti-oestrogen drug, was introduced for treating early breast cancer almost three decades ago. But about 50 per cent of the patients relapsed after the treatment. Of course, each subset of early breast cancer patients experienced a different relapse rate, reinforcing the fact that cancer is a very heterogeneous disease.

Later, many more and effective chemotherapy agents such as Doxorubicin, paclitaxel and docetaxel were developed. Hormonal therapy with greater efficacy and less side effects based on the aromatase inhibitors (anastrozole, letrozole, exemestane), was introduced in the late 1990s.

Trastuzumab is a highly effective targeted therapy. It was initially shown to work very well in advanced breast cancer. A 50 per cent response rate was obtained and lives were prolonged. It was naturally inferred that it should work even better in early breast cancer cases where the tumour load is much smaller.

Yet, four randomized clinical trials were conducted at a cost of over US $1 billion to know if this drug will also work in cases of early breast cancer. The findings of these trials conclusively proved that Trastuzumab works very well in early breast cancer. It targets tumours in 20 per cent of women whose breast cancer expresses the HER2 receptor. It was introduced only a few years ago. Today, the overall relapse rate for early breast cancer has come down to 30 per cent. The advent of new technologies and biotechnological advances has led to the development of improved treatments such as monoclonal antibodies (MAbs). MAbs, that bind only to cancer cell specific antigens and induce an immunological response against the target cancer cells, provide a good treatment option.

The hallmarks of cancer and the principles of tumour development are well-known: self-sufficiency in growth signals, insensitivity to anti-growth signals, evading apoptosis, limitless potential to replicate, induction of angiogenesis, invasion and metastasis. Recent researches have thrown light on how tumours become resistant to targeted therapy (Weinberg, 2006).

Weinberg described a good example of the inhibition of pancreatic cancer and medulloblastoma growth (through targeting of the signalling protein Hedgehog), starting with the story of sheep flocks grazing on corn lily, whose offspring developed malformations including cyclopia. This led to the isolation of cyclopamine and the subsequent discovery of mutations in the *patched* and *sonic hedgehog* genes, as well as new analogues of cyclopamine that inhibit these. The tumour's microenvironment (including the interactions between the seed and the soil) became an independent hallmark of cancer, along with immunoediting, the crosstalk between tumour niche and host immunity. The master regulators of certain processes of development (Slug and Twist) were linked to cancer metastases (Boshoff, 2006).

In some cases, alterations in glycolytic pathways and mitochondrial respiration are involved in tumourigenesis. Epigenetic changes could also be involved in cancer, as also the role of cancer micro RNAs in tumour development, diagnosis and classification. Autophagy (a vacuolar process of cytoplasmic degradation) sometimes contributes to oncogenesis.

Some notable challenges and problems ahead are: for example, if micro metastases are attracted to an environment where they can flourish, why are recurrences of renal cancer not centred on the other kidney? How can we relieve the elevated interstitial pressure inside tumours, which has hindered attempts to deliver therapeutics effectively? And, despite the potential of mechanism-based therapeutics and pharmacogenetics, the best predictor of survival after treatment of lung cancer with an anti-EGFR inhibitor is the 'still smoking status' (Boshoff, 2006).

We are now on the verge of advancing from cancer treatment that uses toxic chemicals to kill malignant cells, a strategy that causes great havoc to the patient's physiology, towards a more specific and gentler, patient-tailored approach. Converting cancer into a chronic, controllable illness is becoming a definite possibility. However, this will still take some more time to become a reality. In the meanwhile, the best preventative strategy is to avoid smoking and eat only healthy diets based mostly on plants, vegetables, fruits and herbs. The right diet may not cure cancer but it can certainly prevent it in healthy individuals.

French fries, car exhaust, and noxious fumes from diesel-operated generators can contain dangerous compounds that cause breast cancer. A new two-part database from the Silent Spring Institute, Newton, Massachusetts, lists various suspect chemicals and lifestyle factors, including obesity, that may be involved in breast cancer.

Researchers analysed toxicity data to compile a roster of 216 compounds that trigger mammary tumours in animal tests. For chemicals such as acrylamide, a byproduct of cooking starchy foods, the site offers information on uses, routes of exposure, and health risks. The database also summarizes and appraises the methodology of 450 studies on links between human breast cancer and non-genetic factors (see *sciencereview. silentspring. org*).

Carcinogenicity and Epidemiology

The term 'carcinogen' denotes an exposure that can increase the incidence of malignant neoplasms. The induction of benign neoplasms can, under certain circumstances, contribute to the judgement that the exposure is carcinogenic. The terms 'neoplasm' and 'tumour' are often used interchangeably.

Several epidemiological and experimental studies have indicated that different agents may act at different stages in the carcinogenic process. Also, several different mechanisms can be involved in this process.

Three types of epidemiological investigations of cancer are involved in assessing carcinogenicity in humans—cohort studies, case-control studies, and correlation or ecological studies. Occasionally, results from randomized trials may be considered.

Cohort and case-control studies relate individual exposures under study to the occurrence of cancer in individuals and give an estimate of relative risk (measured as the ratio of incidence/mortality in people exposed, to incidence/mortality in those not exposed) as the chief parameter of association.

Correlation studies are usually conducted on whole populations in a particular geographical area at a particular time, and cancer frequency is related to a summary value of the exposure of the population to the agent, mixture or exposure condition being investigated (see IARC, 1994).

Most human carcinogens that have been critically studied in some experimental animals have also produced positive results in one or more animal species. For some agents (e.g., aflatoxins, n-aminobiphenyl, betel quid with tobacco, chlorambucil, coal-tar pitches, coal-tars, mustard gas, nonsteroidal oestrogens, solar radiation, thiotepa and vinyl chloride, etc.), carcinogenicity in experimental animals was established or strongly suspected before epidemiological studies confirmed the carcinogenicity in humans (Vainio et al., 1994).

Quite often, exposures are to some extent complex and include both occupational and industrial exposures. For these, chemical composition and the potential contribution of carcinogens known to be present need critical consideration. The extent to which the materials tested in experimental systems are related to those to which humans are exposed also needs to be determined.

Finally, all the available evidence should be considered holistically. This will allow an overall evaluation of the carcinogenicity to humans of an agent, mixture or circumstance of exposure. Some chemical compounds have already been evaluated and found to be carcinogenic. Some others that are related to these carcinogens may also possibly be carcinogenic, even though there may be no direct evidence of capacity to induce cancer either in humans or in animals. An agent, mixture or exposure circumstance can then be classified into one of the following groups:

Group I : The agent (mixture) is carcinogenic to humans. The exposure circumstance entails exposures that are carcinogenic to humans.

Group II : Agents, mixtures and exposure circumstances for which, at one extreme, the evidence of carcinogenicity in humans is *almost* sufficient, as well those for which, at the other extreme, there are no human data, but for which there is evidence of carcinogenicity in experimental animals.

Group II A : The agent or mixture is *probably* carcinogenic to humans. The exposure circumstance entails exposures that are *probably* carcinogenic to humans.

Table 1.1 Evaluation of 14 industrial chemicals for possible carcinogenicity (after IARC, 1994).

Agent	Degree of evidence of carcinogenicity		Overall evaluation of carcinogenicity to humans
	Human	Animal	
Ethylene	I	I	3
Ethylene oxide	L	S	1[b]
Propylene	I	I	3
Propylene oxide	I	S	2B
Isoprene	I[a]	S	2B
Styrene	I	L	2B[b]
Styrene-7,8-oxide	I[a]	S	2A[b]
4-Vinylcyclohexene	I[a]	S	2B
4-Vinylcyclohexene diepoxide	I[a]	S	2B
Venyl toluene	I[a]	ESL	3
Acrylamide	I	S	2A[b]
N-Methylolacrylamide	I[a]	L	3
Methyl methacrylate	I	ESL	3
2-Ethylhexyl acrylate	I[a]	L	3

S, sufficient evidence; L, limited evidence; I, inadequate evidence; ESL, evidence suggesting lack of carcinogenicity

[a] No data available

[b] Other relevant data taken into account in making the overall evaluation

Group II B : The agent (mixture) may *possibly* be carcinogenic to humans. The exposure circumstance involves exposures that are *possibly* carcinogenic to humans.

Group III : The agent (mixture or exposure circumstance) is not classifiable as to its carcinogenicity to humans.

Group IV : The agent (mixture) is *probably not* carcinogenic to humans.

Table 1.1 gives a summary of carcinogenicity evaluations made on 14 different industrial chemicals.

Molecular Oncology

Although the rate of mortality from cancer has changed very little over the past half a century, the picture has started improving. Targeted cancer therapies, cancer biomarkers, and genomic medicine are now undergoing a transition from hype to clinical reality. Cancer may soon be described in molecular terms which could well improve the ways in which cancers are detected, classified, monitored, and treated. The molecular description of cancer could soon form the basis of a new patient-centred model of cancer care.

Current efforts suffer from some limitations to identify and validate molecularly based biomarkers for cancer diagnosis and treatment, and new molecular imaging technologies can potentially empower future models of cancer care (see Varmus, 2006; Weissleder, 2006).

Unfortunately, the impact of the new generation of molecularly targeted therapies on overall cancer mortality rates is at present negligible—imatinib is effective only in CML and a few other relatively uncommon cancers. The new therapies are often called 'targeted', but in fact are no more targeted than the conventional chemotherapies that interfere with DNA replication, DNA repair, or mitotic machineries, or radiotherapies that damage DNA in a focused field. The new class of treatments are usually highly specific for individual cancers, reflecting the particular mutations responsible for that tumour or variations in gene expression—distinctive molecular attributes that are increasingly used to subdivide cancers assigned to the same standard histopathological subtype (Bild et al., 2006).

Some of these attributes are the presence or absence of receptors that bind to hormones or to derivative antagonists; the efficient expression of genes encoding cell surface proteins recognized by antibodies that may inhibit cancer cells; or the activation of intracellular signalling pathways by mutant proteins that are sensitive to molecule-specific drugs (Varmus, 2006).

Cancer Mutation Discovery

Considerable progress has occurred in identifying the molecular genetic events which underlie cancer. For most malignancies, the accumulation of somatic mutations within specific genes results in neoplastic development; usually the effect is erratic inactivation of tumour suppressors or constitutive activation of oncogenes (see Bodmer, 2006). In fact, the accumulation of mutations not only causes cancer in many cases but also contributes to cancer phenotype, such as, a general aggressiveness as found in recurrence and resistance to molecular targeted therapies. These cancer-related genes have many functions, e.g., growth regulation, adhesion, cell cycle control, DNA repair processes, and other cellular processes mediated by various signal transduction pathways (Dahl et al., 2007).

Mutations that lead to drug sensitivity or resistance have been discovered in such specific kinases as the EGFR gene (Paez et al., 2004). Further work on comprehensive mutation discovery from individual genomes will enhance our understanding of the genetics underlying any individual tumour's phenotype. This mutation profile could potentially translate into valuable prognostic and predictive genetic biomarkers (Dahl et al., 2007).

Dahl et al. have developed a procedure for massively parallel resequencing of multiple human genes by combining a highly multiplexed and target-specific amplification process with a high throughput parallel sequencing technology. The amplification process is based on oligonucleotide constructs, called selectors, which guide the circularization of specific DNA target regions. The circularized target sequences are then amplified in multiplex and analysed by using a highly parallel sequencing-by-synthesis technology. Parallel resequencing of 10 cancer genes covering 177 exons with average sequence coverage per sample of 93 per cent was also demonstrated. Seven cancer cell lines and one normal genomic DNA sample were studied with multiple mutations and polymorphisms identified among the 10 genes. Mutations and polymorphisms in the *TP53* gene could be confirmed by traditional sequencing.

Already, massively parallel sequencing technologies have been proposed for making fast and cost-efficient mutation scans of complete human genomes. Dahl et al. have now proposed to combine such technologies with methods for sequence-specific multiplex amplification to resequence genomic regions of particular interest as, for instance, the coding sequences of cancer-related genes. For various applications, this concept may prove useful including lower cost and greater sequencing depth per target than whole-genome sequencing (Dahl et al., 2007).

Attacking Cancer Cells Indirectly

A clear understanding of the tissue environment in which cancers grow is generating novel opportunities to develop therapies that are not targeted at the tumour cells themselves. The best example of these approaches is the anti-angiogenic strategy, for which drugs and antibodies have already been approved by the US Food and Drug Administration (Ferrara and Kerbel, 2005).

There is also considerable potential for other approaches that address the tumour's milieu: (i) by interfering with growth-promoting signals supplied by non-neoplastic ,stromal cells, that surround a tumour; (ii) by inhibiting specific proteases that adjust a tumour's environs to promote the dangerous escape of tumour cells into circulation or by using those proteases to activate molecules that are useful for imaging tumours; and (iii) by promoting an immune response against tumour cells, for example, by inactivating factors, such as the T cell surface protein (CTLA-4), that restricts the immune response to cancer cells (see Grimm et al., 2005).

Despite these optimistic developments, however, it will take several years before they enter clinical practise. Until then, surgery, chemotherapy, radiation, histopathology, and conventional imaging may continue to be the staples of cancer care. Fortunately, they too are becoming more effective, even without any molecular advances, through image-guided and minimally invasive surgery, positron emission tomography—computed tomography scanning, dose-modulated radiotherapy, and other technologies (Varmus, 2006).

Some other methods to prevent or control cancer have also been developed, improved, or popularized. Important strategies for prevention are exemplified by smoking cessation programmes, vaccines against cancer-promoting viruses (hepatitis B and papilloma viruses), and methods for detection of pre-malignant lesions and early cancers (e.g., colonoscopies, mammography, and PAP smears). Neurotropic medications are used to control the ancillary symptoms of cancer, most obviously pain and nausea; haematopoietic growth factors can be employed to weaken the side effects of cytotoxic treatments, such as anaemia and leucopenia; and psychosocial methods can likewise be used to manage the response of patients and families to the diagnosis and treatment of cancers.

Autophagy

Some emerging research areas are attracting much attention. Researchers are now re-examining an old idea to determine how tumours fuel their own growth with a view to finding new ways to cut off their energy supply.

Garber (2006) described how an old discredited idea—that tumour cells depend on glycolysis for energy—has been revived and is catalysing the development of new anti-cancer drugs. Cells rely on autophagy to recycle their components. Some evidence suggests that this "self-eating" suppresses tumour development. But other data suggests that autophagy promotes tumour development and actually protects cancer cells from treatments. Marx (2006) critically reviewed the debate over whether the cellular recycling process called autophagy is a tumour suppressor or promoter. Autophagy means the degradation of unwanted, surplus or defective cell components. It not only acts as a part of a cell's normal routine activities but also as a response to various stresses. It is linked with cellular life-and-death decisions and with cancer (Levine, 2007).

The need for autophagy arises when cells have to 'self-cannibalize' or degrade their constituents. Suitable levels of autophagy appear to occur in most normal cells for preventing the accumulation of protein aggregates and defective cellular substructures. Some environmental stimuli (e.g., starvation, high temperature, low oxygen, etc.) or intracellular stresses (damaged organelles, accumulation of aberrant proteins, or microbial invasion) trigger signalling pathways that stimulate autophagy by a mechanism that is not clear.

Once the cell gets a specific signal, the autophagy-execution proteins activate a series of reactions that result in membrane rearrangements to form a double-membrane-bound vesicle termed an autophagosome. This vesicle fuses with a lysosome whereafter lysomomal digestive enzymes are released into the lumen of the resulting autolysosome. The sequestered cytoplasmic contents are degraded inside the autolysosome into free nucleotides, amino acids and fatty acids, which can be reused by the cell in macromolecular synthesis and to fuel energy production. Although the nutrient recycling and housekeeping functions of autophagy promote cell survival, in some circumstances autophagy may also promote cell death (Fig. 1.1).

Autophagy (self-cannibalism) is like a cellular recycling system that protects cells against stresses such as starvation and eliminates defective cellular constituents, including the energy-generating mitochondria. In autophagy, the cell breaks down its own components. Cells can then recycle the resulting breakdown products and use them to provide energy and cellular building blocks necessary for their survival.

The cancer connection has emerged more recently—autophagy appears to suppress tumour development in animals. Some tumour-suppressor genes stimulate autophagy and certain cancer-causing oncogenes inhibit it. Such work suggests that boosting autophagy will prevent or treat cancers, but the situation is not very clear. Some tumours may exploit autophagy in order to survive. The process is known to operate when cells face nutrient shortages. And if cancer cells in a growing tumour find themselves short of needed nutrients, inducing autophagy may enable them to address the problem (Marx, 2006). In some cases, autophagy seems to help cancer cells fight off chemotherapeutic drugs, but in others it may be part of the drugs' killing mechanisms.

Autophagy does not stop protein synthesis. Rather, through protein recycling, it helps maintain the synthesis of essential proteins when external nutrients are limited. Some stress stimuli (e.g., starvation) which induce autophagy turn off general protein synthesis. They also turn on the synthesis of specific stress-response proteins, including autophagy-execution proteins. In this context, the cell employs a coordinated strategy—it shuts down general protein translation and activates autophagy to ensure that it has enough amino acids to synthesize the proteins that are essential for its survival (Gozuacik and Kimchi , 2004; Hippert et al., 2006; Levine, 2007).

Although many cancer therapies are supposed to kill tumour cells by inducing apoptosis, researchers are now reporting signs of autophagy in tumour cells exposed to che-

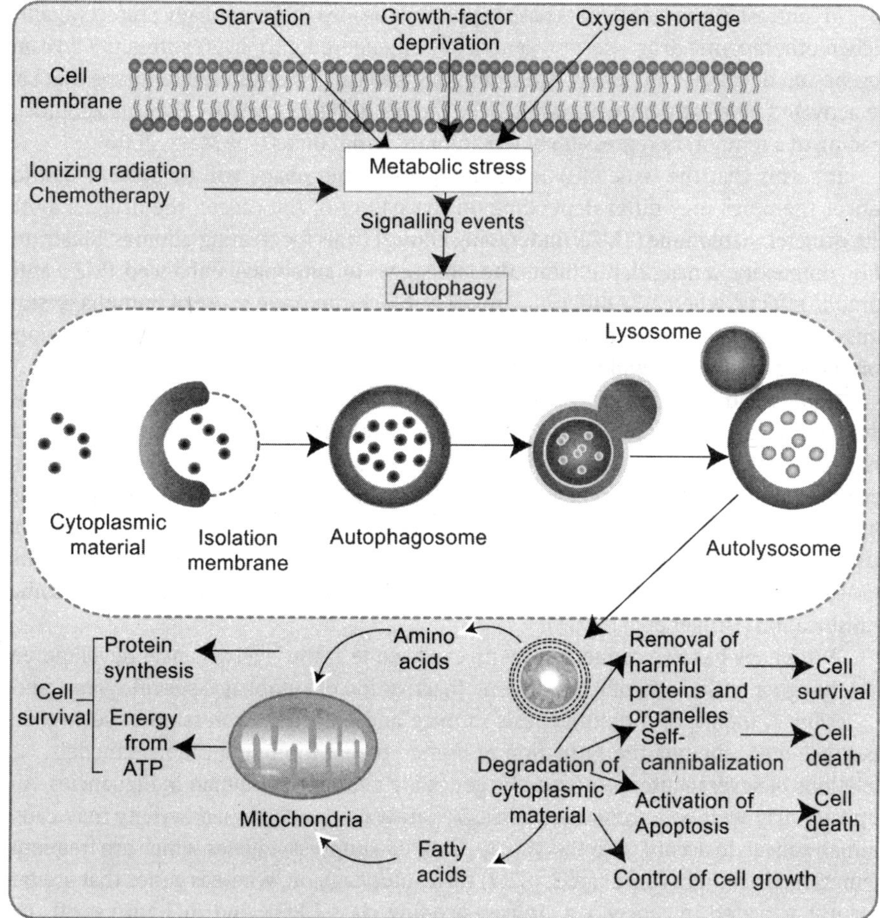

Fig. 1.1 AUTOPHAGY PATHWAY AND ITS VARIOUS CELLULAR FUNCTIONS: Both metabolic stress and cancer therapies activate signalling pathways that stimulate autophagy. The process involves the sequestration of cytoplasmic material by an autophagosome, which then fuses with a lysosome to form an autolysosome. The degradation of cytoplasmic material within the autolysosome promotes cell survival either by generating free fatty acids and amino acids, which can be reused by the cell to maintain energy production and protein synthesis, or by eliminating harmful proteins and organelles. It can also promote cell death independently through self-cannibalization or together with apoptosis. Further, the turnover of proteins and organelles by autophagy may contribute to the control of cell growth (After Levine, 2007).

motherapy or radiation. Some chemotherapeutic drugs that seem to trigger autophagy are tamoxifen, rapamycin, and arsenic compounds.

Many treatments induce autophagy rather than apoptosis. But the crucial question is whether autophagy helps kill tumour cells or instead protects them from the therapies' cell-damaging effects. There is evidence on both sides. One example of a cancer-killing role for autophagy relates to the chemotherapeutic drug rapamycin. The rapamycin sensitivity of cells derived from highly malignant brain tumours called gliomas correlates with the drug's ability to induce autophagy, and drugs that increase autophagy boost rapamycin's ability to kill glioma cells.

In contrast, some researchers have supported the idea that autophagy protects against a chemotherapeutic drug—certain genetically engineered mice overexpress the *myc oncogene* and develop lymphomas. These animals also carried an altered *p53* gene that can be activated by treatment with tamoxifen. The resulting *p53* activity induces apoptosis, leading to a temporary regression of the animals' lymphomas (see Marx, 2006).

It seems that the issue of whether inducers of autophagy will be good or bad for cancer therapies may differ depending on the nature of the cancer, the drug, or both. The drug temozolomide (TMZ), undergoing clinical trials for treating gliomas, illustrates this complexity: a drug that inhibits the late stages of autophagy enhanced TMZ's antitumour effects, whereas a different drug that blocks an early stage of autophagy suppressed them. There is need to understand all the players to predict whether a therapy (promoting autophagy) will protect the cells or kill them.

Understanding the genetic and biochemical mechanisms by which cancers arise and behave can lead to improvements in the way we detect, classify, monitor, and treat these diseases. A variety of new and less toxic agents such as hormones, antibodies, and enzyme-inhibitory drugs can be employed for treating cancers. One very effective drug, imatinib (Gleevec), is a "molecule-specific" agent that induces nearly complete and sustained remissions in most patients in the early stages of chronic myeloid leukaemia (CML), by blocking a protein-tyrosine kinase activated by a well-studied chromosomal translocation (Druker et al., 2001).

Autophagy has two connections with cancer, one at the level of cancer development and the other at the level of its treatment. Inactivation of autophagy-specific genes, such as *becline 1*, increases tumourigenesis in mice and enforced expression of such genes (*beclin 1, atg5*) inhibits the formation of human breast tumours in mouse models. Net deletions of several autophagy-specific genes are common in human malignancies. Autophagy may well be a tumour-suppressor pathway—its decreased activity may cause human cancer. In accord with this theory, tumour-suppressor genes which are frequently mutated in human cancer (*p53, pTEN*) turn autophagy on, whereas genes that are frequently activated in cancer, e.g., those encoding class I PI3K and AKT turn it off. The opposing pro-survival and pro-death functions of autophagy complicate the connection to cancer treatment. The pro-survival function probably helps cancer cells to survive in nutrient-limited environments, and to resist ionizing radiation and chemotherapies (see Fig. 1.1). But the pro-death function may prove lethal to cancer cells, either spontaneously or when they are exposed to radiation or chemotherapy. These paradoxical functions prompt the question: Is autophagy cancer's friend or foe?

Signalling Pathways and Cancer Treatment

Considerable emphasis is being currently placed on tumour-specific, molecularly targeted agents in cancer therapy, with less reliance on drugs that kill tumour as well as host cells. Most current focus on cancer treatment is on disrupting the fundamental signalling pathways that tumours depend upon to grow and survive. The diversity of targets giving rise to the new generation of anti-cancer drugs has increased substantially, but the complex interactions of signal-transduction pathways have greatly complicated the customization of cancer treatments to target single mechanisms. Nevertheless, even though there is much uncertainty over precise or dominant mechanisms of action, especially for compounds targeting multiple gene products, emerging agents exemplify significant

Table 1.2 The eight kinase-targeted oncology agents that have been clinically approved by the FDA for use in the USA since 1998 (After Sebolt–Leopold and English, 2006).

Drug	Known targets
Small molecules	
Imatinib (Gleevec)	Abl, PDGFR, c-Kit
Gefitinib (Iressa)	EGFR
Erlotinib (Tarceva)	EGFR
Sorafenib (Nexavar)	VEGFR, PDGFR, FLT3, c-Kit, B-raf, Raf-1
Sunitinib (Sutent)	VEGFR, PDGFR, FLT3, c-Kit
Biologics	
Trastuzumab (Herceptin)	ErbB2 (HER-1/neu)
Cetuximab (Erbitux)	EGFR
Bevacizumab (Avastin)	VEGF

N.B.: Abl, Abelson leukaemia virus; EGFR, epidermal growth factor receptor; PDGFR, platelet-derived growth factor receptor; VEGFR, vascular endothelial growth factor receptor.

therapeutic advances against a broad range of human cancers (Sebolt-Leopold and English, 2006).

The critical analysis of the signal-transduction network involved in neoplastic transformation has prompted rationally designed cancer therapeutics that target specific molecular events. Recent years have witnessed several drug discovery programmes that, if successful, could substantially decrease our reliance on DNA-directed chemotherapeutic agents with low therapeutic indices as the mainstay of cancer treatment. With a focus on kinase targets, Sebolt-Leopold and English (2006) have described the development of small-molecule inhibitors from both multi-targeted and truly selective classes of agents. Table 1.2 lists eight kinase-targeted oncology drugs or agents and their known targets.

The PI3K Signalling Pathway and Cancer Viability

The reports published by Cantley (2002) and Engelman et al. (2006) have pointed at the crucial importance of the phosphoinositide 3-kinase (PI3K) signalling pathway for the viability of many cancers. Whereas PI3K inhibitors block cancer cell growth and survival, some genetic changes such as loss of the PTEN tumour suppressor enhance PI3K activity in cancer cells. Samuels et al. (2004) discovered that *PIK3CA*—the gene encoding the PI3K catalytic subunit (p110α)—is mutated in cancers. These mutant p110α proteins showed constitutive PI3K activity as well as the capacity to transform normal cells into cancer cells (Vogt et al., 2007). Although mutations in *PIK3CA* occur throughout p110α, there are two hotspot regions (the helical and kinase domains) that make up more than 80 per cent of the mutations. Miled et al. (2007) showed how one of the hotspot mutations increases PI3K activity. This work reveals a new mechanism for activating PI3K and suggests new possibilities for therapeutic agents that target this enzyme. The details of the mechanism were described by Miled et al. briefly—PI3K localizes to the plasma membrane, where it phosphorylates the membrane lipid phosphatidylinositol 4,5-bisphosphate (PIP_2) to produce phosphatidylinositol 3,4,5-triphosphate (PIP_3). This activates downstream signalling pathways that control cell growth and survival (Lee et al., 2007).

Critical and thorough structural information about the enzyme implicated in many cancers has yielded valuable insights into how certain mutations promote the growth and survival of cancer cells. In light of structural findings, two classes of p110α oncogenic mutations were examined, the prevalent helical domain mutations and the less common ABD mutations. Several mutations in the helical domain result in an amino acid of opposite charge, such as a glutamic acid (negative charge) to lysine (positive charge) change at position 545 (E545K). Intensive biochemical studies prompted the authors to suggest that important charge-charge interactions occur between the p110α helical domain and p85 nSH2 domain. They then mutated all nSH2 basic residues to acidic ones. They identified two important residues in p85 (Lys^{379} and Arg^{340}) that are needed to inhibit p110α. When the charge on these basic residues was reversed by mutating to glutamates, the mutant p85 nSH2 domain effectively inhibited p110α E545K but not wild-type p110α. Thus, the authors proposed that p110α E545K is oncogenic because it is not inhibited by the p85 nSH2 domain.

The issue of how the E545K mutant promotes cell growth and survival in the absence of growth factors has aroused some interest. The fact that mutation does abrogate intermolecular inhibition but fails to explain its membrane localization is inspiring researchers to examine whether the p85 nSH2 domain, unencumbered by interaction with the p110α helical domain, may continue to be more tightly associated with receptors and adaptors. This in turn protects critical tyrosine residues from dephosphorylation and prolongs PIP3 production. Another possibility may be that the mutant PI3K localizes to the membrane through membrane-bound Ras protein (p110α has a Ras-binding domain) or random encounters with membrane lipid substrate.

PI3K inhibitors are now undergoing clinical trials. The success of drugs that block kinases–trastuzumab in *HER2*-amplified breast cancers, imatinib in Philadelphia-chromosome chronic myelogenous leukaemia, and gefitinib in *EGFR*-mutant lung cancers, is prompting researchers to determine whether cancers with genetic activation of PI3K signalling might be susceptible to PI3K inhibitors. Thus, cancers with *PIK3CA* mutations (or *PTEN* loss) deserve critical investigation for sensitivity to PI3K inhibitors. It is conceivable that the p110α E545K mutant could be susceptible to compounds that bind to its unique helical domain surface. Such a specific therapy might inhibit wild-type PI3K, thus minimizing undesirable side effects (Lee et al., 2007).

Autophagy-specific Genes

These genes are needed for the execution of the autophagy pathway. They code for proteins that are components of kinase complexes, which regulate the activity of proteins and lipids by the addition of a phosphate group. Alternatively, they code for components of protein-conjugation systems, which attach either to each other or to membrane lipids to make the membrane of the autophagosome. If an autophagy-specific gene is deleted, it blocks autophagy. The genes may also possibly be involved in other cellular processes.

Distinction between Autophagy and Apoptosis

Both these processes used to be classified as different forms of programmed cell death. But while apoptosis invariably leads to cell death, autophagy (in spite of its frequent occurrence in dying cells) usually promotes cell survival! If autophagy-specific genes in cells of diverse organisms are removed, it not only increases cell death during development, but also susceptibility to starvation and other apoptotic stimuli. This does not imply that autophagy cannot be a death programme. However, it seems to assume this function primarily when the cellular apoptotic machinery is damaged or when autophagy is induced so greatly that cells literally eat themselves to death (Levine, 2007).

While these scenarios may not be relevant to normal development or to physiological adaptations of cells and tissues to stress, they may be applicable to the development of cancer and to cancer therapy. Cancer cells can have mutations that make them resistant to apoptosis, and many toxic chemotherapeutic agents can induce high levels of autophagy (Levine, 2007).

The relationship between autophagy and apoptosis is complex. It appears to vary depending on the biological context. The two pathways are regulated by common factors, share common components, and can have overlapping functions. One route may regulate and modify the activities of the other. Many signals (e.g., sphingolipids, death-receptor signalling molecules, serine/threonine death kinases and mitochondrial-associated cell-death proteins) that activate apoptosis also activate autophagy. Conversely, signalling pathways such as class I PI3K/Akt signalling pathway and the stress-activated NF-kB signalling pathway that inhibit apoptosis also inhibit autophagy.

Autophagy and apoptosis are not mutually exclusive. They usually occur in the same cell, both when autophagy is trying to keep cells alive and when it contributes to cell death (see Levine, 2007). This coexistence can have different consequences. In certain circumstances, including starvation and treatment with certain DNA-damaging agents, autophagy delays the onset of apoptosis. In others, such as HIV infection, autophagy is needed for the onset of apoptosis in uninfected lymphocytes. During mammalian embryo development, autophagy neither delays nor promotes apoptosis, but it is required for the dying cells to generate signals that can efficiently eliminate dead cells.

Autophagy is linked to both health and disease. Normally, it contributes to adaptation to cellular stress, to development and differentiation, to immunity and to longevity. Excessive or deficient autophagy can contribute to certain cardiac- and skeletal-muscle diseases, liver diseases, infectious diseases, neurodegenerative disorders and cancer.

Autophagy and Prevention of Cancer

Autophagy may prevent cancer in different ways. One involves suppression of tumourigenesis through its death-promoting effects. Another view postulates that autophagy prevents DNA damage, possibly through its cellular housekeeping role in eliminating sources of oxidative stress such as defective mitochondria or endoplasmic reticulum. This theory interconnects the tumour-suppressor and anti-ageing functions of autophagy and accounts for the increased incidence of cancer as people age when their underlying housekeeping levels of autophagy decline. A third possibility is that autophagy negatively regulates cell growth. Not only changes in protein degradation mediated by a proteasome complex contribute to the development of cancer, but imbalances between autophagy-dependent protein degradation and synthesis might also be involved. It seems that the effects of autophagy on cell growth, rather than its potential pro-death effects, have a crucial role in tumour suppression (Levine, 2006).

As discussed above, autophagy also sometimes promotes cancer in various ways. In eukaryotic organisms, autophagy-specific genes promote the survival of normal cells during nutrient starvation. Autophagy may also increase the survival of rapidly growing cancer cells that have outgrown their vascular supply and face oxygen deficiency or metabolic stress.

According to Levine, it may be the crutch used by tumour cells to survive the deficiency of energy and nutrients. It might also enhance the survival of cancer cells by targeting damaged mitochondria and other organelles for lysosomal degradation, thereby buffering oxidative stress that can be triggered by activated cancer-causing genes or by cancer treatments (Levine, 2006).

The crucial question to be asked here is: Should autophagy be turned on or off to kill a tumour cell? The answer is: either action may be correct. The absence of autophagy promotes death when cells confront stressful conditions. High levels of autophagy, or its prevalence in cells with damaged or apoptotic machinery, can also cause cell death. But it cannot be concluded that one should attempt to kill tumour cells by turning autophagy either on or off. Whether we take one approach or the other, it may become risky if cell death does not invariably occur. Actions that abolish only some of autophagy's effects could result in loss of its tumour-suppressive function, whereas those that enhance only some of its effects could enhance the survival of tumour cells (Levine, 2007).

In the face of several paradoxes concerning the involvement of autophagy in cell death and cancer, top priority should be given to determine more precisely if, when, and how autophagy prevents or promotes cancer. The issue of whether to turn autophagy on or off may ultimately be resolved by data from clinical trials in cancer patients. Several anti-cancer agents are potent inducers of autophagy; it may be that inducing autophagy is a desirable target for cancer therapy. By contrast, others can argue that autophagy may function as a stress response to counter the toxic effects of anti-tumour drugs, and that such drugs might work even better if coupled with autophagy inhibitors (Levine, 2006). Primarily, all current anti-tumour agents target pathways other than autophagy. It is impossible to dissect the role of autophagy stimulation in their therapeutic action. Novel agents that specifically target autophagy need to be developed and tested to resolve this controversy.

Balance Between Life and Death

Cancerous cells usually possess not only a capacity for excessive proliferation but also a resistance to apoptosis. The oncoprotein c-MYC is an important contributor to many human tumours. It activates the transcription of some genes and represses that of others, hence influencing many target genes that might contribute to the regulation of apoptosis. The binding of c-MYC to the transcription factor MIZ-1 and the inhibition of MIZ-1-dependent transcription are important for promoting apoptosis. In human fibroblasts, a form of c-MYC (c-MYCV394D) that does not interact with MIZ-1 does not induce apoptosis. When the level of MIZ-1 is reduced in these cells, the apoptotic effect of c-MYCV394D is restored. MIZ-1 activates the transcription of many genes; a search of target genes in micro-arrays has yielded a promising candidate—the gene encoding the anti-apoptotic protein BCL2. Indeed, expression of BCL2 was decreased by c-MYC but not by c-MYCV394D, and inhibiting BCL2 expression enabled c-MYCV394D to promote apoptosis. Previous studies have shown that BCL2 and c-MYC appear to work together in promoting cancer. These important findings indicate that transcription of the *BCL2* gene is regulated through c-MYC and MIZ-1 (see J. Biol. Chem. 282: 5, 2007).

Inflammation

Chronic inflammation has clear linkages with cancer. Inflammation can drive tumour progression and, in the case of mice, the disruption of endogenous anti-inflammatory mechanisms can lead to tumour development (see Balkwill and Coussens, 2004; Lawrence, 2007). While inflammation is normally self-limiting, it can become chronic if an inflammatory stimulus persists or if endogenous anti-inflammatory mechanisms are not properly regulated (Lawrence et al., 2002). The resolution of inflammation is an active and coordinated 5-step process that depends on the expression of specific anti-inflammatory mediators (Gilroy et al., 2004); the termination of pro-inflammatory signalling pathways; as well as the effective clearance or migration of inflammatory cells. The five steps involved in this coordinated process are as follows:

1. The release of endogenous anti-inflammatory mediators;
2. The inhibition of pro-inflammatory signalling pathways;
3. Apoptosis and phagocytic clearance of inflammatory cells, which is also linked to the inhibition of pro-inflammatory signalling and the release of anti-inflammatory mediators;
4. The migration of macrophages and APCs to the draining lymphatics (this is an important requirement for macrophage clearance and for priming adaptive immune responses); and, in the event of infection, the inflammatory response results in
5. The generation of immunological memory by priming adaptive immunity (Lawrence, 2007).

If any of these processes is disrupted, it can cause chronic persistent inflammation and tumour growth. The mediators and mechanisms that drive inflammation are now fairly well characterized but the endogenous mechanisms that limit the inflammatory response, and particularly their role in cancer, are not clear. There is considerable potential for drug discovery and the development of new therapeutic strategies that target tumour-associated inflammation and the mechanisms of chronic inflammation (Lawrence, 2007).

Karin et al. (2006) reviewed what is known about the mediators and mechanisms that limit inflammation and innate immunity and that drive the resolution of inflammation. The involvement of these mechanisms in cancer has been outlined by Lawrence (2007). Tumours are not composed simply of transformed cells; as much as 80 per cent of the tumour mass can be made of stromal cells and inflammatory cells that have no genetic lesions. Both stromal cells and bone marrow-derived leukocytes are needed for the establishment and maintenance of tumours in mice (Lin et al., 2001). Inflammation and activation of innate immune system play a significant role in the progression of cancer (Karin et al., 2006). Tumour-associated macrophages (TAMs) seem to have an important role in tumour progression and metastasis (Pollard, 2004).

The chronic activation of innate immunity and inflammation seem to drive tumour initiation and growth. There are indications that defects in endogenous anti-inflammatory mechanisms that promote the resolution of inflammation could be a critical factor in the progression of cancer.

The evidence in support of the connections among activation of the innate immune system, inflammation and cancer is mostly based on the promotion of cell survival and proliferation by pro-inflammatory cytokines. Also, specific cytokines and chemokines seem to promote the invasion and metastasis of tumours. Cells of the immune system play an extrinsic role in tumour promotion in animal models. Appropriate pharmacological manipulation of the immune system can potentially benefit cancer therapy—chronic administration of non-steroidal anti-inflammatory drugs such as aspirin is known to decrease the incidence of cancer. New biological therapies that target certain pro-inflammatory mediators are being tested in cancer patients. The idea is to block the tumour-promoting action of inflammation. However, it should be noted that the chronic inhibition of innate immunity can have serious implications for those cancer patients who might be specially vulnerable to opportunistic infections. Perhaps, a better strategy may be to target the tumour-specific mediators and mechanisms that prevent the resolution of inflammation, which might leave the innate immune system intact (Lawrence, 2007).

Triangular Interaction

Recent researches have revealed an interesting triangular interaction between signals induced by sex hormones, inflammation and cancer (Mantovani, 2007). Unexpected windows have opened to show the relationship between gender differences and cancer, suggesting that the inflammatory response, which is mediated by the innate (nonspecific) immune system, might be an essential element of the action of sex steroid hormones.

Hepatocellular carcinoma, a common and deadly cancer of the liver, is much more likely to occur in men than in women. It is a frequent outcome of chronic inflammation triggered by hepatitis due to viral infection (Balkwill and Mantovani, 2001). Working on a mouse model in which liver cancer develops due to exposure to some carcinogenic agent, Naugler et al. (2007) proposed a molecular basis for this phenomenon that can be explained by the action of the female hormone oestrogen and its ability to inhibit responses in the liver. Oestrogen inhibits secretion of interleukin-6 (IL-6) by liver macrophages called Kupffer cells. Production of IL-6 depends on the signalling adoption protein MyD88, which seems to be produced from dying cells in the injured liver.

In vitro work and *in vivo* studies on mice have revealed that carcinogen-induced tissue damage results in the release of debris, which in turn causes MyD88-dependent activation of Kupffer cells in the liver (Fig. 1.2A). These cells act like a macrophage, a main player in the innate immune response. The cellular debris seems to act via Toll-like receptors. The Kupffer cells produce IL-6, which aggravates liver injury, inflammation, compensatory cell proliferation, and carcinogenesis. In females, however, oestrogen steroid hormones act through gene transcription factors to inhibit IL-6 production in Kupffer cells, thereby protecting female mice from cancer. Strangely, tumour-necrosis factor, another cytokine, has been implicated in liver carcinogenesis but is not involved in this gender difference.

Other researchers have shown the role of innate immune signalling in carcinogenesis. Mice deficient in MyD88 are relatively resistant to intestinal cancer, and this resistance is associated with altered expression of NF-kB-dependent modifier genes (Rakoff-Nahoum and Medzhitov, 2007). In other similar studies, mice deficient in an inhibitor of Toll-like-receptor signalling were highly susceptible to cancer involving inflammation of the colon. It appears that oestrogens interfere with carcinogenesis by acting on an endogenous tumour promoter that is activated by MyD88-dependent signalling in the innate immune system (Mantovani, 2007). Zhu et al. (2006) also have demonstrated the interplay between sex steroid hormones and inflammation in prostate cancer, a clas-

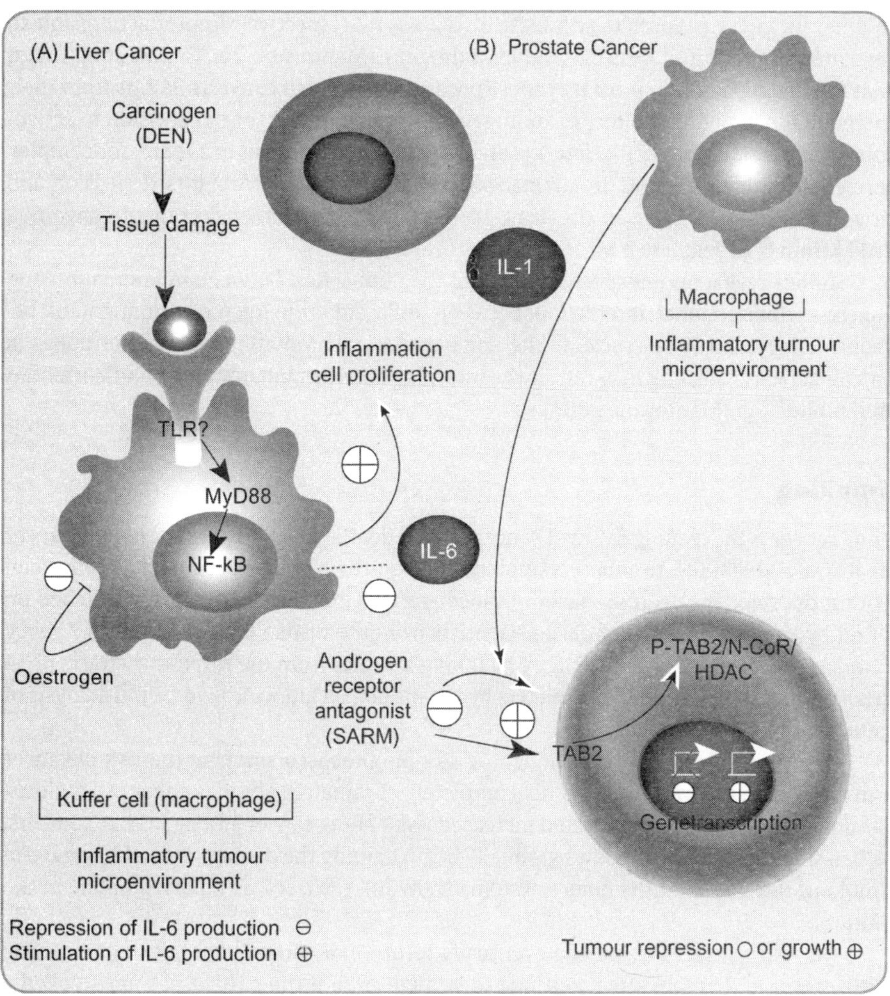

Fig. 1.2 SEX STEROID HORMONES, INFLAMMATION AND CANCER: A. In the liver, a carcinogen (diethylnitrosamine, DEN) causes tissue damage that (presumably acting via Toll-like receptors, TLR) activates the MyD88-NF-kB signalling pathway in Kupffer cells. These cells, a macrophage, produce interleukin-6 (IL-6), which in turn promotes inflammation, tissue damage, cell proliferation and tumour formation. Oestrogens interfere with NF-kB activity and IL-6 production, so females tend to be protected against liver cancer. B. In prostate cancer, macrophage-derived IL-1 converts an androgen-receptor antagonist (a steroid androgen receptor modulator, or SARM) into an agonist that stimulates gene transcription. The molecular sensor for the IL-1 inflammatory signals is TAB2, which on phosphorylation releases the TAB2/N-CoR/HDAC repressor complex from the gene promoter sequence, activating gene transcription. A SARM is thus converted from a tumour inhibitor to a tumour promoter (after Naugler et al., 2007; Zhu et al., 2006; and Mantovani, 2007).

sic hormone-stimulated tumour. They examined the actions of macrophages in prostate cancer cells in vitro. The activity of androgens (male sex hormones) is modulated by 'selective androgen-receptor modulators' (SARMs), which act as weak agonists or antagonists (so amplifying or blocking hormone action). Their counterparts for oestrogen are 'selective oestrogen-receptor modulators' (SERMs). Each type of molecule functions in different circumstances to stimulate or repress its respective receptor action, and so regulates the action of oestrogens and androgens (Mantovani, 2007). Zhu et al. found that the macrophages in prostate cancer produce IL-1, which converts SARMs from their intended function of inhibitors of androgen-receptor-induced gene expression to activators of expression (Fig. 1.2B). Here a protein TAB2 is a component of a repressor complex termed TAB2/N-CoR/HDAC. Inflammation of phosphorylated TAB2 lifts repression and drives gene transcription. In this way, an inflammatory microenvironment converts a SARM from 'a Dr Jekyll to a Mr Hyde' (Mantovani, 2007).

Studies reveal an unexpected aspect of the connection between inflammation and cancer—a bidirectional interaction between inflammatory microenvironment of tumours. They seem to be crucial in the link between inflammation and sex hormones in carcinogenesis. This link may reflect the interplay between inflammation and hormones in reproduction (Mantovani, 2007).

Smoking

Lung cancer is the leading cause of cancer related deaths. Over 80 per cent of lung cancer deaths are attributed to tobacco smoking. But quitting the tobacco habit, even when young, does not always reset harmful cancer-related genes that have been switched on or off by smoking in the first place. Scientists from the British Columbia Cancer Agency (Canada) have analysed gene activity by taking samples from the respiratory tracts of 24 smokers, non-smokers and ex-smokers by means of a technique called "serial analysis of gene expression" (SAGE).

The results showed that although by stopping tobacco smoking the risk of cancer can be significantly reduced, it is not completely eliminated. This has enhanced molecular understanding of the continued increased risk of lung cancer among former smokers. When smokers quit, their bodies gradually begin to undo the damage caused by cigarette smoking. But not all of the body's systems show full recovery, as reported online in the *Nature*.

The risk of heart disease can eventually return to a non-smoker but that of getting lung cancer and emphysema continue to be high even if the patient has not smoked a cigarette in decades. It appears that those functions which fail to revert to normal levels upon smoking cessation could possibly throw light on why former smokers still maintain a risk of developing lung cancer.

Researchers Wan Lam and Stephen Lam also identified several genes which were previously not associated with smoking that are switched on in active smokers. *CABYR* is a gene that enables sperms to swim. It is associated with brain tumours and has a role in bronchial repair.

Careful investigation of genes involved in regeneration of the respiratory passageways has led to classification of the genes into three classes; some, e.g., *CABYR* and *TFF3*, which encode a structural component of mucus are reversible, while others are only partially reversed. Others, such as *GSK3B*—associated in earlier studies with lung cancer—remained in their altered condition even long after smokers had quit.

In total, more than three million SAGE tags representing over 110,000 potentially unique transcripts were generated in the study and represented the largest human SAGE study to date. While tobacco smoking accounts for over 80 per cent of lung cancers, former smokers account for half of those newly diagnosed with the disease.

Alcohol

The *British Journal of Cancer* has recently reported that alcohol consumption may lower the risk of developing kidney cancer. Dr Alicja Wolk (Karolinska Institute, Stockholm) investigated the association of different types of alcoholic beverages and of total alcohol consumption with the risk of kidney cancer in a large population-based study in Sweden. The work was done on 855 patients of kidney cancer and 1204 'controls' without cancer. Their alcohol consumption was recorded in terms of standard portion sizes—a glass of beer, 200 millilitres; a glass of wine, 100 ml, and a glass of strong wine or hard liquor of 40 ml. The alcohol content of different beverages was rated as follows: medium-strong beer had 2.8 g alcohol per 100 g; red wine had 9.9 g per 100 g; and hard liquor had 32 g alcohol per 100 g. The odds of developing kidney cell cancer were about 40 per cent lesser among those who consumed 620 g ethanol per month as compared to teetotalers—those who did not drink at all. Drinking more than two glasses of red wine per week was associated with a 40 per cent reduction of risk of kidney cell cancer as compared with drinking no red wine.

Cancer Incidence in India

Tobacco or cigarette smoking is associated with about 50 per cent of all cancers, mostly of the neck, head, lung and oesophagus. More than one million people die of tobacco-related cancers annually. Cancer is a silent killer.

According to the Indian Council of Medical Research (National Cancer Registry Programme data), every hour, cancer kills around 50 people in India and about 100 other people are diagnosed with cancer. Annually, around 440,000 cancer patients die in the country, while 700,000 to 900,000 are diagnosed with various cancers. At any given instant, there are some 2.5 million cancer patients in the country. Cancer is the fourth biggest killer disease in the country.

Some parts of India have the world's highest incidence of cancers of the gall bladder, mouth and pharynx. Among women living in cities, breast cancer has replaced cervical cancer as the leading cancer. In metropolitan urban areas of Mumbai, Kolkata and Delhi, lung cancer is the commonest cancer in men. Dietary factors and obesity can increase risk of cancers of the breast, uterus, stomach, colon and kidney. Habitual and frequent chewing of paan (betel leaves) containing tobacco and cigarette smoking greatly increases the risk of certain cancers, such as oral (for paan) and lung (for cigarette smoke).

Excessive intake of alcoholic drinks can cause several cancers, notably of liver, oesophagus, pharynx, larynx and breast. The leading cause of most cancers and the single most important risk factor for cancers is tobacco smoking. In fact, as many as one half of deaths from cancer can be prevented simply by avoiding smoking. About three-fourths of cancer cases are detected when the disease has already advanced so much that treatment becomes ineffective.

Classification

There are two systems of classifying cancer; (i) by the type of tissue in which it originates (histological type); and (ii) by primary site, or location in the body where it first appeared. The histological classification is based on the International Classification of

Diseases for Oncology. Histologically, there are hundreds of different cancers, grouped into five major categories: carcinoma, sarcoma, myeloma, leukaemia, and lymphoma. Also, there are some cancers of mixed types.

Carcinoma

This refers to a malignant neoplasm of epithelial origin or cancer of the internal or external lining of the body. Malignancies of epithelial tissue account for 80–90 per cent of all cancers. Epithelial tissue, which is distributed throughout the body, is present in the skin, the covering, and lining of all organs. Two major subtypes are adenocarcinoma (develops in an organ or gland) and squamous cell carcinoma (originates in the squamous epithelium). The former generally occurs in mucus membranes and first appears as a thickened plaque-like white mucosa. It spreads easily through soft tissue. Squamous cell carcinomas can occur in many areas of the body. Most carcinomas affect secretory organs or glands such as breasts, lungs, colon, prostate or bladder.

Sarcoma

This originates in supportive and connective tissues such as bones, tendons, cartilage, muscle, and fat. Generally occurring in young adults, the commonest sarcoma usually grows as a painful mass on the bone. Sarcoma tumours often resemble the tissue in which they grow. Notable examples of sarcomas are osteosarcoma or osteogenic sarcoma (bone), chondrosarcoma (cartilage), leiomyosarcoma (smooth muscle), rhabdomyosarcoma (skeletal muscle), mesothelioma (membranous lining of body cavities), fibrosarcoma (fibrous tissue), angiosarcoma or haemangioendothelioma (blood vessels), liposarcoma (adipose tissue), glioma or astrocytoma (neurogenic connective tissue of the brain), myxosarcoma (primitive embryonic connective tissue), and mesenchymous or mixed mesodermal tumour (mixed connective tissue types).

Myeloma

This originates in the plasma cells of bone marrow. It is the plasma cells which produce some of the essential proteins found in blood.

Leukaemia

Leukaemias ('liquid cancers' or 'blood cancers') affect the bone marrow which is the site of blood cell production. The disease is usually associated with the overproduction of immature white blood cells which cannot function properly. Consequently, the patient becomes prone to infection. Leukaemia also affects red blood cells and adversely affects blood clotting. Specific examples of leukaemia are:

- Myelogenous or granulocytic (malignancy of the myeloid and granulocytic white blood cells);
- Lymphatic, lymphocytic or lymphoblastic (malignancy of the lymphoid and lymphocytic blood cell series);
- Polycythemia vera or erythremia (malignancy of various blood cell products, but with red cells predominating).

Table 1.3 Tissues commonly affected by various tumours.

Tumour type	Tissues
Blastoma	Germ/precursor cells
Carcinoma	Epithelial/connective
Hepatoma	Liver
Leukaemia	Leukocytes
Lymphoma	Lymphoid
Melanoma	Skin
Myeloma	Bone marrow
Sarcoma	Bone, cartilage, muscle

Lymphomas

These affect the glands or nodes of the lymphatic system, a network of vessels, nodes, and organs (specifically the spleen, tonsils, and thymus) that purify body fluids and produce infection-fighting white blood cells (lymphocytes). Whereas leukaemias are sometimes called 'liquid cancers', lymphomas are termed 'solid cancers'. Lymphomas can also appear in the stomach, breast or brain, and these are termed extra-nodal lymphomas. The two categories of lymphomas are: Hodgkin and Non-Hodgkin. The presence of Reed–Sternberg cells in Hodgkin lymphoma distinguishes Hodgkin from Non-Hodgkin lymphoma in diagnostics.

Table 1.3 shows some tumour types and tissues affected by them.

Melanoma (Skin Cancer)

Skin cancer is one of the commonest cancers all over the world. Over 75 per cent cases of skin cancer can be easily prevented through 'sun-safe' strategies like wearing sunscreen and limiting exposure to intense sunlight between 9 am and 5 pm. Older people who did not know about the utility of the sun-safe strategies or sunscreens until late in life, are particularly vulnerable. In the past 30 years, in the USA, death rates for melanoma, the most serious skin cancer, have risen by more than 50 per cent in old women (over 65) and over 150 per cent in old men (over 65).

If detected early, 95 per cent of melanoma cases can be cured. What is more, an emerging technology may help doctors catch melanoma before it kills. One of the prototypes is a device called MelaFind. It is a hand-held painless probe that captures images of a suspicious mole or skin spot and then transmits them to a computer that analyses the cell's physical changes. For clinical diagnosis, this device has been more successful than human experts in identifying melanoma. And because it can measure the depth of a malignancy, its use can potentially simplify treatments.

This device (MelaFind) was invented by Marek Elbaum, founder of Electro-Optical Sciences Company in the USA. Conceivably, MelaFind could find a melanoma, and if it is localized in the epidermis, the physician could safely remove it in a single visit. Similar devices are being developed in Europe and Australia, although MelaFind was the first to hit the US market.

What about people whose melanoma has already reached a life-threatening stage? Researchers at Penn State University's Milton Hershey Medical Centre have identified a gene called *PTEN* that seems to play a role in up to 60 per cent of malignant melanomas. Animal experiments have shown that by inserting a chromosome containing *PTEN* from healthy cells into melanoma cells, the spread of tumours can be temporarily stopped.

Novel Breast Cancer Susceptibility Loci

Breast cancer is one of the few cancers that can generally be detected at an early stage. From 1998 to 2002, only 50 per cent of Malaysian women survived the disease as compared to 80 per cent among the Chinese and Indians, according to Dr (Ms) Nur Aishah M Taib of the University of Malaya, Department of Surgery.

Early breast cancer survival can often be 100 per cent, but when women come with stage IV cancers, there is no more than 20 per cent chance of survival. This makes it essential to get breast cancer treated at the earliest possible.

According to CGHFBC (2001), breast cancer is about twice as common in the close relatives of women with the disease as in the general population, consistent with variation in genetic susceptibility to the disease.

Two major susceptibility genes for breast cancer, BRCA1 and *BRCA2*, were identified by Miki et al. (1994) and Wooster et al. (1995). Mutations in these genes increase the risk of breast and other cancers (Antoniou et al., 2003). Breast cancer susceptibility appears to be largely 'polygenic', that is, it is conferred by a large number of loci, each with a small effect on breast cancer risk (Pharoah et al., 2002). However, our understanding about the relevant loci is quite low.

Familial aggregation seen in breast cancer patients is consistent with variation in genetic susceptibility to the disease. Known susceptibility genes account for less than 25 per cent of the familial risk of breast cancer, and the residual genetic variance is likely to be due to variants conferring more moderate risks.

To identify further susceptibility alleles, Easton et al. (2007) conducted a two-stage genome-wide association study in 4,398 breast cancer cases and 4316 controls, followed by a third stage in which 30 single nucleotide polymorphisms (SNPs) were tested for confirmation in 21,860 cases and 22578 controls from 22 studies. They used 227,876 SNPs estimated to correlate with 77 per cent of known common SNPs in Europeans at $r^2 > 0.5$. SNPs in five novel independent loci showed robust evidence of association with breast cancer ($P < 10^{-7}$). Four of these contain plausible causative genes (*FGFR2, TNRC9, MAP3K1* and *LSP1*).

At the second stage, 1,792 SNPs were significant at the $P < 0.05$ level as compared to an estimated 1,343 that would be expected by chance, indicating that many additional common susceptibility alleles may be identifiable by this approach (Easton et al., 2007). The work of Easton et al. successfully identified five novel breast cancer susceptibility loci, and proved that some of the variation in breast cancer risk is due to common alleles. None of the identified loci had been previously reported in association studies. Most of the previously identified breast cancer susceptibility genes are involved in DNA repair, and many association studies in breast cancer have focused on genes in DNA repair, sex hormone synthesis, and metabolism pathways.

However, none of the associations reported by Easton et al. appear to relate to genes in these pathways—three of the five loci contain genes related to control of cell growth or to cell signalling; only one (FGFR2) had a clear prior relevance to breast cancer. These results can potentially open new windows for further research.

Herceptin and Dimercept

Herceptin is one of the blockbuster targeted therapeutics that has already achieved commendable record for a subset of breast cancer patients. Some patients who take it live longer and the size of their tumours is better controlled than if they had received standard chemotherapy alone. This drug was developed by Genentech and approved for release in 1998. The company researchers critically studied the molecular workings of a cancer cell.

Some breast cancer cells stud their external surface with receptors that join in pairs to trigger a cascade of signals that cause the cells to replicate uncontrollably, become resistant to chemotherapy and encourage the growth of blood vessels that promote the spread of tumour cells (Bazell, 1998; Stix, 2006).

Unfortunately, Herceptin (generic name trastuzumab) is aimed only at about 25 per cent of breast cancer patients—those whose tumour cells have excessive numbers of a receptor known as *HER2* on the surface. It is also not effective against other cancers.

Another potential new drug called Dimercept couples with a receptor on a cancer cell and inhibits signals that inform the cell to replicate. Cancer cells often display more cell-surface receptors of the HER family than normal cells do. When something causes receptor molecules to pair up, the 'dimerization' induces the receptors to transmit signals that induce cancer cells to divide uncontrollably and metastasize.

Herceptin is a monoclonal antibody that acts on breast cancers with a surfeit of *HER2* receptors which can dimerize with copies of themselves. Binding by Herceptin curbs signalling primarily by *HER2–HER2* pairs.

Dimercept inhibits both *HER2* and other receptors in its family by joining with them at the site where they usually form dimers with copies of themselves or other family members. This prospective drug was originally called Herstatin, and later named Dimercept because it 'intercepts' dimerization. The molecule moves up along a receptor. The amino acids coded by an intron appear to initiate contact. A tiny arm that projects laterally from the protein interacts with a similar protuberance on the receptor and prevents the receptor from joining to another, so inhibiting the chain of signals.

Dimercept exerts the same effect not only on *HER2* but also on other receptors in the same family (the epidermal growth factor receptor family): *HER1*, *HER3* and, possibly, *HER4*. The interesting protein Dimercept is made naturally in humans and is present mostly in foetal liver and kidney tissue. It probably serves as a growth inhibitor in early development (see Stix, 2006). By inhibiting dimerization, this coupling can prevent all known permutations of *HER* receptor pairs from emitting cell-replication signals into cells. Both the breast cancer drug Herceptin and the experimental drug Dimercept target solid tumours by hampering those signals which they get in different ways.

Herceptin and Dimercept stop the *HER2* receptor but the two molecules are quite different. The Genentech drug is a monoclonal antibody—an immune molecule that binds to only a single target or antigen.

Monoclonals are made by cultivating antibody-producing cells in mice and are extracted from their spleen. These antibodies are then humanized so as to avoid immune reactions in human patients.

In contrast, Dimercept is a protein found naturally in the body, and hence does not arouse concerns about immunogenicity. Another potential new monoclonal antibody-based drug called Omnitarg (pertuzumab) is now undergoing clinical trials. It impedes the *HER2* receptor from dimerizing with other *HER* receptors, possibly providing some of the same benefits as those from Dimercept in treating a range of solid tumours.

The potentially useful molecules exhibit promising anticancer activity in mice. However, the formidable barrier to the success of these molecules as drugs will be the development of new techniques to identify the subpopulation of patients who respond to them.

Carcinogenic Viruses

The American Cancer Society has estimated that 17 per cent of all cancer cases, i.e., over 1.8 million per year, are caused by viruses and other pathogens. One such pathogen is the human papillomavirus, responsible for almost half a million cases of cervical cancers diagnosed annually. This virus enables host cells to divide long after normal cells would stop; it also prevents them from repairing mutations in their DNA.

Papillomaviruses are found in most vertebrates, in whom they usually cause only warts and other benign growths. Yet when *Homo sapiens* first emerged, our ancestors already carried a number of strains that could infect only our species and no other animal, and these included cancer-causing types (Xi et al., 2006).

Later, after some 100,000 years, *Homo sapiens* migrated out of Africa to other continents, taking the viruses with them. As the human population became isolated from one another, these papillomaviruses also got isolated. Certain benign papillomaviruses evolved to cause cancer. Vaccines may soon be introduced against these viruses. The Federal Drug Administration (FDA) of the USA has already approved a vaccine against the most dangerous human papillomavirus strain known as H16.

Evolutionary studies indicate that on rare occasions, human papillomavirus types have traded genes involved in triggering cancer. The global HIV epidemic might raise the risk of this gene swapping. As HIV weakens a person's immune system, more types of human papillomaviruses can invade and coexist. This mingling could conceivably give rise to a new cancer-causing strain for which today's vaccines would not be quite effective (Zimmer, 2007).

Uterine Cervical Cancer

Cervical cancer is the commonest cause of cancer deaths in developing countries, even when the disease is preventable. Cervical cancer figures second only to breast cancer in most cancer registries in India. Women between around 30 to 60 years of age face the highest risk of cervical cancer and need to be screened by various screening tests.

Vaccines based on human papillomavirus (HPV) are undergoing trials in some countries to evaluate their efficacy in preventing cervical cancer. In fact, long-term effectiveness of HPV vaccine may be a good opportunity for global control of cervical cancer. According to Lehtinen and Paavonen (2003), the HPV vaccine may be effective in the control of cervical cancer, especially in developing countries. According to Satyanarayana and Asthana (2007), the Institute of Cytology and Preventive Oncology of the Indian Council of Medical Research has started vaccine trials and is interested in developing a low-cost DNA vaccine against HPV for use in the prevention of HPV-associated cancer.

2 Tumours and their Metastasis

Introduction

Cancer cells have generally been considered as a problem that is innate to their host, but they may sometimes become infectious agents and can be transmitted between individuals (Dingli and Nowak, 2006).

As per the current view of cancer development, normal cells get transformed into tumour cells by sequential mutations which either activate cancer-promoting 'oncogenes', or inhibit genes that would otherwise suppress tumours, or trigger genetic instabilities. Every tumour arises as the result of a unique evolutionary process as the cancer cells adapt to out-compete their neighbours. This process initiates in its individual host and terminates when the tumour is eliminated or the host dies. Pearse and Swift (2006) suggested that some tumour cells can behave like infectious agents and move from one animal host to another.

There is no evidence yet that infectious transmission of cancer occurs between people, involving direct person-to-person transmission of tumour cells during normal social contact. The only known physiological route for tumour cell transmission in humans is through pregnancy. In the USA, every year about 3,500 pregnant women also have a malignancy, and transplacental transmission of acute leukaemia, lymphoma, melanoma and carcinoma from the mother to the foetus has been reported (Tolar and Neglia, 2003). These authors could transfer acute leukaemia cells between foetuses in mothers with a multiple pregnancy, followed by the development of disease in both the foetuses.

Another possible route of tumour cell transmission between people is organ transplantation. The immunosuppressive therapy needed to ensure survival of the transplanted organ weakens the immune surveillance that might otherwise recognize and react against donor-derived tumour cells (Dingli and Nowak, 2006). However, the development of donor-derived tumours is rare: only 0.04 per cent of solid organ transplant recipients develop a cancer that was transferred from their donor (Kauffman et al., 2002), and according to Sala-Torra et al. (2006), only 0.06 per cent of recipients of haematopoietic stem-cell transplants develop blood cancer from the transferred cells. The chief culprit appears to be malignant melanoma which remains undetected in the donor at the time of harvesting the organ. One troublesome issue is why cancer is generally not transmissible between people? The primary reason could be tissue graft rejection caused by the so-called major histocompatibility complex (MHC) incompatibility—in humans as well as other vertebrates, the immune system uses cell-surface proteins called MHC antigens to differentiate 'self' from 'non-self' cells as these proteins vary between individuals. The immune system then reacts against those cells that show non-self MHC antigens. Such reactions may conceivably buffer some protection against tumour cell engraftment by eliminating implanted cells (Dingli and Nowak, 2006).

MHC incompatibility means that the cancer cells of a donor would be expected to induce a robust immune response in a healthy recipient. In fact, tumour transfer in mice can only take place between animals that share the same MHC, or if the recipient is severely immuno-suppressed. Murgia et al. (2006) postulated the interesting idea that the chief reason for MHC diversity in humans and other vertebrates may be to ensure that cancer is not normally an infectious disease. Should this hypothesis be true, it would imply that certain cancers have developed mechanisms to bypass these safeguards.

Circulating Tumour Cells

Both in solid and haematological malignancies, changes in oncogenes and suppressor genes are critical steps in carcinogenesis and tumour progression. Therapeutic strategies that interfere with the functional pathways regulated by these genes exemplify targeted therapy, e.g., imatinib in chronic myelogenous leukaemia and trastuzumab in breast cancer (Slamon et al., 2001; O'Brien et al., 2003).

Meng et al. (2006) have raised interesting possibilities for exploring circulating tumour cells (CTCs) to personalize targeted therapy of cancer in the future. As discussed by Yarden and Sliwkowski (2001), members of the ErbB family of receptors alter frequently in breast cancer. *HER-2* (also known as *erbB-2* or *neu*) is a proto-oncogene that encodes a 185-kDa tyrosine kinase glycoprotein. Its amplification is crucial in the pathogenesis of breast cancer and is associated with a poor prognosis in patients suffering from axillary node-positive breast cancer. Treatment with the humanized monoclonal antibody (Herceptin) directed against the extracellular domain of *HER-2/neu*, has significantly improved clinical responses to chemotherapy and outcomes in primary and metastatic breast cancer (Piccart-Gebhart et al., 2005; Romond et al., 2005). The *HER-2/neu* status of tumour cells detected in metastatic sites, bone marrow, or peripheral blood of patients with advanced diseases sometimes differs from the original primary tumour, suggesting either a clonal selection or a genetic instability (Lorinez et al., 2006). Also, the presence of concomitant alterations of certain other oncogenes better defines biological subsets of the disease and facilitates appropriate decisions on treatment selection. This points to the need for a 'real time' testing of *HER-2* status and other abnormally functioning genes in tumour cells, either from tissue or from peripheral blood (Cristofanilli and Mendelsohn, 2006). These analyses also help to identify additional molecular markers useful in selection of therapeutic targets.

It is possible to detect and isolate CTCs from the peripheral blood of women suffering from breast malignancy, including women with no current sign of disease—'tumour dormancy'.

CTCs found in patients with both localized and metastatic breast cancer are significantly associated with the worse outcome (Cristofanilli and Mendelsohn, 2006). Meng et al. (2006) analysed CTCs from the blood of patients with newly diagnosed, advanced breast cancer and from those with recurrent breast cancer. The objective was to assess the utility of measuring gene status in CTCs as compared with cancer cells in the primary tumour tissue and to explore amplification of the uPA (urokinase plasminogen activator) receptor gene.

The results obtained by Meng et al. raise the possibility that circulating tumour cells may be representative of cells in tumour tissue. This would greatly enhance our capacity to monitor the presence of genetic abnormalities and changes that occur during the course of the disease. Meng et al. concluded that TPs (tumour touch preps) can be used to determine the status of certain concerned genes in patients.

Heterogeneity of gene copy number and expression was observed among the CTCs from single patients, confirming heterogeneity among breast cancer cells from a single patient but leaving open the issue of whether the set of CTCs came from one or many sites in a single tumour mass or from one or many sites throughout the body. This question is important in view of the general belief that cancer cells that have spread to different metastatic sites express different genes and may harbour different genetic abnormalities.

Second, the CTCs studied by Meng et al. came from patients with recurrent disease and from others with progressive advanced breast carcinoma who were in their initial episode. In all cases, the comparison made was with the original primary cancer. It would be advisable to use this method for comparing the status of genes in CTCs with genes in the primary tumour in patients that initially have progressive advanced disease and, separately, in patients with recurrence of disease, to address the question of changes in gene expression between initial presentation and development of recurrence (Cristofanilli and Mendelsohn, 2006).

It now seems feasible that clinical trials testing correlations between gene status data obtained from CTCs before treatment and the responses of patients to various therapeutic regimens could possibly lead to diagnostic tests that can select the therapy most likely to be effective for an individual patient.

In fact, CTCs provide valuable access to samples of a patient's cancer for performing several biological analyses, including gene copy number by FISH, gene expression at the level of mRNA, and gene expression at the protein level by immunohistochemistry (Speicher and Carter, 2005). Their use as potential noninvasive tools for improving selection of individualized cancer therapy deserves to be explored.

Indeed, a thorough analysis of the properties of CTCs may provide new insights into the biology of breast cancer and also help in defining novel treatments, especially development of more 'tailored' and personalized therapies (Cristofanilli and Mendelsohn, 2006).

Chromosome Instability, Chromosome Transcriptome and Tumour Cell Populations

Although chromosome instability and aneuploidy are important characteristics of cancer, not much is known about how changes in the chromosomal content of a cell leads to malignant phenotype. Highly proliferative tumour cells and their revertants have been isolated from highly invasive tumour cell populations, indicating how phenotypic shifting might contribute to malignant progression (Gao et al., 2005). Gao et al. (2007) showed that chromosome instability and changes in chromosome content occur with phenotypic switching. Also, changes in the copy number of each chromosome proportionally alters the chromosome transcriptome ratio. This correlation also applies to sub-chromosomal regions of derivative chromosomes.

Another contribution of Gao et al. is that the changes in chromosome content and transcriptome favour the expression of several genes which are appropriate for the specific tumour phenotype. Chromosome instability generates the necessary chromosome diversity in the tumour cell populations and, therefore, the transcriptome diversity to allow for environment-facilitated clonal expansion and clonal evolution of tumour cell populations.

Both invasion and proliferation are important requirements for tumour progression, and Gao et al. have studied these steps in glioblastoma tumour cells. Glioblastoma cells invade normal brain tissue; after surgical resection, residual invasive cells regain a proliferative phenotype and progress to become a more aggressive tumour. As glioblastomas rarely spread from the CNS, the sequential selection of invasive and proliferative tumour cells is the primary factor involved in the tumour's progression (Maher et al., 2001). This is why it is important to understand the molecular mechanisms that permit high-frequency phenotypic switching and control tumour cell proliferation and invasion.

Glioblastomas typically exhibit extensive regional cytogenetic heterogeneity. Conceivably, this diversity could be responsible for tumour evolution and progression. Gao et al. (2007) showed that distinct changes in karyotype from chromosome instability accompany phenotypic switching. These changes, in turn, produce changes in the chromosome transcriptome that provide the expression of individual genes essential for conversion between the invasive and proliferative phenotypes.

Dysfunctional Mitochondria and Tumour Development

The role of aberrant mitochondrial function in tumour development has been suspected since long. Recent studies have implicated mitochondrial DNA (mtDNA) mutations in various solid tumours (Fliss et al., 2000; Wallace, 1999). Many of these investigations have been restricted to the mitochondrial non-coding D-loop region, and the mutation frequency and pattern in the entire mitochondrial genome are not well defined for specific tumours because of the limited sample sizes (Zhou et al., 2007). While mitochondrial genomic mutations are fairly common in various human cancers, the frequency of mtDNA mutations in coding regions is poorly defined, and the functional effects of mitochondrial mutations seen in primary human cancers are not well described.

One popular hypothesis for the role of mtDNA mutations in primary cancers postulates that these mutations enhance generation of reactive oxygen species (ROS), which in turn alters signal transduction pathways and either activates oncogenes or inactivates tumour-suppressor genes. However, mitochondrial genes cannot be directly cloned into conventional expression vectors because direct translation of mitochondrial sequences produces multiple amino acid alterations or premature truncation due to differences in translation between the mitochondrial and nuclear genetic code. That is why, even though mtDNA mutations have been widely reported, only a few studies have explored the biological mechanism of these mutations in cancer. Murine studies with knockout of MnSOD have shown increased DNA damage and cancer incidence, pointing to a role of ROS in tumour development (see Zhou et al., 2007). Petros et al. (2005) demonstrated the potential for mtDNA mutations to influence tumour development: ATP/6 mutant cybrids induce an increase in ROS generation with increased tumourigenicity when placed into prostate cancer cell lines.

Zhou et al. have developed an oligonucleotide micro-array (MitoChip version 2.0) for rapid and accurate sequencing of the entire mitochondrial genome. Using MitoChip, they sequenced the whole mitochondrial genome in 83 head and neck squamous cell carcinomas. Forty-one of 83 (49%) tumours contained mtDNA mutations. Mutations occurred within non-coding (D-loop) and coding regions. A non-random distribution of mutations was found throughout the mitochondrial enzyme complex components. Sequencing of margins with dysplasia demonstrated an identical non-conservative mitochondrial mutation (A76T in ND4L) as the tumour, suggesting a role of mtDNA mutation in tumour progression. Analysis of *p53* status showed that mtDNA mutations correlated positively with *p53* mutations ($P < 0.002$). To characterize biological function of the mtDNA mutations, they cloned NADH dehydrogenase subunit 2 (ND2) mutants based on primary tumour mutations. Expression of the nuclear-transcribed, mitochondrial-targeted ND2 mutants resulted in increased anchorage-dependence and independent growth, which was accompanied by increased ROS production and an aerobic glycolytic metabolic phenotype with hypoxia-inducible factor (HIF)-1α induction that is reversible by ascorbate. This means that cancer specific mitochondrial mutations may contribute in the development of a malignant phenotype by direct genotoxic effects from increased reactive oxygen species production as well as induction of aerobic glycolysis and growth promotion (Zhou et al., 2007).

Angiogenesis

The growth of new blood vessels in an embryo from existing ones occurs through the active process of angiogenesis. In adults, blood vessels in most organs are quiescent, except during the growth of solid tumours, when embryonic signalling pathways direct new blood vessels to grow around and into the tumour. The vascular endothelial growth factor (VEGF) and Notch signalling pathways are the two important players in this process. Of the two, the latter has been the focus of much recent research (Siekmann and Lawson, 2007; Gridley, 2007). Knowledge of the role of Notch pathway during the formation of blood vessels in both embryos and tumours has greatly enhanced. Recent work has even revealed a new drug target for disrupting tumour angiogenesis.

VEGF is a secreted glycoprotein that is a strong inducer of angiogenesis both in embryos and tumours (see Coultos et al., 2005). The Notch pathway is an intercellular signalling system in which both the signalling (ligand) and receiving (receptor) molecules are attached to the cell surface, thereby restricting signal transmission to adjacent cells. This pathway is usually involved in regulation of cell differentiation. Gale et al. (2004) had shown that the Notch ligand Delta-like 4 (Dll4) is essential for vascular development in mice. The recent researches of Hellström et al. (2007) and Siekmann and Lawson (2007) have not only identified previously unknown role for Dll4/Notch signalling during vascular development but also verified the mechanism responsible for the vascular defects that result from reduced Notch signalling.

Different research teams analysed blood-vessel development in three different experimental systems: the zebrafish embryo, the retina of the mouse-eye, and solid tumours growing in mice. Being transparent, developing zebrafish embryos are ideal for high-resolution imaging studies of blood-vessel development. The advantage of the mouse retina is that blood vessels develop mainly after birth in a highly reproducible spatial and temporal pattern and the retinal vasculature is readily accessible for observation as well as for experimental administration of drugs or other agents.

All the studies found that inhibition of Notch signalling led to increased sprouting and branching of blood vessels. The Notch pathway regulates sprouting and branching behaviours by influencing the formation of vascular 'tip cells'—specialized endothelial cells found at the leading edge of vascular sprouts. The tip cells have protrusions, called filopodia, that sense the local environment and direct growth of these sprouts along gradients of VEGF protein. In both mouse retina and zebrafish embryo, Dll4/Notch signalling regulated the formation of tip cells. Weaker Notch signalling increased the number of tip cells, extension of filopodia and branching of vessels. Conversely, any experimental manipulations that blocked VEGF function retarded both Dll4 expression and blood-vessel sprouting (Ridgway et al., 2006). This suggests that the suppression of tip cell formation and angiogenic sprouting by Notch signalling occurs downstream of the VEGF signal.

Growth and metastasis of solid tumours require the recruitment of host blood vessels. Many solid tumours express the angiogenesis-promoting VEGF. Anti-VEGF therapies can effectively block growth of solid tumours (Ridgway et al., 2006). Although Notch signalling is essential for angiogenesis in embryos (Gale et al., 2004; Ferrara and Kerbel, 2005). It does not seem to have any big role in maintaining established blood vessels in adults. So protein components of the Notch pathway, particularly if their expression and function are confined to the vascular system, could possibly provide drug targets during tumour angiogenesis (Gridley, 2007).

Ridgway et al. identified the Dll4 protein as just such a drug target. Systemic administration of either neutralizing antibodies against Dll4 protein that had been modified to block Dll4/Notch signalling (Noguera-Troise et al., 2006) inhibited growth of various different solid tumours in mice. Anti-Dll4 treatment increased the sprouting and branching of blood vessels, and led to a marked increase in blood-vessel density in tumours. However, new vessels functioned inefficiently and were not connected functionally to the vascular network of the tumours, leading to an overall inhibition of tumour growth.

Unfortunately for many cancer patients, individual therapies can be ineffective against specific tumours, and tumours that do respond initially to drugs can later become resistant to them. Both Ridgway et al. and Noguera-Troise et al. reported that anti-Dll4 treatment inhibits tumour growth better when combined with anti-VEGF treatment than when given alone, and is also effective even against those tumours which do not respond to anti-VEGF therapies. Anti-Dll4 treatment may therefore be a good option for alternative or combinatorial therapy for those solid tumours which are resistant to anti-VEGF therapies.

Mosaic Tumour Vessels for Molecular Diagnosis of Cancer ?

There is considerable evidence to support the view that tumour growth is angiogenesis-dependent (see Streit et al., 1999; Carmeleit and Jain, 2000). A switch to the angiogenic phenotype is critical in tumour progression. Before this switch occurs, most tumours are very small. Early *in situ* carcinoma exemplifies this—neighbouring microvessels are quiescent and mature, and metastases virtually do not exist (Folkman, 2002). But after the angiogenic switch, for example in late stages of in situ breast carcinoma, neovascular sprouts break through the basement membrane, and tumour cells can grow around new capillary vessels, enter the circulation, and metastasize. Indeed a single endothelial cell may support as many as about 100 tumour cells. Importantly, this finding has made the microvascular endothelial cell recruited by a tumour an important second target in cancer therapy. Treating both the cancer cell and also the endothelial cell in a tumour could be more effective than treating the cancer cell alone (Folkman, 2002). Consequently, angiogenesis inhibitors have appeared as a new class of drugs which selectively or specifically inhibit proliferation or migration of activated endothelial cells, or induce their apoptosis. Tumour growth is either inhibited, or tumours undergo regression. Angiogenesis inhibitors are being tested in clinical trials separately and also together with chemotherapy or radiotherapy (Folkman, 2002).

Chang et al. (2000) used elegant methods to quantify traffic of tumour cells traversing new microvessels. Tumour cells in transit to the vascular lumen may reside temporarily in the microvessel wall and fill up to 4 per cent of the total vascular surface area. Around 15 per cent of vessels in a human colon carcinoma in mice contain tumour cells that share space in the vessel wall with endothelial cells. These are called 'mosaic' vessels. Almost half of the tumour cells exposed to the vessel lumen are shed into the circulation in a given day; this rate of tumour cell intravasation is consistent with previous reports that up to one million cells are shed per gram of tumour per day.

These findings have far-reaching implications for cancer therapy. Endothelial cells stimulated by mitogens such as basic fibroblast growth factor (bFGF) or vascular endothelial cell growth factor (VEGF), secrete metalloproteinase-2 (gelatinase A) which promotes degradation of basement membrane in microvessel walls (Folkman, 2002). Such a breakdown in the vascular basement membrane could possibly facilitate extravasation of endothelial cells during the formation of neovascular sprouts, as well as intravasation of tumour cells into the lumen.

The angiogenesis inhibitor endostatin is now undergoing clinical trials for use in patients suffering from advanced metastatic cancers. It inhibits endothelial cell and tumour cell invasion by blocking the catalytic activities of both metalloproteinase-2 and membrane type-1 metalloproteinase.

Besides the fairly small number of tumour cells in transit across the microvessel wall, another subpopulation of cells, viz., progenitor endothelial cells circulating from bone marrow may also enter the wall of new microvessels (see Folkman, 2002). Under typical tumour angiogenesis, when endothelial cells in the tumour bed have been largely recruited from the local neighbourhood, only a tiny fraction of these endothelial cells, if any, are derived from bone marrow progenitor endothelial cells. But, when a tumour cannot recruit endothelial cells from its local neighbourhood, the bone marrow may contribute these cells. It appears that the endothelial cell lining is continuously migrating, whereas at the same time tumour cells in transit to the lumen are residing temporarily in the microvascular wall and a few progenitor endothelial cells may be reaching the angiogenic site from the bone marrow. In contrast, little or no endothelial cell turnover or tumour cell traffic would be seen within the walls of mature, quiescent microvessels covered with pericytes and contained by a stable nondegraded basement membrane. Angiogenesis inhibitors may effectively prevent growth of neovasculature or cause regression of neovasculature, but have little or no effect on mature microvasculature (Folkman, 2002).

Lung Cancer

Lung cancer is the leading cause of cancer deaths throughout the world, with an annual fatality of more than one million. Non-small-cell lung cancer (NSCLC) accounts for about 80 per cent of all lung cancer cases. Soda et al. (2007) have discovered a gene associated with human NSCLC. A mutation involving positional rearrangement of genes along chromosome 2p activates the expression of the gene *ALK*, which encodes the *ALK* tyrosine kinase. Tyrosine kinases act as molecular switches which regulate the activity of other proteins by attaching phosphate groups to their tyrosine amino-acid residues. These enzymes seem to be involved in many cancers; they block the activity of *ALK* kinase which could lead to a powerful therapy for patients whose cancers bear this rearrangement (Meyerson, 2007).

Inhibiting protein products of activated oncogenes is an effective strategy in cancer therapy (Sawyers, 2004). Many early successes involved enzymatic blockade of tyrosine kinases. One example of this is the kinase inhibitor imatinib (Gleevec) which prolongs the lifespan of patients with chronic myelogenous leukaemia, which is caused by chromosomal rearrangements that activate the ABL tyrosine kinase (see Druker et al., 2001).

Unfortunately, the gene-targeted therapy has attracted limited application because only a few of the oncogenes that support the growth and survival of any given cancer type have been identified. Also, therapeutic strategies to disrupt gene function are not always available even for known oncogenes. In this context, the work of Soda et al. (2007) on a new oncogene for a common cancer is important. The molecular structure of this oncogene's product makes it well suited for enzymatic inhibition.

Soda et al. worked on a lung tissue specimen from a smoker NSCLC patient, isolated its total messenger RNA pool, and amplified it by generating a library of complementary DNA sequences to the mRNA transcripts, followed by analysing the oncogenic activity of the complementary DNA sequences using a classic transformation assay. They then searched for genes that could transform mouse 3T3 fibroblasts, that is, genes whose expression could confer certain properties of tumour cell on these cells. They identified a complementary DNA sequence derived from a fusion mRNA transcript as the sequence that could transform 3T3 cells. The first part of this sequence consisted of a portion of

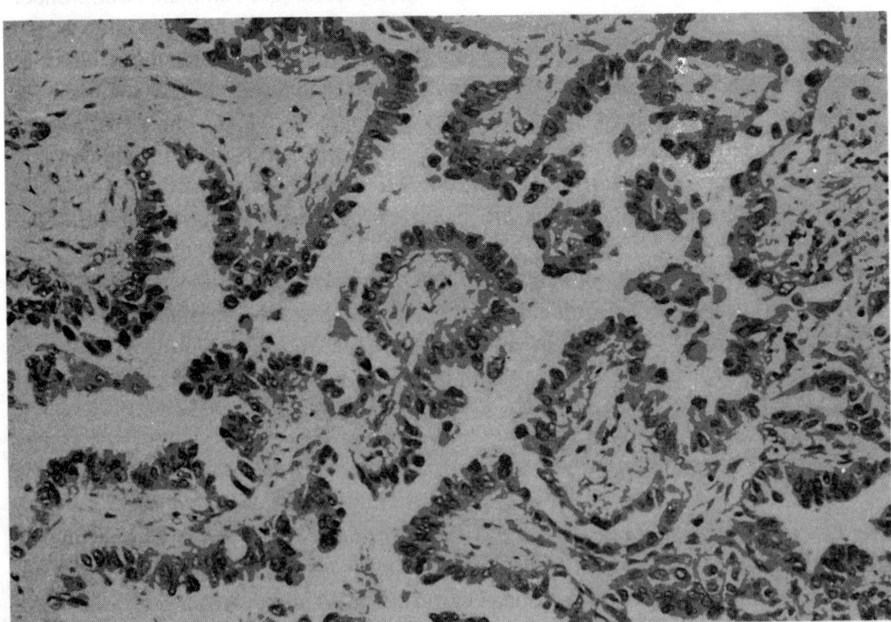

Fig. 2.1 Apical portion of human lung adenocarcinoma stained by the peroxidase technique. The cancerous cells are positively stained with monoclonal antibody YH206 (IgM). Figure provided by Drs A Yachi and K Imai (see Yachi et al., 1986).

the *EML4* gene, while the second consisted portions of the *ALK* gene. Some mutations cause portions of two genes to fuse together and form a hybrid gene. These mutations are quite frequent in blood-related cancers. *ALK* had been earlier identified through its role in anaplastic large-cell lymphoma (a blood-derived cancer); the finding of its activation in lung cancer is surprising.

Most NSCLCs, especially lung adenocarcinomas (see Fig. 2.1) the commonest type, activate a molecular signalling pathway mediated by some receptor tyrosine kinases and their downstream Ras and Raf oncogenes (Sharma et al., 2007). This points to the possibility that activated *ALK*, like EGFR/Erbb2, might constitutively switch on the Ras-Raf signalling pathway (Meyerson, 2007).

Soda et al. also searched for the *EML4-ALK* fusion gene in 75 Japanese NSCLC patients; among them, five had this oncogene. Till today, the tyrosine kinase inhibitors gefitinib (Iressa) and erlotinib (Tarceva) are the only effective targeted therapies for lung cancer. These drugs prove effective in the treatment of NSCLC patients with *EGFR* mutations (Paez et al., 2004), *ALK* inhibition is physiologically feasible, and mouse BA/F3 cells that were transformed with the *EML4-ALK* fusion gene are specifically killed with an *ALK* inhibitor. The potential therapeutic use of these inhibitors would be interesting if the *EML4-ALK* fusions are often found in smoker NSCLC patients. Gefitinib/erlotinib are most effective for non-smoker NSCLC patients whose tumours are most probably due to *EGFR* mutations.

Activated fusion genes associated with chromosomal rearrangements may be both common and important in solid tumours. Developing systematic genome-wide approaches for discovery and diagnosis by using these gene fusions could conceivably enhance our understanding of the causes of solid-tumour cancers.

Renal Cancer: Wilms' tumour

Wilms' tumour, a cancer of the kidney, occurs mostly in children and sometimes runs in families (Rivera and Haber, 2005). Genetic changes in these tumours usually cause mutations in the protein β-catenin that forms part of a signalling pathway controlled by the secreted morphogen *WNT*. *WNT*-β-catenin signalling is crucial during animal development. Some tumours not only have mutations in the gene encoding β-catenin, but also lack a normal tumour-suppressor gene, *WT1*. In many cases of Wilms' tumours there are no mutations in either gene. Rivera et al. (2007) reported another tumour-suppressor gene in Wilms' tumour, *WTX*, and Major et al. (2007) showed that *WTX* operates through □-catenin activation.

Moon et al. (2007) also reported that mutations in the gene *WTX* cause cancerous growth in Wilms' tumour, a type of kidney cancer that mostly affects children. This gene has been linked to the cancer. By means of proteomic techniques, Moon et al. have shown that the *WTX* protein forms part of a complex that normally promotes destruction of β-catenin, a key signalling protein. β-catenin is involved in the *WNT* signal transduction pathway, which plays an important role during embryo development and tissue repair.

Mutations in *WTX* lead to increased levels of β-catenin. This, in turn, promotes cell proliferation.

Rivera et al. (2007) identified deletions in the gene *WTX*; this gene becomes defunct in about one-third of Wilms' tumours, at the somatic-cell level. Interestingly, *WTX* is inactivated by a monoallelic 'single-hit' mutation and hence differs strikingly from the inactivation of most tumour-suppressor genes, which are biallelic, that is, one allele is inactivated in the germ line, followed by mutation of the second allel at the somatic-cell level (Nusse, 2007).

A single hit can produce phenotypic effect when the gene is located on the X chromosome (X-linked); indeed, *WTX* mutations occur on the single X chromosome in tumours from males and the active X chromosome in tumours from females. Tumours with mutations in *WTX* do not show *WT1* mutations. The important point about this pattern of exclusive mutations is that it may point to separate pathways leading to a similar end point in causing cancers, viz., that the WNT signalling pathway is activated because the nuclear translocation and activity of β-catenin are critical in WNT signalling (Nusse, 2007).

By now, several different components of the *WNT* signalling pathway have been shown to be involved in human tumours or experimental cancer models. One of these is adenomatous polyposis coli (APC), first isolated as a tumour-suppressor in human colon cancer. Further, activating mutations in the human gene encoding β-catenin have been reported in human colon cancer and melanomas, as well as in Wilms' tumour.

According to Major et al., WTX is a new component of the protein complex that sequesters β-catenin in the cytoplasm and blocks its gene-regulatory activity. *WTX* satisfies all the criteria of being another negative regulator of β-catenin—overexpression of *WTX* reduces *WNT*-β-catenin signalling, whereas inhibiting *WTX* enhances β-catenin activity in the nucleus, both in cultured cells as well as in animals. *WTX* is a tumour-suppressor gene in Wilms' tumours because its normal function is to control β-catenin activity (Nusse, 2007).

Besides Wilms' tumour, some pointers to β-catenin activity have been seen in other human cancers, mostly in terms of the nuclear presence of the β-catenin protein. In many such cases, there is still no evidence that the known components of the *WNT* signalling pathway are mutated, suggesting that β-catenin becomes activated without any genetic alterations. But the work of Major et al. has generated speculation that *WTX* could in fact be mutated in these cancers.

Metastasis

The complex phenomenon of metastasis involves an array of genetic changes and coordination of many positive and negative factors leading to motile cells that enter and travel through the bloodstream, forming secondary tumours elsewhere in the body. Metastasis is a selective, nonrandom and inefficient process that significantly contributes to morbidity and mortality of cancer patients and is a major challenge in cancer therapeutics (Inoue et al., 2007). The vast majority of all cancer deaths occur due to the metastatic spread of primary tumours.

Although various processes are involved in carcinogenesis, local invasion and the formation of metastases are the clinically most relevant processes. These two processes are the least well understood at the molecular level (Christofori, 2006). Understanding their mechanisms is crucial for cancer research. Recent experimental work has led to the identification of several molecular pathways and cellular mechanisms that underlie the multistage process of metastasis formation. These include tumour invasion, tumour-cell dissemination through the bloodstream or the lymphatic system, colonization of distant organs and, finally, fatal outgrowth of metastases.

Our understanding of the genetic and epigenetic events involved in early events of cancerogenesis has considerably improved in recent years. In contrast, there continues to be a woeful paucity of therapies that could efficiently prevent metastasis. Multiple signal-transduction pathways, changes in the adhesive, migratory capabilities of tumour cells and the tumour microenvironment play crucial roles in malignant tumour progression. It is at this stage of tumour development that tumour cells migrate into and invade the surrounding tissue either as single cells or in clusters, thereby forming an invasive front. Christofori (2006) has summarized new insights into the molecular mechanisms that underpin tumour invasion and metastasis. Critical elucidation of the interactions and relationships between these processes at various levels will not only enhance our understanding of the system involved but also hopefully lead to new cancer therapies.

Although solid tumours are sometimes considered as a malignant mass of epithelial cells, they contain such normal cells as fibroblasts and the endothelial and smooth muscle cells that make up tumour blood vessels. The molecular interactions between malignant cells and these stromal cells can markedly affect tumour growth. This has made stromal cells possible targets for cancer therapy. In contrast to tumour cells, stromal cells appear to be genetically stable and hence are not likely to develop resistance to therapy.

Pelham et al. (2006) explored the possibility that tumour-associated stromal cells, like their malignant neighbours, tend to be genetically changed during tumour progression. They used highly sensitive DNA copy-number analysis to study human breast and colorectal tumours that had grown in mice for one to five months. This experimental design allowed the stromal components to be easily identified on the basis of their mouse origin. The stromal cells were found to have undergone amplification or deletion of several genes, some of which might be linked to tumourigenesis.

Increased cell motility is an early manifestation of metastatic cancers and involves concerted reorganization of the actin cytoskeleton that regulates cell shape and motility through spatio-temporal activation of Rho-family GTPases (Etienne-Manneville and Hall, 2002), but the molecular mechanisms and its upstream regulators, the potential targets of metastasis, have not been clearly defined. Several approaches can be adopted to identify 'metastasis genes'. Fok et al. (2006) employed a functional interference of proteins by expression of intracellular antibodies, also called 'specific functional ablators' and 'functional therapeutical molecules' (see Inoue et al., 2007).

Inoue et al. developed a loss-of-function screening system on the basis of intracellular expression of single-domain antibodies and demonstrated its use in identification of potential targets of metastasis of human cancerous cells. Randomized intracellular antibodies were expressed in highly metastatic cells, and a derivative pool of cells with loss of migration phenotype in chemotaxis assay was isolated. Isolation of antibodies from cells with loss of migration phenotype and identification of their target proteins revealed the involvement of the heterogeneous nuclear ribonucleoprotein K (hnRNP-K), a multifunctional signalling protein, in metastasis. The cytoplasmic accumulation of hnRNP-K is critical for its role in metastasis. The above results demonstrate: (i) the advantages of our functional interference screening over the gene-knockouts and gene-silencing, (ii) hnRNP-K as a potential target of metastasis, and (iii) a potential anti-metastasis peptide validated in *in vitro* cell migration assays (Inoue et al., 2007).

Breast cancer usually spreads to several different organs such as lymph nodes, bone, lungs, brain, and liver; the most frequent site of metastasis is the bone, which occurs in approximately 80 per cent of patients with advanced diseases (Jemal et al., 2004).

Tumour metastasis can be better understood by developing animal models that reliably reproduce the metastatic process. This view is supported by the work of Welm et al. (2007) who, by modifying an existing mouse model of breast cancer, discovered that macrophage-stimulating protein (MSP) promotes breast tumour growth and metastasis to several organs. A special feature of this work was the occurrence of osteolytic bone metastases, which are conspicuous in human breast cancer. To explore the clinical relevance of this model, Welm et al. examined expression levels of three genes involved in activation of the MSP signalling pathway (*MSP*, *MT-SP1*, and *MST1R*) in human breast tumours. Overexpression of these three was found to be a strong independent indicator of both metastasis and death in cancer patients and significantly increased the accuracy of an existing gene expression signature for poor prognosis. These data suggest that signalling initiated by MSP contributes to metastasis of breast cancer and can be an independent biomarker for assessing the prognosis of females suffering from breast cancer.

Macrophage infiltration is typical of invasive cancers and is associated with poor prognosis in breast cancer (Lin and Pollard, 2004). Macrophages are involved in lung metastasis in mice from which Welm et al. obtained the tumours used in their studies (see Lin et al., 2001). Since MSP activates macrophages, it may be that the effects of MSP occur through a mechanism involving inflammation. The *in vitro* data reported by Welm et al. show that recombinant MSP can suffice to stimulate mammary epithelial cells to invade extracellular matrix, indicating that these cells directly respond to MSP. The effect of MSP is augmented, however, when macrophages are co-cultured with the epithelial cells (see Welm et al., 2007). Whether or not macrophages play a role in MSP-induced metastasis *in vivo* is not known.

Use of time lapse microscopy has thrown light on how tumours degrade and invade the protein matrix around healthy cells to spread through the body.

P Friedl et al. (see *Nature Cell Biol.* 9: 893-904, 2007) studied fibrosarcoma and breast cancer cells as the cells invaded three-dimensional blocks of collagen in a lab dish. They identified two crucial steps. First, single cells rearrange collagen fibres that are blocking their way into tube-like holes. Then, groups of cells behind the leading cells expand the tubes to clear away larger areas of the matrix with the help of enzymes including membrane-type-1 matrix metalloproteinase.

Epithelial-mesenchymal Transition

Approximately 90 per cent of cancers originate from epithelial tissue. The most striking morphological change during the transition from a benign tumour to a malignant and metastatic one is that tumour cells change from a highly differentiated epithelial morphology to a migratory and invasive phenotype. Metastatic tumour cells then enter the basal lamina barrier and invade the neighbouring tissue. During this epithelial-mesenchymal transition (EMT), cells progressively redistribute or down-regulate their apical and basolateral epithelial-specific tight and adherens junction proteins (including E-cadherin and cytokeratins) and re-express mesenchymal molecules (such as vimentin and N-cadherin) (Thiery, 2002; Huber et al., 2005). Cell-cell contacts are lost and cell motility is gained; these changes are necessary for invasion. EMT can be induced by several growth factors, produced either by tumour cells themselves or by stromal cells, and include transforming growth factor-β (TGF-β), hepatocyte growth factor (HGF), epidermal growth factor (EGF), insulin-like growth factors (IGFs) and fibroblast growth factors (FGFs), and also by the upregulated proteolytic activity of matrix metalloproteases (MMPs). However, in most cancers, full EMT—the complete loss of epithelial markers and the gain of mesenchymal markers—is rarely observed. Indeed, the presence of certain epithelial markers, such as cytokeratins, is routinely used to detect and characterize metastatic epithelial cancers in patients (Christofori, 2006).

TGF-β plays a dual role during tumour progression: repressing tumour growth during the early phases of tumourigenesis by inducing cell-cycle arrest and apoptosis, but promoting EMT, tumour invasion and metastatic dissemination of tumour cells during the late phases of carcinogenesis (Siegel and Massague, 2003). In keeping with its tumour-suppressor functions, several components of the TGF-β-mediated signalling pathways are found to be impaired in various human cancer types, including ovarian, breast and pancreatic cancers, colorectal and lung cancers. TGF-β promotes tumour progression by exerting an immunosuppressive function. It represses the expression of major histocompatibility complex (MHC) class II and adversely affects antigen-presenting cells.

HGF, produced mainly by stromal cells and the *c-Met* receptor tyrosine kinase (RTK) (its cognate receptor on tumour cells), are important mediators of invasive growth during embryonic development and tumour progression (Corso et al., 2005). Germline and somatic mutations, and amplifications of the *c-Met* gene that lead to increased c-met activity, are common in various cancer types.

TGF-β and HGF-induced signalling have a critical part in tumour progression – they provide functional connections among several molecular players implicated in the metastatic process. Indeed, they are first-line targets for the development of anti-metastasis therapies. Yang et al. (2002) reported that lifetime exposure of mice to a soluble version of TGF-βRII prevents the formation of metastases.

Tumour Progression

An elegant expression-cloning approach has recently identified TrkB, a neurotrophic RTK for brain-derived neurotrophic factor (BDNF), as a suppressor of cell death induced by the lack of cell-matrix adhesion (anoikis) (Douma et al., 2004). TrkB seems to confer survival on cells that would otherwise die when dislodged from their substrate. Instead, they migrate and invade new sites, and form metastases. TrkB and BDNF are frequently expressed in metastatic human cancers. The IGF-1 receptor (IGF-1R) is also highly expressed in many types of human cancers. It has been shown to promote tumour invasion and metastasis in a transgenic mouse model of pancreatic β-cell carcinogenesis (Douma et al., 2004). IGF-1R can impair E-cadherin function and induce tumour-cell migration and invasion. IGF-1R may be an excellent multipurpose target for the development of cancer therapies (see Garcia-Echeverria et al., 2004).

The so called hedgehog signalling pathway, essential in developmental patterning, has been implicated in the origin of many types of cancer. In the prostate, for example, sustained hedgehog signalling induces tumour formation and metastasis by a process that relies on the presence of the hedgehog signal transducer 'smoothened'. As this 'smoothened' is not expressed in benign prostate epithelial cells, it may serve as a molecular marker to distinguish between benign and malignant prostate cancer (Karhadkar et al., 2004).

Tumour hypoxia induces tumour angiogenesis and also modulates the expression of certain genes involved in tumour metastasis. A good example is the hypoxic induction of *c-Met* gene expression, which amplifies HGF signalling by sensitizing cells to HGF signalling. Hypoxia may affect tumour cells in two ways: induces angiogenesis and locally adapts the tumour environment for optimal tumour growth. By stimulating *c-Met* signalling and favouring tumour-cell migration and invasion, it facilitates metastatic dissemination, for example, in breast cancer invasiveness and organ-specific metastasis (Matteucci et al., 2005).

Members of the immunoglobulin superfamily play crucial roles in tumour progression. The cell-adhesion molecule (CAM) L1 has been shown to be a direct target of *WNT*-β-catenin signalling in colorectal cancer cells (Gavert et al., 2005). It is highly expressed at the invasive front of colorectal cancers, and promotes motility, transformation and tumourigenicity in experimental cell systems. Similarly, neuronal CAM (NrCAM) is a bona fide target of *WNT* signalling and confers tumourigenicity and motility on various tumour-cell types. It is highly upregulated in colorectal cancers as well as in melanomas (Conacci-Sorrell et al., 2002). By contrast, neural CAM (NCAM) is down-regulated in various types of cancer, and its loss results in the formation of lymph node metastases in a transgenic mouse model of pancreatic β-cell carcinogenesis (Perl et al., 1999). According to Cavallaro et al. (2001), NCAM and L1 (like N-cadherin) bind to and activate FGFR (fibroblast growth factor receptors) in neurons and tumour cells, thereby modulating β_1 integrin-mediated cell-matrix adhesion, neurite outgrowth and cell migration.

Recent results from the cellular and molecular dissection of tumour progression have generated the view that, besides the cellular processes and molecular pathways operating in tumour cells themselves, an equally important contribution to malignant tumour progression may come from cells and components of the tumour microenvironment. These include endothelial cells and mural cells of blood or lymphatic vessels, tumour fibroblasts, infiltrating cells of the immune system and the tumour's extracellular matrix (Bissell and Labarge, 2005).

Carcinoma-associated fibroblasts The demonstration that fibroblasts of malignant cancers are not identical to fibroblasts of the corresponding normal organ points to the contribution of stromal fibroblasts to tumour progression. Non-tumourigenic prostate epithelial cells co-implanted with carcinoma-associated fibroblasts (CAFs) into immunocompromised mice develop tumours, whereas normal fibroblasts can adversely affect the growth of malignant tumour cells (Hayward et al., 2001). CAFs isolated from breast carcinomas also promote the growth of breast cancer cells (Orimo et al., 2005). CAFs can also stimulate tumour angiogenesis by attracting endothelial precursor cells (EPCs).

Cells of the immune system The immune system has two functions in modulating tumour progression: repression of tumour growth by the adaptive immune system (immunosurveillance) and support of tumour progression by the innate immune system (inflammatory response). This view has recently been challenged (see de Visser et al., 2005): the presence of T and B cells is usually taken as a sign of active immunosurveillance of the tumour and hence, good prognosis. But the work of de Visser et al., using a transgenic mouse model of skin carcinogenesis, shows that T and B cells are actually required for tumour malignancy.

The role of innate immune system in tumour progression is also dual. The presence of macrophages, granulocytes, neutrophils and mast cells is indicative of good prognosis in some cancers, but seems to act negatively in many others. In particular, monocytes and their differentiated/activated derivatives, infiltrating tumour-associated macrophages (TAMs), are found in large numbers in tumours (Pollard, 2004; Joyce, 2005). On the one hand, they secrete cytokines that support the immune response, and also promote antigen processing and presentation, resulting in an anti-tumour immune response. On the other hand, many reports claim that the balance of secreted factors tilts towards a cytokine/chemokine milieu that promotes tumour progression—for example, by angiogenic factors, inflammatory cytokines and matrix metalloproteases (MMPs) (Dranoff, 2004).

Infiltrating cells of the immune system, together with CAFs and tumour cells themselves, may provide many pro-invasive factors, such as proteases, survival factors and angiogenic factors. Surprising indications about the strong role of proteases in tumour progression have come through the transgenic expression of MMPs in breast epithelial cells which, unexpectedly, resulted in full-fledged cancer. For example, MMP3 expression results in transcriptional upregulation of the small GTPase Rac1b and upregulated levels of reactive oxygen species (ROS) which, in turn, induce genomic instability and tumour progression (Radisky et al., 2005). MMPs also promote tumour-cell invasion and metastatic dissemination by activating the protease-activated receptor 1 (PAR1), a G-protein-coupled receptor implicated in metastasis of several cancers (Christofori, 2006).

Metastatic Dissemination

The formation of new blood vessels during tumour progression is a must for tumour outgrowth. It contributes to malignant tumour progression on the basis of two main observations (Folkman, 2002; Bergers and Benjamin, 2003). First, angiogenesis can be induced by transforming signals which promote tumour progression and directly upregulate the expression of angiogenic factors. Second, ongoing angiogenesis and the ensuing increase in microvessel density along with the presence of inflammatory sites, make it possible for invasive tumour cells to intravasate and disseminate through the bloodstream.

Conversely, there are indications that the outgrowth of new lymphatic vessels can directly promote the formation of lymph node metastases, chiefly at the draining regional lymph nodes of a tumour (Achen et al., 2005).

Both angiogenesis and lymphangiogenesis contribute not only to primary tumour growth but also to the metastatic dissemination of tumour cells. Together, they constitute appropriate targets for the development of anti-metastatic therapies. The first angiogenesis inhibitors have entered clinical use but we should await results on the combinatorial inhibition of angiogenesis and lymphangiogenesis and its specific effects on tumour metastasis (Christofori, 2006).

One puzzling and little-understood aspect of tumour metastasis is the specificity with which certain cancer types metastasize to specific organs. The anatomy of the bloodstream and lymphatic drainage do explain some patterns of metastasis but it appears that they do not tell the whole story—other guiding cues seem to be involved (Zeelenberg et al., 2003; Christofori, 2006).

Gene-expression profiling studies with breast cancer cell lines metastasizing to specific target organs have revealed many interesting genes and factors. Significant genes that are expressed in breast cancer cell lines colonizing bone include IL-11, connective-tissue growth factor (CTGF), CXCR4 and osteopontin. Their combinatorial expression induces bone metastasis in cells that would not otherwise colonize bone (Kang et al., 2003). Genes that direct breast cancer cells to the lungs include SPARC (secreted protein, acidic, cysteine-rich), Id1 (inhibitor of DNA binding 1), MMP1, MMP2, VCAM1 (vascular cell-adhesion molecule 1), IL-13Rα (interleukin 13 receptor-α), COX2 (cyclooxygenase 2) and CXCL1 (Minn et al., 2005). It is their combinatorial expression that enables them to metastasize to the lungs; combinatorial ablation of their expression impairs lung-specific metastasis. Besides the above, some pathophysiological changes in the target organs also influence organ-specific metastasis. Another possibility, the interaction between specific receptors on the surface of disseminating tumour cells and the target organ endothelium may also explain organ-specific metastasis. Kaplan et al. (2005) showed that bone-marrow-derived vascular endothelial growth factor receptor (VEGFR1)-positive cells play an enigmatic part in directing metastatic tumour cells to a specific target organ: metastatic tumour cells secrete previously unknown factors which induce expression of fibronectin specifically in the metastatic target organs. In turn, VEGFR1 cells are recruited to these sites where they prepare the metastatic niche for the arrival of tumour cells. Finally, the outgrowth of secondary tumours may offer another approach to the design of anti-metastatic therapies, because after dissemination to specific organs, tumour cells need to adapt to and communicate with the new environment and induce angiogenesis (Chambers et al., 2002).

Role of Isozymes in Cancer

Some drugs that interfere with the DNA topoisomerase II enzyme (Top2) effectively treat cancer but can sometimes cause secondary malignancies. Azarova et al. (2007) reported that the β form of Top2 is mostly responsible for these secondary cancers, whereas the α form is most susceptible to chemotherapy. The authors examined the effects of the drug VP-16 etoposide on skin cancer rates in mice and observed that mice with the Top2β gene showed a higher incidence of skin cancer than those with no Top2 gene. It was also found that DNA rearrangements and double-strand breaks caused by VP-16 depend on the presence of Top2β. It was possible to inhibit the carcinogenic action of VP-16 by adding a proteasome inhibitor. This suggests that processing of Top2β-DNA complexes by proteasome is critical in VP-16-induced DNA rearrangement and carcinogenesis. In cells with both forms of Top2, it was found that the α form is chiefly responsible for causing cell death in VP-16-treated cells. Drugs that act specifically on Top2α may, therefore, be more effective anticancer agents, with less chance of causing secondary cancers.

Metastasis Micromanagement

MicroRNAs are naturally occurring short RNA sequences that were discovered in the early 1990s. They have many regulatory functions, including mediation of cancer metastasis. To spread successfully, a tumour cell has to perform many complex processes, such as invasion, survival and arrest in the circulatory system, and colonization of foreign organs (Steeg, 2007). Ma et al. (2007) proposed that microRNAs (miRNAs), which regulate levels of messenger RNAs, coordinate some of the intricate gene-expression programmes implicated in cancer metastasis. Tumour metastasis is undoubtedly one of the most complex processes known. Just consider a tumour cell's movement. The leading edge of the cell protrudes because of cytoskeletal change and adherence to the extracellular matrix, whereas the trailing edge gets detached from the matrix. It is not known how many separate gene-expression programmes are involved in simple motility, let alone the many more requirements of metastasis. But miRNAs seem to be prime candidates for coordinating the complex gene-expression events that lead to metastasis.

Ma et al. studied the complex role of the transcription factor called Twist in tumour-cell motility. They found that Twist induces the transcription of microRNA-10b (miR-10b), which inhibits translation of, *inter alia*, the mRNA for the transcription factor HOXD10 by binding to its three untranslated region. This, in turn, increases both the expression of RHOC and cell motility. However, not all of Twist's known downstream effects leading to metastasis are regulated by the miR-10b-mediated pathway (Ma et al., 2007; Steeg, 2007).

It appears that some other miRNAs also contribute to metastasis. For instance, the miR-17-92 cluster of miRNAs regulates the expression of connective-tissue growth factor and thrombospondin-1 (Dews et al., 2006), which are important for the formation of new blood vessels. Other candidate miRNA-regulated mRNAs, whose expression is thought to mediate metastasis, may include mRNAs for proteins involved in different aspects of metastasis, such as adherence, invasion, motility, angiogenesis and protein degradation (Dalmay and Edwards, 2006). This prompts the question whether individual miRNAs can contribute to various events associated with metastasis and, if so, how are they regulated in a cellular context? Should different miRNA pathways control various aspects of metastasis, therapeutic strategies for targeting miRNAs implicated in other pathological processes (such as those suggested by Hammond, 2006) may also be applicable to preventing cancer spread (Steeg, 2007).

Future Scope

The various stages of development of fatal metastasis involve many different cellular and molecular mechanisms. Hopefully, many of the molecular pathways and compounds that are causally involved could be suitable targets for the development of efficient anti-metastatic therapies. Yet, the identification of these players and routes has just begun and their functional contributions are being explored. Table 2.1 lists some common tumour markers that are currently being used. New technologies such as the high throughput

Table 2.1 Common tumour markers currently in use*.

Tumour markers	Cancers of	What else?	When/How used?
AFP	Liver, germ cells of ovaries or testes	Also elevated during pregnancy and in hepatitis	To diagnose, monitor treatment, and determine recurrence
CA 15-3	Breast, lung, ovarian	Also elevated in benign breast conditions	Stage disease, monitor treatment, and determine recurrence
CA 19-9	Pancreas, bowel and bile ducts	Also elevated in pancreatitis and inflammatory bowel disease	Stage disease, monitor treatment, and determine recurrence
CEA	Bowel, lung, breast, thyroid, pancreas, liver, cervix, bladder	Elevated in conditions such as hepatitis, colitis, pancreatitis, and in cigarette smokers	Monitor treatment and determine recurrence

Contd...

Contd...

Tumour markers	Cancers of	What else?	When/How used?
Oestrogen receptors	Breast	Increased in hormone-dependent cancer	Determine prognosis and guide treatment
hCG	Testicles and trophoblasts	Elevated in pregnancy, testicular failure	Help diagnose, monitor treatment and determine recurrence
HER-2/neu	Breast	Oncogene that is present in multiple copies in 20–30% of invasive breast cancer	Determine prognosis and guide treatment
Monoclonal immuno-globulins	Multiple myeloma and Waldenstrom's macroglobulinemia	Overproduction of an immunoglobulin or antibody, detected by protein electrophoresis	Help diagnose, monitor treatment and determine recurrence
Progesterone receptors	Breast	Increased in hormone-dependent cancer	Determine prognosis and guide treatment
PSA	Prostate	Elevated in benign prostatic hypertrophy, prostatitis, and with age	Help diagnose, monitor treatment, and determine recurrence

*(Sampling is on blood for # 1–4, 6, 8, 9; tissue # 5, 9; urine 6, 8).
Source: Lab Tests Online UK

quantitative genomic and proteomic approaches combined with appropriate computational power, novel highly sensitive and quantitative measurements of the ever-growing number of metabolic parameters and finally, the improvement of animal models to mimic malignant human disease should facilitate unravelling the complexity of the processes involved (Christofori, 2006).

3 Carcinogenic Risks of Exposure to Solar and Ultraviolet Radiation

Introduction

Carcinogenic risks associated with human exposure to solar and ultraviolet (UV) radiation from medical and cosmetic devices, general illumination and industrial sources have been evaluated (see IARC, 1992). Solar radiation is largely optical radiation (UV, visible and infrared), although both shorter wavelength (ionizing) and longer wavelength (microwaves and radiofrequency) radiation is present. UVR lies in the interval 100–400 nm and is further subdivided into UVA (315–400 nm), UVB (280–315 nm) and UVC (100–280 nm) (Kumar and Häder, 1999).

The UV part of terrestrial radiation from the sun makes up about 95 per cent UVA and 5 per cent UVB; UVC is absorbed from extraterrestrial radiation by stratospheric ozone. Earlier around AD 1900, the sun was essentially the only source of UVR. The advent of artificial sources increased the opportunity for additional exposure, not only to UVA and UVB but also to UVC ever since. The potential of UVR for causing damage to biomolecules, cells, tissues and organisms varies greatly over the spectral region from 250 to 400 nm.

The UVA radiation is a component of solar emissions as well as of emissions from medical lamps and lamps used for cosmetic purposes.

The UVB radiation is present in solar emissions, from lamps used in medicine and for cosmetic purposes, and in certain lamps used for general illumination, such as unshielded fluorescent and tungsten-halogen lamps. It causes sunburn quite easily and is immunosuppressive; it can also cause ocular cataracts. The possibility that the UVB component of solar radiation will increase as a result of depletion of the ozone layer has generated considerable concern (see Häder et al., 2007; McKenzie et al., 2007).

Exposure to UV Radiation

The quality (spectral distribution) and quantity (total UV irradiance) of UVR reaching the earth's surface depend on the radiated power from the sun and the transmitting properties of the atmosphere. UVC in the extra-terrestrial solar spectrum is completely filtered-out by the ozone layer in the atmosphere. UVB radiation represents about 5 per cent of the total solar UVR that reaches the Earth. It is the most biologically significant part of the terrestrial UV spectrum. The levels of UVB radiation reaching the Earth's surface, although heavily attenuated, are also mostly controlled by the ozone layer.

Factors Influencing Terrestrial UVR Levels

1. Variations in stratospheric ozone with latitude and season.
2. **Time of day** In summer, about 20–30 per cent of the total daily amount of UVR is received between 11:00 and 13:00 hours and 75 per cent between 9:00 and 15:00 hours (Diffey, 1991; Table 3.1). Although the amount of visible light falling on the ground in the summer may vary by only 30 per cent between 12:00 and 15:00 hours (local solar time), the short-wavelength component of the UVB spectrum undergoes a marked change during this period. At a wavelength of 300 nm, the spectral irradiance decreases tenfold from approximately 1.0 to 0.1 μW (cm² × nm).
3. **Season** Seasonal variation in terrestrial UV irradiance, especially UVB, at the Earth's surface is quite significant in temperate regions but is much less nearer the equator.
4. **Geographical latitude** Annual UVR exposure dose decreases with increasing distance from the equator.
5. **Clouds** They reduce UV ground irradiance. Changes in UVR are smaller than those of total irradiance because water vapour in clouds attenuates solar infrared radiation more than UVR. Even with heavy cloud cover, the scattered UVB component of sunlight is seldom less than 10 per cent of that under clear sky; however, very heavy cloud cover can virtually eliminate UVB even in summer. Light clouds scattered over a blue sky make little difference in sun-burning effectiveness unless they directly cover the sun. Complete light cloud cover prevents about 50 per cent of UVB energy, relative to that from a clear sky, from reaching the surface of the Earth (Diffey, 1991).
6. **Surface reflection** The importance of reflected UVR to an individual's total UVR depends on several factors (Table 3.2). A grass lawn scatters about 3 per cent of incident UVB radiation. Sand reflects about 10–15 per cent—sitting under an umbrella on the beach can lead to sunburn both from scattered UVB from the sky and reflected UVB from the sand. Fresh snow can reflect up to 90 per cent of incident UVB radiation, although reflectance of about 30–50 per cent is probably more typical. Ground reflectance is important, because parts of the body that are normally shaded are exposed to reflected radiation.
7. **Altitude** Generally, each 300 m increase in altitude increases the sun-burning effectiveness of sunlight by about 4 per cent. Conversely, places on the earth's surface below sea level have lower UVB exposures than nearby sites at sea level.
8. **Air pollution** Tropospheric (ground level) ozone and other pollutants can decrease UVR, particularly in urban areas.

Table 3.1 Percentage of daily UVB and UVA radiation received during different time periods on a clear summer's day. Solar noon is assumed to be at 12:00 hours, i.e., no allowance is made for daylight saving time (after Diffey, 1991).

Latitude (°N)	UVB		UVA	
	11:00–13:00 hrs	9:00–15:00 hrs	11:00–13:00 hrs	9:00–15:00 hrs
20	30	78	27	73
40	28	75	25	68
60	26	69	21	60

Table 3.2 Representative terrain reflectance factors for horizontal surfaces measured with a UVB radiometer at 12:00 hours (290–315 nm) in the USA (after Sliney, 1986).

Material	Reflectance (%)
Lawn grass, winter, Maryland	3.0–5.0
Soil, clay/humus	4.0–6.0
Sidewalk, light concrete	10–12
Asphalt roadway, two years old (grey)	5.0–8.9
House paint, white, metal oxide	22
Sea surf, white foam	25–30
Snow, fresh	88
Snow, two days old	50

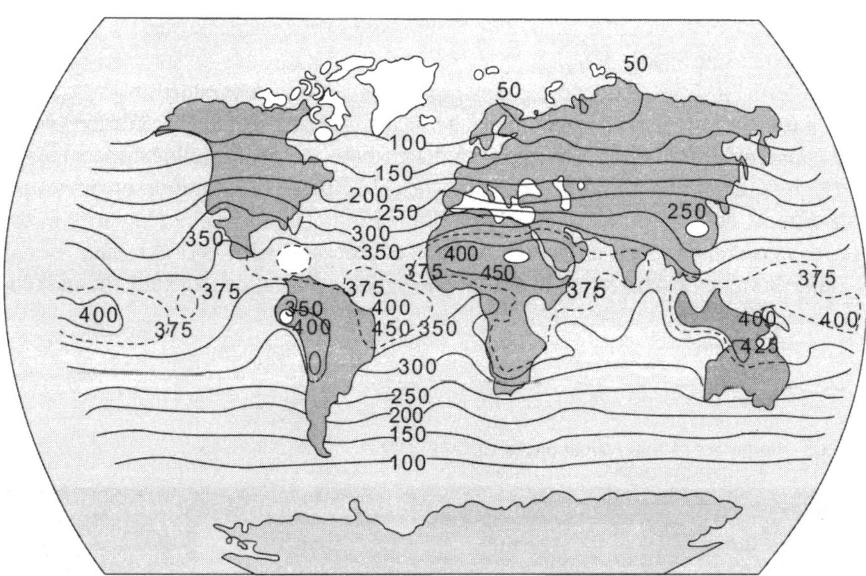

Fig. 3.1 Global distribution of ultraviolet radiation (after Schulze, 1970).

A map of annual UVR exposure as shown in Figure 3.1 was compiled for epidemiological studies of skin cancer and other diseases (Schulze, 1970). However, its interpretation in relation to human exposure is complicated by three factors: (i) the considerable variation in UVB spectral irradiance with solar position throughout the day and with season; (ii) the effect of the geometry of exposure of individuals; and (iii) variation between humans in outdoor exposure and the parts of their bodies that are exposed (IARC, 1992).

Carcinogenicity Assessment

Carcinogenicity assessment involves such considerations of qualitative importance as: (i) the experimental conditions under which the test was performed, including route and schedule of exposure, species, strain, sex, age, duration of follow-up, etc.; (ii) the consistency of the results, for example, across species and target organ(s); (iii) the spectrum of neoplastic response, from pre-neoplastic lesions and benign tumours to malignant neoplasms; and (iv) the possible role of modifying factors (IARC, 1992).

When benign tumours occur together with and originate from the same cell-type in an organ or tissue as malignant tumours in a particular study, and seem to represent a stage in the progression to malignancy, it is advisable to combine them in assessing tumour incidence. The occurrence of lesions suspected to be pre-neoplastic may in certain instances help in assessing the biological plausibility of any neoplastic response observed. If an agent or mixture induces only benign neoplasms which appears to be end-points that do not readily undergo transition to malignancy, it should nevertheless be suspected of being a carcinogen and it should be further investigated.

The probability that tumours will occur usually depends on the species, sex, strain and age of the animal, the dose of the carcinogen, and the route and length of exposure. Evidence of an increased incidence of neoplasms with increased level of exposure strengthens the inference of a causal association between the exposure and the development of neoplasms (IARC, 1992).

The form of dose-response relationship varies widely, depending on the specific agent and the target organ. Since many chemicals require metabolic activation before being converted into their reactive intermediates, both metabolic and pharmacokinetic aspects are crucial in determining the dose-response pattern. Saturation of steps such as absorption, activation, inactivation and elimination can produce nonlinearity in the dose-response relationship, as could saturation of processes such as DNA repair.

Table 3.3 gives a short summary of carcinogenicity evaluations for sunlight and other types of radiations.

Table 3.3 Summary of final evaluations (after IARC, 1992).

Agent	Degree of evidence of carcinogenicity		Overall evaluation of carcinogenicity to humans
	Humans	Animals	
Solar radiation	S	S	1
Broad-spectrum ultraviolet radiation		S	
Ultraviolet A radiation		S	2A
Ultraviolet B radiation		S	2A
Ultraviolet C radiation		S	2A
Fluorescent lighting	I		3
Sun-lamps and sun-beds, use of	L		2A

S, sufficient evidence; L, limited evidence; I, inadequate evidence.
1–3A refers to groups or categories.

Solar Radiation and Cancer

Non-melanocytic skin cancer is classified into two major histological types: basal-cell carcinoma (BCC) and squamous-cell carcinoma (SCC). BCC is the commoner type in white populations.

Xeroderma pigmentosum (Xp) is a rare autosomal-recessive genetic disease in which there is an excision repair defect. Patients show cellular and clinical hypersensitivity to UVR. The disease incidence is about one in 250,000 people in the USA and Europe, and as much as 1 in 100,000 or even 1 in 40,000 people may be affected in Japan (see Cleaver and Kraemer, 1989).

The occurrence of non-melanocytic skin cancer according to host factors, such as race, provides indirect evidence that sunlight is a cause.

In most white populations, non-melanocytic skin cancer occurs more commonly in men than in women. Populations with greater skin pigmentation tend to have low rates of non-melanocytic skin cancer.

The majority of cases of skin cancer recorded in several cancer registries and in special surveys in the USA occurred on the head and neck. SCC occurred mostly on exposed sites.

One distinctive feature of the site distribution of BCC is a virtual absence on the dorsa of the hands and infrequent occurrence on the forearms as compared with the distribution of SCC. BCC also occurs frequently on parts of the face that receive comparatively little sun exposure.

Non-melanocytic skin cancer incidence and mortality tend to increase with increasing proximity to the equator; there is usually a negative correlation between incidence of non-melanocytic skin cancer in various countries and latitudes. Several authors have correlated non-melanocytic skin cancer incidence (or mortality) with estimates of UVR (see IARC, 1992).

The fact that UVR by itself can produce tumours, makes it a 'complete' carcinogen and it may also be involved in co-carcinogenicity. Several researchers have attempted to find whether UVR has tumour 'initiating' and/or tumour 'promoting' activity when tested in a traditional two-stage protocol.

A 'tumour initiator' can be defined as an agent that, at a stated amount and upon administration, is incapable of causing tumours in the population of animals unless the skin is subsequently treated with a 'tumour promoter'.

A 'tumour promoter' is defined as an agent that, under stated conditions is incapable of causing tumours unless the skin was previously treated with a 'tumour initiator'. The test systems used may cover several variables. For example, UVR has also been shown to influence the immune system, and that polycyclic aromatic hydrocarbons are photochemically active.

Administration with Polycyclic Aromatic Hydrocarbons

Many animal studies have demonstrated that UVR has a co-carcinogenic action with other carcinogens (e.g., 3,4-Benzopyrene). There is also additional information on co-carcinogenesis, on photolysis of polycyclic aromatic hydrocarbons and on other interference with chemical carcinogenesis (see Clark, 1964; Ito, 1966; Stenbäck, 1975; Roberts and Daynes, 1980; Gensler and Welch, 1992; IARC, 1992).

Administration with Other Agents with Promoting Activity

Some studies (on mice, involving the use of croton oil) were designed to evaluate the action of UVR as a tumour initiator. Groups of 15–53 male and 9–30 female 'random-bred' hairless mice, 9–12 weeks old, received a single exposure to UVB for 30 seconds or no exposure at all, followed a fortnight later by applications to the dorsal skin of 0.1 ml croton oil in acetone twice a week for 18 months. Neither UVB exposure nor croton oil alone produced any skin tumour over the course of the study. The group of 79 mice that received both UVB exposure and croton oil had eight persistent skin tumours (one per mouse). Table 3.4 summarizes genetic and related effects of UVA radiation.

UV-B Radiation and Skin Cancers

Excessive solar UV-B radiation (280–315 nm) resulting from stratospheric ozone depletion can cause an inflammatory sunburn to people exposed to it. By being directly exposed to solar radiation, the skin is vulnerable to cancer development as the main negative health effect of excessive UVR exposure (see van der Leun and de Gruijl, 2002). Although human skin is adapted to the ambient UVR, the sunburn reaction shows that excessive exposures can severely stress defensive mechanisms or even exceed them and cause pain and blister formation. Fair-skinned people are most susceptible to sunburn, and run a higher risk than dark-skinned people of long-term adverse effects, such as skin cancer. Norval et al. (2007) have reviewed the relationship between various types of skin cancer and solar UVR.

Skin cancer is the commonest form of cancer among fair-skinned populations and its incidence has increased significantly over the last century. Many skin cancers manifest themselves early and so can be effectively treated. This limits the morbidity and mortality caused by them. For many skin cancers, the 'non-melanoma' skin cancers (NMSC) consisting of basal cell carcinomas (BCC) and squamous cell carcinomas (SCC), the malignant potential is quite low. This also reduces mortality. But this is not the case for melanoma, the most malignant form of skin cancer that arises from pigment cells (melanocytes), and is responsible for most of the deaths from skin cancer.

Molecular Genetics of Human Skin Cancers

Mutations in DNA isolated from tumours and relevant to carcinogenesis can point to a causal link with exposures to carcinogens, but two important qualifications must be borne in mind. Firstly, the changes detected may have arisen late in tumour development (whether or not the tumour is the result of exposure to UVR) and may not be involved in initiation or other early steps. Secondly, the spectrum of mutations observed may be limited to those changes that can lead to a functional gene product. This qualification applies, for example, to mutations that activate *ras* genes but to only a lesser extent to tumour-suppressor gene mutations in which inactivation of gene function is involved.

Experimental studies indicate that UV-induced mutations have a distinctive pattern of base-substitution mutations. Virtually, all mutations occur at dipyrimidine sites, especially 5'TC and 5'CC sequences; the majority of the base- substitution mutations involve cytosine with the C→T transition predominating; and tandem 5'CC→5'TT mutations occur.

Table 3.4 Genetic and related effects of ultraviolet 'A' radiation (after IARC, 1992).

Non-mammalian Systems													Mammalian Systems																											
Prokaryotes		Lower eukaryotes				Plants			Insects				*In vitro*																*In vivo*											
													Animal cells								Human cells								Animals							Humans				
D	G	D	R	G	A	D	G	C	R	G	C	A	D	G	S	M	C	A	T	I	D	G	S	M	C	A	T	I	D	G	S	M	C	DL	A	D	S	M	C	A
	+	+											$+^{1}$	+	$+^{1}$		$+^{1}$				+	+														$+^{1}$				

Table 3.5 Genetic and related effects of ultraviolet B radiation (after IARC, 1992).

Non-mammalian Systems													Mammalian Systems																											
Prokaryotes		Lower eukaryotes				Plants			Insects				*In vitro*																*In vivo*											
													Animal cells								Human cells								Animals							Humans				
D	G	D	R	G	A	D	G	C	R	G	C	A	D	G	S	M	C	A	T	I	D	G	S	M	C	A	T	I	D	G	S	M	C	DL	A	D	S	M	C	A
	+							$+^{1}$					+	+	$+^{1}$				+		+	+					$+^{1}$		+							+				

A, aneuploidy; C, chromosomal aberrations; D, DNA damage; DL, dominant lethal mutations; G, gene mutation; I, inhibition of intercellular communication; M, micronuclei; R, mitotic recombination and gene conversion; S, sister chromatid exchange; T, cell transformation.

In completing the tables, the following symbols indicate the consensus of the Working Group with regard to the results for each endpoint:

+ considered to be positive for the specific endpoint and level of biological complexity

$+^{1}$ considered to be positive, but only one valid study was available to the Working Group; sperm abnormality in mouse

– considered to be negative

$-^{1}$ considered to be negative, but only one valid study was available to the Working Group

? considered to be equivocal or inconclusive (e.g., there were contradictory results from different laboratories; there were confounding exposures; the results were equivocal

Primary melanomas, metastases and cell lines derived from melanomas which developed at body sites characterized as exposed 'rarely', 'intermittently' or 'continuously' to the sun have been analysed for the presence of N-*ras* mutations (see IARC, 1992). Of 37 cutaneous melanomas, seven had N-*ras* mutations; all were from 'continuously' exposed sites. All mutations in the N-*ras* gene were at TT or CC sites, which are potential locations for mutagenic UV photoproducts, suggesting a role of sun exposure in N-*ras* mutation. In several investigations, base-substitution mutations were found in Ha-, Ki- and N-*ras* gene in human skin melanomas and in SCC and BCCs from exposed and normal patients.

p53 Gene Mutations

Brash et al. (1991) reported *p53* mutations at various codons in 14 out of 24 (58 per cent) invasive SCCs from sun-exposed skin (Table 3.6). The mutations found were predominantly C→T (5 of 14 total mutants, 36%) and CC→TT (3 of 14, 21%) transitions, exclusively at tandem pyrimidine stretches. This finding is in accord with the hypothesis that these mutations are induced by UV irradiation. CC→TT double-base change in the *p53* gene has not been found in tumours in any internal organ. These results suggest that solar radiation can induce *p53* gene mutations (IARC, 1992).

Pierceall et al. (1991) found *p53* mutations in exon 7 in two out of ten SCCs carcinomas from sun-exposed body sites; one was a C→T transition and the other a C→A transversion.

Melanoma

Cutaneous malignant melanomas are related to sun exposure in early life, to episodes of severe sunburn, and to the number of moles (nevi), which in turn are related to sun

Table 3.6 Depicts *p53* tumour-suppressor gene mutations in human squamous-cell carcinomas that developed at sites subject to sun exposure (after Brash et al., 1991).

Codon	Nucleotide sequence	Base-substitution mutation	Incidence[a]	Site of tumour origin
7	TCT	TGT; C→G	1/14/24	Preauricular
56	*TT*CA	TAA; C→A	1/14/24	Chest
104/105	*C*G *CC*T	Deletion of a C	2/14/24	Preauricular/ temple
151	*CCC CC*	CAC; C→A	1/14/24	Scalp
152	*CC CCC*	CAC; C→T	1/14/24	Hand
179	A *CC*A	CAA; C→A	1/14/24	Scalp
245	G *CC*G	CAG; C→A	1/14/24	Cheek
247/248	A*C C*G	T T; CC→TT	1/14/24	Nose
248	G*CC*	GAC; C→A	1/2/10	Face
258	*T TCC*	TTC; C→T	1/14/24	Face
285/286	T*C CT*	T T; CC→TT	1/14/24	Face
286	T*C CT*	CTT; C→T	1/14/24	Forehead

Italics indicate potential pyrimidine dimer site.

[a] Number of specific mutations/number of total mutations found/Total number of samples tested only from sites continuously exposed to the sun.

exposure in early life. In many countries, the incidence of cutaneous melanoma (CM) has been rising at the highest rate for any form of cancer.

Although CM is not so common in individuals under the age of 20, its incidence in teenagers in the USA increased by 2.9 per cent per year between 1973 and 2003, and was higher in those areas of the country where sun exposure was greater (Lange et al., 2007).

In recent years, genetic changes have been identified in melanoma cells, and their functional importance for melanoma development has been demonstrated in genetically modified mice.

Like cutaneous melanoma, many countries also witnessed significant annual increases in the incidence of non-melanoma skin cancers (NMSC) (Brewster et al., 2007). In fact, the incidence of NMSC in Australia in 2002 was five times greater than that of all other cancers combined, and its treatment and diagnosis costs were also the highest. In 2002, almost 2 per cent of the white Australian population had to be treated for NMSC.

Residence in areas exposed to high ambient solar UV-B during the first two decades of life appears to be associated with an increased risk of mutations in an oncogene (*BRAF*) commonly found in melanomas. This finding highlights the need to protect children from excessive exposure to solar UV radiation (see Lange et al., 2007).

Genetic risk factors Well-established genetic factors confer susceptibility to melanoma—notably inherited mutations in the cell-cycle control gene, *p16INK4a*, and in the 'hair-colour' gene which codes for the melanocortin 1 receptor (MC1R). The *MC1R* gene contributes to the control of pigmentation in hair and skin and is an important risk factor for all types of skin cancer, including melanoma (Sturm, 2002).

UVR damages DNA which can then give rise to gene mutations that contribute to skin cancer formation (see below). This makes repair of damage all the more important. The solar UV-B induced DNA damage (mainly cyclobutane pyrimidine dimers, CPDs) is removed by a 'cut-and-paste' type of DNA nucleotide excision repair. A complete dysfunction in one of the enzymes in this repair system sharply increases risk of skin cancer, including melanoma.

More subtle genetic variations (polymorphisms) in the repair enzymes can modify the efficacy of DNA repair, and so affect skin cancer risk. Table 3.6 summarizes genetic and related effects of UV-B radiation.

Oncogenic alterations Melanomas from chronically exposed, intermittently exposed and unexposed skin sites show different molecular signatures (Grimm and Wei, 2006). The melanomas from intermittently exposed skin have a high frequency of activating mutations in a critical signaling molecule, *B-RAF. MC1R* variants, which are associated with enhanced risk of melanoma, are strongly associated with *B-RAF* mutations. Sunburning UV-B exposure of adults may also contribute to melanoma development by stimulating the proliferation of melanocytes (van Schanke et al., 2005).

Immunity The presence of immune mechanisms against melanomas in humans is suggested by the occasional spontaneous regression of some pigmented skin lesions. Immune responses against melanoma antigens can be detected in patients and immunotherapy is currently being used for melanoma treatment (Overwijk and Restifo, 2000; Steitz et al., 2006).

Non-melanoma Skin Carcinomas (NMSCs)

Whereas SSC is associated chiefly with chronic and life-long accumulated sun exposure, BCC, like melanoma, is more closely associated with early-life and intermittent exposures resulting in episodes of severe sunburn. SCCs occur on body sites most regularly exposed to the sun, such as the face; whereas, BCCs are also found frequently on sites exposed intermittently to sunlight. The genetic alterations identified in SCC and BCC are also quite different.

Epidemiology The incidence of both SCC and BCC has been increasing with disproportionately high increases in BCC in young females on the lower limbs (Pearce et al., 2003; Christenson et al., 2005). Sunbathing is associated with a fivefold rise in the risk of BCC on the trunk (Lovatt et al., 2005).

BCC is locally invasive. It is usually a slow growing, not very aggressive tumour; superficial BCC on the trunk is sometimes misdiagnosed and confused with eczematous skin lesions.

One interesting finding is that in patients of skin cancer, whose cancer is strongly linked with solar UV-B radiation, the risk of developing many other cancers is reduced, and they also have a lower risk of osteoporotic fractures.

The risk of individuals developing an internal solid cancer following the diagnosis of skin cancer was significantly decreased for BCC and SCC in sunny countries, such as Australia, as compared to less sunny countries, such as Finland. Analysis of data on second cancers that had developed following a diagnosis of NMSC revealed that the relative risks of several internal cancers such as cervical, oesophageal and gastric were reduced (see Norval et al., 2007; pers. commun.). Similarly, skin cancer patients in the south-east region of the Netherlands had a lower risk of developing prostate cancer as compared with the general population. Furthermore, the risk of advanced prostate cancer was reduced by 27 per cent. These and other studies strongly point to the possibility that UV radiation not only lowers the chances of developing several internal cancers, but also protects against osteoporotic fractures in later life (see Norval et al., 2007; pers. commun.).

The most interesting point emerging from several recent studies is the suggestion that the protective factor induced by solar UV radiation is vitamin D. While it has long been known that exposure of the skin to solar UV-B is associated with reduced risk of certain cancers and autoimmune diseases, the possibility that vitamin D, synthesized in the skin exposed to UV-B radiation playing a protective role, has emerged only recently. However, optimization of vitamin D levels requires special consideration in view of the fact that indiscriminate overall increases in UV exposures can often accentuate skin cancer incidence without significantly increasing beneficial effects.

Genetic risk factors UV-B inflicts characteristic DNA damage (mainly CPDs) whose repair in human skin diminishes with age (Yamada et al., 2006). Such damage tends to cause specific 'point mutations' in the *p53* tumour-suppressor gene in NMSC. NMSC also show frequent crude chromosomal aberrations which are already abundantly present in the benign precursor lesions of SCC, the actinic keratoses (AKs). Complete double strand breaks (DSBs) in the DNA cause these gross chromosomal losses and duplications. Variants in genes involved in thc repair of DSB in DNA may be related to NMSC risk, but not to melanoma risk (Han et al., 2004). The association between NMSC and DSB repair is consistent with the finding that UV-B-exposed blood cells from patients with skin carcinomas are more prone to develop chromatid breaks than equivalent cells from melanoma patients and control subjects (Wang et al., 2005).

Oncogenic alterations Although less efficient than UV-B, long-wave UV-A can also cause the same type of DNA damage as UV-B, and so lead to 'UV-B-like' mutations in the *p53* tumour-suppressor gene. However, oxidative damage contributes much at these longer wavelengths and causes different p53 mutations from those induced by UV-B (Besaratinia et al., 2005; Kramata et al., 2005).

Vitamin D

Exposure to solar UVR produces many adverse health effects in humans but one beneficial effect is its contribution to vitamin D status. In an individual, this status can be estimated by measuring the serum or plasma concentration of 25-hydroxyvitamin D [25(OH)D]. The active form of vitamin D, 1,25-dihydroxyvitamin D [1,25$(OH)_2$D] is synthesized in the last step of the metabolic pathway. The levels of 1,25$(OH)_2$D are maintained even when 25(OH)D levels fall. Currently, the serum levels of 25(OH)D considered excessive, sufficient, insufficient and deficient are less than 250, 50–250, 25–50 and more than 25 nmol L^{-1}, respectively (Holick, 2004; Grant and Holick, 2005; Wolpowitz and Gilchrest, 2006). According to Bischoff-Ferrari et al. (2006), serum concentration of 25(OH)D for a number of health endpoints lies between 90–100 nmol L^{-1}.

For most people, more than 90 per cent of their vitamin D requirement is met from exposure to solar UVR. In human skin, synthesis occurs most effectively following exposure to the UV-B waveband. As solar UVB is reduced to almost zero in winter months at latitudes above 50° North or South, vitamin D status varies considerably with season and location. Many people living in high latitude areas tend to be vitamin D-insufficient. Vitamin D is essential for good bone health and protects against certain cancers and autoimmune diseases.

There is an inverse correlation between sun exposure (usually estimated from latitude, weather stations and the UV Index) and the incidence or mortality from several internal cancers (for examples, see Brewster et al., 2007).

Certain groups of people, such as those with dark skin, veiled women, the elderly, and those who live at high latitudes in winter months, face special risk of vitamin D deficiency and may need to take vitamin D supplements.

For some healthy individuals, however, even abundant sun exposure may not increase their vitamin D status above what is considered insufficient—prolonged sun exposures may not necessarily result in vitamin D adequacy in all subjects, possibly due to their inability to synthesize precursors of active vitamin D. This suggests that such individuals should take vitamin D supplements rather than opt for abundant sun exposure to attain optimal vitamin D status. An added merit of this strategy is that it would avoid the enhanced risk of skin carcinogenesis from longer solar UV-B exposure. Large dietary intakes of vitamin D, especially in winter months, can maintain vitamin D levels in people living at high latitudes (69°N). This shows that diet alone can compensate adequately for lack of sun exposure.

One other complicating factor is that while regular use of sunscreens has been widely promoted because they protect against skin cancers, it could also retard or inhibit vitamin D synthesis in those individuals for whom sun exposure is the major source of this vitamin.

Many people, even those living in countries with high solar UVR, may have inadequate vitamin D status (see Brock et al., 2004; MacFarlane et al., 2004; Andersen et al., 2005). Melanin, because of its ability to absorb UV-B in the skin, can also decrease vitamin D status but, with sufficient UV-B, adequate vitamin D status is achieved.

Vitamin D is an important hormone required for general health. It has a substantial role in the growth, development and maintenance of bones, with deficits leading to low bone mineral density resulting in an increased risk of osteoporosis and fractures in adults and rickets in children.

Adequate vitamin D status prevents several non-skeletal disorders also, including some internal cancers, autoimmune diseases, and hypertension. It can affect the immune system by suppressing T-cell proliferation; down-regulating antigen presentation, stimulating the generation of T_{reg} cells and Th2 cells, and activating macrophage function (see Mathieu et al., 2004).

When it was discovered that $1{,}25(OH)_2D_3$ is synthesized in the skin following UVR, it was suggested as a mediator of UV-induced immunosuppression. This is best illustrated by its inhibitory effects on the ability of Langerhans cells (which form a dendritic cell network in the outermost layers of the skin and survey the skin for any foreign challenges) to present antigens (Meindl et al., 2005).

4 Genetics, Epigenetics and Cancer

Introduction

Mendel had ingeniously unraveled the laws of inheritance without knowing anything about the process of development, and most geneticists followed this path thereafter. Many embryologists and developmental biologists concentrated on their own studies, and spared no thought for the manner in which genes might control the unfolding of the developmental program. JBS Haldane, inspired by the earlier work of Garrod (1909) on inborn errors of metabolism, was one geneticist who got interested in the way genes controlled metabolism. In the 1940s, Beadle and Tatum formulated their famous concept of one gene-one enzyme.

There were two other geneticists who were also deeply interested in embryology, and who believed that sooner or later the two disciplines would come together; Ernst Hadorn studied development in *Drosophila*, and CH Waddington first introduced the term epigenetics (Waddington, 1939). In general terms, this was the study of the manner in which genes controlled and directed the developmental program. Epigenesis referred to the process whereby more and more complex structures emerged during development (Holliday, 2002).

Cancer as a Genetic Disease

Cancers arise by accumulation of structural or functional changes in cellular DNA. Many of these changes involve mutations of proto-oncogenes, tumour-suppressor genes, and DNA repair genes. About 30 tumour-suppressor (recessive) oncogenes and more than 100 dominant oncogenes have been identified. Some cancers are initiated by germ-line mutations of these genes which are heritable. These cancers are termed familial or inherited cancers.

The proportion of cancers that can be directly attributed to inherited genes in populations is quite low; only about 1 per cent of all cancers are truly inherited. Another 5 to 10 per cent of common cancers that occur in smaller familial clusters may have a genetic predisposition. Strong cancer-predisposing genes (e.g., *APC* and *RB1*) arise as new germ-line mutations or deletions during gametogenesis, without any family history (see Kumar, 2004).

Table 4.1 gives some selected examples of inherited syndromes that cause genetic predisposition to cancer.

According to Vogelstein and Kinzler (2004), cancer is a genetic disease caused by sequential accumulation of mutations in oncogenes and tumour-suppressor genes. Can-

Table 4.1 Selected examples of inherited syndromes that cause genetic predisposition to cancer (after Mohandas, 2001).

Cancer syndrome	Major cancer	Other cancer	Genes
Hereditary breast/ ovarian	Breast, ovary	Colon, prostate	*BRCA1, BRCA2*
Familial prostate	Prostate	—	*HPC1*
Juvenile polyposis	Colorectal cancer	Pancreas	*MADH4*
Familial gastric	Stomach, breast		*CDH1*
Hereditary non-polyposis colon carcinoma (HNPCC)	Colon and rectum	Endometrium, stomach, ovary, pancreas	*MSH2, MSH6, MLH1, PMS1, PMS2*
Familial retinoblastoma	Retinoblastoma	Breast, sarcoma, lung	*RB1*
Familial Wilms' tumour	Wilms' tumour	Hepatoblastoma	*WT1*
Lung	Small cell lung cancer	—	*SCLC1*
Ataxia telangectasia	Leukaemia, lymphoma	Ovary, stomach, brain	*ATM*
Bloom	Leukaemia	Tongue, colon, oesophagus, Wilms' tumour	*BLM*
Xeroderma pigmentosum	Skin	—	Several
Cutaneous melanoma	Skin	—	*CDKN2A*
Gorlin	Basal cell cancer	Brain tumour	*PTCH*

cer somatic mutations appear to be more frequent than initially suspected. Extensive sequencing work directed toward human colorectal and breast cancer DNA gene coding domains as well as exon-intron boundaries has identified 1,307 novel confirmed somatic mutations (Sjoblom et al., 2006). The subset of affected genes varies both with cancer type and within the same cancer type with individual tumours. Thus, the heterogeneity of cancer somatic mutations is definitely established (Brulliard et al., 2007).

Table 4.2 lists some oncogenes and tumour-suppressor genes and their alterations in cancers.

The heterogeneous nature of most cancer-biological attributes makes it difficult to reconcile results of cancer transcriptome and proteome experiments. Cancer somatic mutations arise at rates higher than suspected, and yet cannot account for all cancer cell heterogeneity. Brulliard et al. (2007) analysed sequence variations of 17 abundantly expressed genes in a large set of human ESTs originating from either normal or cancer samples. (ESTs—Expressed Sequence Tags, are derived from *mRNA* reverse transcribed in cDNA and inserted into a plasmid with a TAG allowing rapid sequencing of cloned bacteria. As a rough approximation, ESTs provide information on the sequence of *mRNA* of the cells from which the library was made). They found that cancer ESTs have greater variations than normal ESTs for >70 per cent of the tested genes. These variations cannot be explained by known and putative SNPs. Furthermore, cancer EST variations are not random, but are determined by the composition of the substituted base (b0) as well as that of the bases located upstream (up to b–4) and downstream (up to b+3) of the substitution event. The replacement base is also not randomly selected but corresponds in about 73 per cent of cases to a repetition of b–1 or b+1. Base substitutions follow a

Table 4.2 Some oncogenes and tumour-suppressor genes and their alterations in cancers (after Zingde, 2001).

Gene type	Gene	TSG/ONC	Alteration in cancer	Some associated cancers
Growth factors	*SIS (PDGF)*	ONC	Over-expression	Astrocytoma, oesteosarcoma
	INT-2, HST-1	ONC	Over-expression	Melanoma, breast, stomach
	IGF 2	ONC	Amplification	Head and neck cancer
	–	–	Methylation	Wilm's tumour
Growth factor receptor				
Transforming growth factor βR2	*TGF βRII*	TSG	Deletion	NSCLC, SCLC
Non-receptor tyrosine kinase	*SRC*	ONC	Mutation	Large intestinal tumours
Transcription factor	*DPC4*	TSG	Mutation or deletion	Colon, neuroblastoma
Transcription factor	*MYC*	ONC	Chromosomal translocation	Burkitt's lymphoma
	–	–	Gene amplification	SCLC, neuroblastoma
Cell cycle				
Transcription factor	*p53*	TSG	Mutation or deletion	Many
CDK inhibitor	*p16/p15*	TSG	Methylation, mutation or deletion	Melanomas, NSCLC
Transcriptional regulator				
	BRCA1	TSG	Mutation or deletion	Breast, ovary (familial)
	BRCA2	TSG	Deletion or mutation	Breast, ovarian (sporadic)
Others				
Dual-specificity phosphatase	*PTEN*	TSG	Mutation	Glioblastoma, prostate, endometrium
DNA repair	*hMLH1, hMSH2*	–	Mutation or deletion	Colon (HNPCC), endometrium
	APC	TSG	Mutation or deletion	Colorectum (familial and sporadic)

NSCLC, non-small cell lung carcinoma; SCLC, small cell lung carcinoma; HNPCC, hereditary non-polyposis colon carcinoma; ONC, oncogene; TSG, tumour-suppressor gene.

specific pattern of affected bases: A and T substitutions were preferentially observed in cancer ESTs. In contrast, cancer somatic mutations (Sjoblom et al., 2006) and SNPs identified in the genes of the study conducted by Brulliard et al. (2007) occurred preferentially with C and G. On the basis of these observations, Brulliard et al. (2007) proposed that cancer EST heterogeneity results primarily from increased transcription infidelity.

Chromosomal Imbalances

Tumour-specific patterns of large-scale chromosomal imbalances characterize many cancers. Work done on neuroblastomas suggests that large-scale chromosomal imbalances may be crucial for tumour pathogenesis and seem to affect the global transcriptional profile of cancer cells. Neuroblastoma is defined as a pediatric tumour derived from precursor cells of the sympathetic nervous system, which accounts for about 15 per cent of all childhood cancer deaths. It appears that some imbalances even initiate cancer, but the genes and genetic pathways that have been dysregulated by such imbalances are not known. Although many genes are affected by the regions of gain and loss, the complex interactions and relationships among these genes hinder their identification. According to Stallings (2007), the study of untranslated RNA sequences, such as microRNAs, which are also dysregulated by chromosomal imbalance, may contribute to pathogenesis. MicroRNAs are 19–22 base pair double-stranded RNA sequences that are processed from larger RNA sequences and regulate gene activity at a post-transcriptional level. MicroRNAs target specific *mRNAs* by base pair complementarity to the *mRNAs* 3' untranslated region, either inhibiting translation of the *mRNA* into protein or by causing the *mRNA* to degrade (Esquela-Kerscher and Slack, 2006; Stallings, 2007).

It is possible to identify the genes that promote an oncogenic effect in balanced reciprocal translocations, through cloning and sequencing of the break-point regions. In contrast, the genes contributing to disease pathogenicity resulting from chromosomal imbalance are lost in vast genomic regions containing many genes. The highly complex effects of such large-scale chromosomal imbalances are presumably mediated by the altered expression of tumour-suppressor and oncogenes.

Aneuploidy and Cancer

Aneuploidy refers to a condition in which a cell has either some extra chromosomes or in which some chromosomes are missing. It is often associated with tumours. Each aneuploid cancer has its own particular abnormal chromosome content, and hence its own special characteristics.

Cells can become aneuploid in two ways (for detailed explanation, see Fig. 4.1): (a) they can develop changes in the number of intact chromosomes (whole-chromosome aneuploidy; it originates from errors in cell division, or mitosis); and (b) they can undergo such rearrangements in chromosome structure as deletions, amplifications or translocations; these rearrangements arise from breaks in DNA and can cause tumour development. In contrast, the contribution of whole-chromosome aneuploidy to cancer is controversial.

Weaver et al. (2007) studied genetically engineered mice that gain or lose whole chromosomes with each cell division. Mutations in mitotic spindle-checkpoint genes can promote aneuploidy as well as tumourigenesis (Kops et al., 2005). Weaver et al. found that mice with compromised CENP-E (the protein of the *cenp-e* gene for centromere protein E) developed cancer which was accompanied by an age-dependent increase in whole-chromosome aneuploidy. In contrast to control strains, at about 20 months of 'old' age, 10 per cent of the *cenp-e*-heterozygous animals developed splenic lymphomas, and were three times more likely to develop benign lung tumours. These findings support Boveri's theory (see Boveri, 1914) that aneuploidy promotes tumourigenesis. But there are some qualifiers. Weaver et al. also found that *cenp-e* heterozygosity inhibited tumourigenesis in those mice which lacked the tumour-suppressor gene *p19/ARF*. *In vitro* experiments reinforced the conclusion that aneuploidy not only inhibits cell growth due to compromised *CENP-E*, but could also increase the frequency of rare transforming events (Pellman, 2007). The above results are consistent with findings of genetic instability and cells' ability to acquire new traits (Rajagopalan et al., 2003). Chromosomal instability tends to increase the frequency both of growth-promoting mutations that could initiate cancer, and of deleterious mutations that could block cell growth or trigger cell death. The final outcome depends on such factors as the population size of the cells at risk, the frequency of growth-promoting mutations relative to deleterious mutations, and the degree of dominance of these mutations. Another similar analogy is the work on telomere attrition—the erosion of the ends of chromosomes (see Maser and DePinho, 2002).

Recent researchers have established that, like other types of genetic instability, cancer is a potential, but not obligatory, outcome of aneuploidy. What is still not clear is how different paths to aneuploidy, different cell types and different genetic contexts interconnect to determine whether aneuploidy leads to cell death or cancer (Pellman, 2007).

DNA Methylation

Development involves many branching processes, whereby a given cell gives rise to two independent cell types. In such a process there is a developmental switch in which one daughter gains a new phenotype, or potential phenotype; whereas, the other retains its original phenotype. This represents a stem cell situation. In other cases both daughter cells may have phenotypes not only different from each other but also different from the parental cell. There is also the stability of differentiated cells, so that lymphocytes, fibroblasts and keratinocytes, etc., retain a stable karyotype through many divisions. These cells contain the same chromosomes, the same genes, and the same DNA sequences, but their patterns of gene expression differ. They may be said to have different epigenotypes.

Cancer is usually characterized through its global hypomethylation and site-specific gene hypermethylation. A better description is that it involves both global and gene-specific hypomethylation and hypermethylation as well as widespread chromatin modifications. Feinberg and Vogelstein (1983) defined the first eigenetic change in tumour as gene hypomethylation. Now, many growth-promoting genes are known to be activated through hypomethylation in various tumours (Wilson et al., 2007). Many cancer/testis genes that are expressed normally in the healthy testis become activated in other cells by hypomethylation in cancer, including the melanoma-associated antigen (MAGE) gene family, which has antigenic and immunotherapeutic value in melanoma and glioblastoma (Feinberg and Tycko, 2004). Activation of the human papillomavirus *HPV16* by hypomethylation affects tumour latency in cervical cancer (Wilson et al., 2007).

In contrast to the above, tumour-suppressor gene silencing seems to be linked to promoter hypermethylation, as described for *RB*, the gene associated with retinoblastoma (Greger et al., 1989), and several other tumour-suppressor genes (Jones and Baylin, 2002). The idea of switching of gene activities, and the somatic inheritance of a given set of ac-

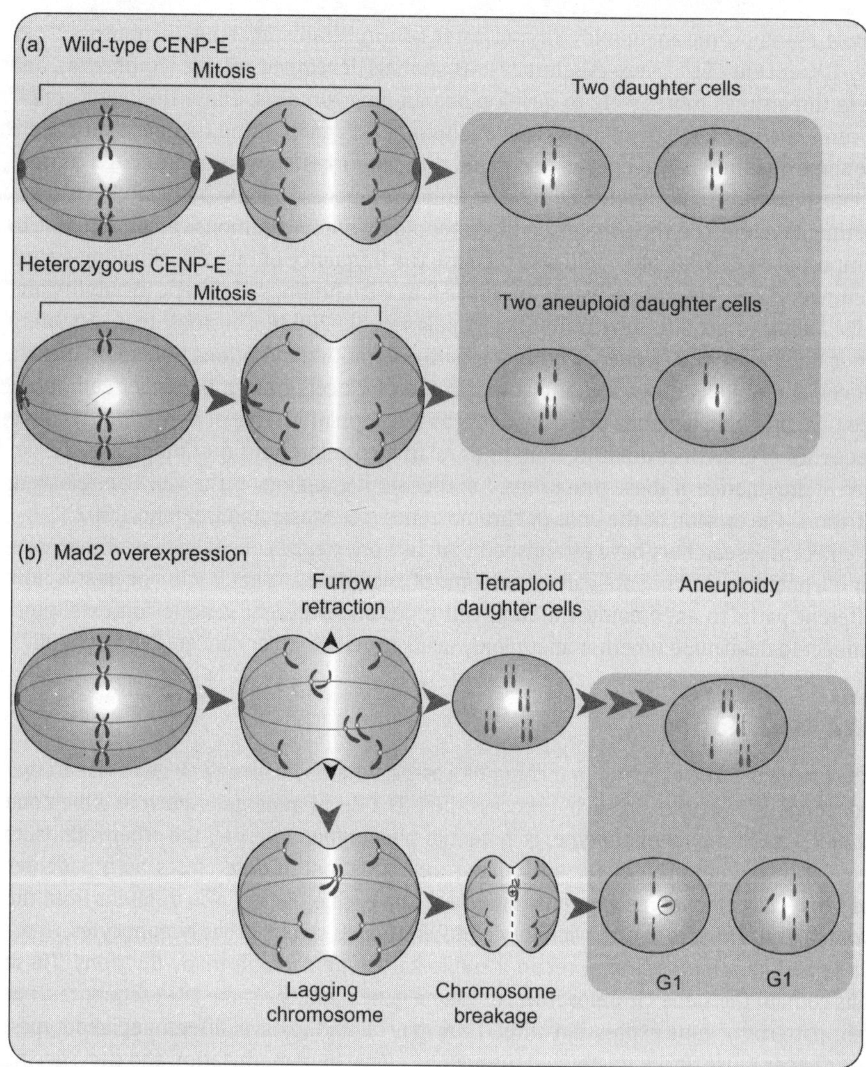

Fig. 4.1 DIFFERENT ROUTES TO ANEUPLOIDY: A. In wild-type cells, each daughter cell inherits one copy of a chromosome after mitosis (top panel). However, in CENP-E-deficient cells, sister chromatids of some chromosomes fail to separate, resulting in whole-chromosome aneuploidy (bottom panel). B. Over-expression of Mad2, which delays mitosis and entrapment of chromosomes in the cleavage furrow, can lead to aneuploidy in two ways. Furrow retraction can result in failure of cytokinesis and thus tetraploidy, with subsequent errors in the division of tetraploid cells causing aneuploidy (top panel). Alternatively, incomplete separation of chromosomes, with a lagging chromosome, might lead to chromosome breakage during cytokinesis (bottom panel); but how frequently this might occur, and the underlying mechanism, is not known (after Pellman, 2007).

tive and inactive genes, formed the basis for a new epigenetic mechanism, namely DNA methylation. 5-Methylcytosine (5-mC) is produced by an enzyme, DNA methyltransferase, which was known to attach a methyl group to the carbon at the 5 position of the pyrimidine ring soon after replication. In mammalian DNA, 2–5 per cent of cytosines are methylated, but not at random because CpG doublets are the major site of methylation, and these doublets are depleted in relation to the cytosine and guanine contents. Possibly, 5-mC has a role in controlling gene expression during development in higher organisms (see Holliday, 1984). Particularly interesting is the X chromosome inactivation in female mammals, where early in development one X chromosome is permanently inactivated in every cell, while the other is active.

In eutherian mammals, both the active and inactive states are subsequently maintained. It appeared that the hemimethylated DNA after replication served as a substrate for a maintenance methylase, which does not act on unmethylated DNA. However, these early papers did not refer to the term epigenetics. The connection between DNA methylation and epigenetics emerged in 1987 when Holliday published a paper titled 'The inheritance of epigenetic defects'. It had become apparent that gene inactivation could not only be due to mutation, but also to DNA methylation. This was actually demonstrated by the use of the potent demethylating agent 5-azacytidine which reactivated, at high frequency, genes that had been silenced by DNA methylation.

The term epimutation had been used previously to refer to heritable changes in phenotype which are not due to any alteration in DNA sequence (Holliday, 1984). Holliday (1979) had also proposed that heritable changes in DNA methylation might be important in carcinogenesis. The 1987 paper (in *Science*) explained the possible role of epigenetic defects or epimutations in cancer and ageing, and also the likelihood that they might be transmitted from one generation to the next; this topic was explored in more detail by Jablonka and Lamb (1995).

The discovery of genomic imprinting in mammalian gametes greatly advanced the study of epigenetics. The paternal and maternal gametes have different information which is superimposed on the chromosomal DNA of one parent but not the other. The two genomes complement each other to produce a normal zygote, whereas zygotes arising from two paternal nuclei or two maternal nuclei give rise to abnormal embryos. Imprinting has been linked to differences in DNA methylation in male and female gametes. Details of how long imprinting persists in the developing organisms are not known but we do know that in the formation of gametes for the next generation, the normal pattern of imprinting is reimposed (Holliday, 2002).

Considerable information about DNA methylation and the epigenetic control of gene activity is available for plants (Martienssen and Colot, 2001). There is also keen interest in the inactivation and methylation of tumour-suppressor genes during tumour progression. Recent studies have related DNA methylation to changes in chromatin proteins, particularly the acetylation and deacetylation of histones (Rountree et al., 2001).

Although in mammalian development no key role for DNA methylation has so far been revealed, it seems highly probable that DNA methylation does play a crucial role in unraveling the developmental program.

Other Epigenetic Mechanisms

While DNA methylation is a major epigenetic mechanism, it is not the only one. The changes in DNA taking place in the assembly of immunoglobulin genes in cell lineages of the immune system constitute an epigenetic mechanism, which depends on the creation of new DNA sequences. According to Holliday, the alternative splicing of gene transcripts that occurs in different cell types also represents an epigenetic mechanism, because it results in the formation of particular polypeptide chains and proteins appropriate for a specialized cell. There also exist some regulatory proteins that stably repress or induce particular genes without any involvement of DNA methylation, but it is not often clear whether these gene activities (or inactivities) are stably inherited through mitosis.

Whether or not a particular process or mechanism should be regarded as epigenetic ultimately depends on the definition of epigenetics (Wu and Morris, 2001). In 1994, Holliday suggested two, namely: (i) the study of the changes in gene expression that occur in organisms with differentiated cells and the mitotic inheritance of given patterns of gene expression; (ii) nuclear inheritance that is not based on differences in DNA sequence.

In contrast, Wu and Morris suggested a single definition: The study of changes in gene function that are mitotically and/or meiotically heritable and that do not entail a change in DNA sequence. Holliday considers this too narrow a definition because it does not encompass changes in somatic cells that should surely be regarded as epigenetic.

It is clear that the rules governing epigenetic processes are completely different from those governing classical genetics. In the 20th century, geneticists confirmed Mendel's results and successfully revealed the basic mechanism of heredity in many eukaryotes, and all the variations that can be imposed on that mechanism. The twenty-first century could reveal many epigenetic mechanisms, and the way they govern or influence the developmental programs of animals and plants. The relative importance of the epigenetic transmission of information from one generation should also become apparent, as also its possible role in evolution.

Epigenetics and Phenotypic Plasticity

Epigenetics refers to information heritable during cell division other than the DNA sequence itself. Developmental processes are regulated largely by epigenetics, because different cell types maintain their fate during cell division even though their DNA sequences are essentially the same (Feinberg, 2007).

Whereas in sick individuals, genetic lesions—sequence changes, breakages and deletions—are easily visualized, the effects of epigenetic lesions have only recently attracted attention. Defects in the epigenome can cause disease and include changes in the localized or global density of DNA methylation, incorrect histone modification, and altered distribution or function of chromatin-modifying proteins that, in turn, leads to abnormal gene expression. The disruption of higher-order loop structure in disease could also be involved.

Epigenetic changes refer to modifications of DNA that affect gene expression without altering DNA base sequences. Common epigenetic changes are cytosine methylation, histone deacetylation, histone methylation and loss of imprinting (LOI).

Epigenetic changes are not only involved in human disease but also may take place during normal development. Feinberg (2007) reviewed the epigenetics of single-gene disorders, cancer and common complex diseases and suggested that a common theme in disease epigenetics is the disruption of phenotypic plasticity, i.e., the ability of cells to change their behaviour in response to internal or external environmental cues.

Disease epigenetics involve defects in phenotypic plasticity—cells' ability to change their behaviour in response to internal or external environmental cues. According to this model, hereditary disorders of the epigenetic apparatus lead to developmental defects: cancer epigenetics involves disruption of the stem-cell programme; and common diseases with late-onset phenotypes involve interactions between the epigenome, the genome and the environment.

A thorough understanding of epigenetic-disease mechanisms can potentially lead not only to disease-risk stratification for targeted intervention but also to targeted therapies. Two main types of monogenic epigenetic diseases are those involving genes that are regulated epigenetically (e.g., imprinted genes), and those that affect the epigenome as a whole (e.g., modifiers of DNA methylation). The first category is exemplified by Beckwith Wiedemann syndrome; it is characterized by prenatal overgrowth, a midline abdominal wall and other malformations, and cancer. Some patients with this syndrome suffer from tissue overgrowth and increased cancer risk (DeBaun et al., 2002).

The other class involves genes that code for components of the machinery that regulates the epigenome. Mutation of these genes causes developmental disorders. In these disorders, mutations in epigenome regulators usually disrupt development and often cause phenotypic changes in multiple organ systems (Feinberg, 2007).

Chromatin

In cancer, chromatin modifications are as widespread and crucial as those in DNA methylation. For example, overexpression of the polycomb group protein EZH2, a H3 lysine-27 histone methylatransferase takes place in metastatic prostate cancer and sometimes causes widespread transcriptional repression (Varambally et al., 2002). Generalized loss of H4 acetylated Lys-16 and trimethylated Lys-20 is seen in lymphoma and colorectal cancer, which could also lead to transcriptional silencing (Fraga et al., 2005). Indeed, both DNA methylation and histone modification are altered in cancer, although they show interdependence in normal development (Terranova et al., 2006).

Aberrant Cytosine Methylation

The commonest epigenetic modification is methylation of the C5 position of cytosine in deoxycytosine. Methylation occurs often in promoter-associated CpG islands and silences genes by interfering with sequence-specific binding of transcription factors or by producing some general effects on chromatin. Many cases of colon cancer with microsatellite instability show promoter hypermethylation of a DNA mismatch repair gene, *hMLH1*. Transcriptional silencing through methylation sometimes occurs along with other inactivating mechanisms such as a combination of hypermethylation and loss of heterozygosity (LOH) of the *BRCA1* in certain breast and ovarian tumours. LOH involves the loss of the functional allele of a gene.

Changes in Histone Acetylation

Modified histone acetylation patterns are seen in several tumours. A good example is acute leukaemia cases in which a fusion of the *MLI* (mixed lineage leukaemia) and histone acetyltransferase (*CBP*) genes disrupts histone acetylation and leads to gene silencing.

Aberrant Histone Methylation

Histone methyltransferases methylate lysines in the tails of histones H3 and H4 which contain a conserved domain. Some colorectal and hepatocellular carcinomas are associated with overexpression of certain methylating enzymes.

Loss of Imprinting (LOI)

This occurs in the gamete and causes differential expression of the two alleles of a gene in somatic cells. The result may contribute to tumourigenesis by activating a transcriptionally-repressed allele or inactivating an expressed allele of an imprinted tumour-suppressor gene. LOI-mediated silencing of expression of the single functional allele can occur in ovarian cancer and breast cancer.

Cancer Epigenetics and Stem Cell Hypothesis

Epigenetic alterations are commonly viewed as substitutes for genetic change in cancer. They could also possibly be important first steps in neoplastic progression and may disrupt the normal stem or progenitor-cell programme, for instance, by stimulating stem-cell proliferation outside their normal microenvironment (Feinberg et al., 2006). As per this 'epigenetic progenitor model', cancer originates in stem or progenitor cells after epigenetic changes. It is supported by the ubiquitous early nature of epigenetic changes observed in cancer and by the demonstration of altered progenitor cells in normal tissues of patients suffering from cancer.

The work of Hochedlinger et al. (2004) on reprogramming of a melanoma genome by nuclear transplantation in mice also supports this model—the mouse melanoma and medulloblastoma nuclei have been successfully cloned to form blastocysts or chimaeric mice; while mice derived from the former were more prone to forming melanomas. Many of the associated tumour properties must be epigenetic in origin while some cells within the tumour are pluripotent.

In breast cancer, extensive epigenetic changes take place in tumour cells, stromal cells and the myoepithelium, pointing to the possibility that the entire tumour microenvironment, including apparently normal cells, could be the target of epigenetic disruption (Hu et al., 2005). Cancers also appear to exhibit greater epigenetic plasticity which may be an inherent property of the stem cells from which they originate; one example is the bivalent nature of adjacent H3K4 and H3K27 methylation occurring at many genomic sites in stem cells but not in somatic cells after differentiation (Bernstein et al., 2006). Polycomb group genes could possibly also be tumour progenitors—they are overexpressed in cancer and repress developmental regulators in embryonic stem cells (Boyer et al., 2006). Epigenetics may be central to plasticity both in development and in tumour cells.

Prospects for Epigenetic Therapy

Identification of several epigenetic mechanisms for human disease is inspiring development of therapies. In fact, some drugs are being used specifically because of their known effects on the epigenome. Two classes of epigenome-modifying agents are currently in clinical trial for cancer, for example, for the treatment of myelodysplasia (Mack, 2006): (i) DNA methyltransferase inhibitors such as decitabine, and (ii) histone deacetylase inhibitors such as suberoylanilide hydroxamic acid.

Some drugs which affect the epigenome are already in common use, but their epigenetic effect has only recently been discovered—valproic acid, a potent histone deacetylase inhibitor, is used to treat seizures, bipolar disorder and cancer (see Phiel et al., 2001). Since epigenetics lie at the core of phenotypic variation in health and disease; it is likely that enhanced understanding and appropriate manipulation of the epigenome could potentially prevent and treat common human illness. Epigenetics also enhances understanding of the involvement of the environment's interactions (see Callinan and Feinberg, 2006) with the genome in causing disease, as also in modulating such interactions to improve human health (Feinberg, 2007).

Targeting Epigenetic Changes in Cancer Cells

Current cancer chemotherapy treatments are based on toxic drugs that kill not only cancerous cells but also healthy cells. Physicians usually adopt the trial and error method to determine the right dose of the right medicine before it is too late. Hopefully, development of new molecular drugs targeting so-called epigenetic phenomena would change that and usher in a new array of cancer prevention strategies that are less toxic to the body (Interlandi, 2007).

'Epigenetics' deals with the study of changes in gene expression that do not involve changes in the genetic code; they include a growing list of subtle molecular modifications that inform cells which genes to activate (or transcribe) and which to suppress. In cancer cells, these small regulatory molecules can turn genes that promote cell growth all the way up and those that suppress tumours all the way down. Comparison of the epigenetic patterns of cancerous cells with those of healthy cells enable researchers to identify the aberrations linked to tumour growth. Indeed, some epigenetic culprits have already been discovered in many cancers, e.g., those of the colon, prostate, breast and blood.

Epigenetic analyses are likely to form an important component of the concept of personalized medicine. By diagnosing the epigenetic characteristics of tumours, physicians could better predict which drugs will work for which patients.

Like genetic mutations, epigenetic changes can pass from one generation of cells to their daughter cells but unlike genetic mutations, they are reversible; this is what makes them a drug target. Rather than killing cells that have become cancerous via epigenetic modifications, therapies that correct such changes could possibly re-establish the affected cells' normal functions. Two molecular switches—methylation and acetylation—have attracted much attention. Methylation turns genes off, whereas acetylation turns them on. The US Food and Drug Administration (FDA) has already approved two compounds that inhibit methylation: Vidaza in 2004 and Dacogen in 2006. Both treat myelodysplastic syndrome, a blood disorder that can lead to leukaemia. Likewise, Zolinza has become the first FDA-approved drug that treats cutaneous T cell lymphoma by enhancing acetylation. Other similar drugs are undergoing clinical trials, and other epigenetic modifications are being identified for potential use in therapy. Epigenetic drugs, however, do not aim to eliminate tumours permanently. Rather the idea is to reach a stage where some cancers can be reduced to a chronic state.

A drug's power may possibly be increased by first assessing epigenetic profiles. Epigenetic drugs might also enhance the efficacy of existing chemotherapies that bind to DNA by helping those drugs gain access to their double-helix targets (Interlandi, 2007).

Cancer and Ageing

It appears that in some ways cancer and ageing may be analogous. A series of critical observations have led to a complex but growing convergence between our understanding of the biology of ageing and the mechanisms that underlie cancer (Finkel et al., 2007). Five aspects of cancer biology that may be particularly informative about normal ageing are: (i) the connection between cellular senescence and tumour formation; (ii) the common role of genomic instability; (iii) the biology of the telomere; (iv) the emerging importance of autophagy in both cancer and ageing; and (v) the central roles

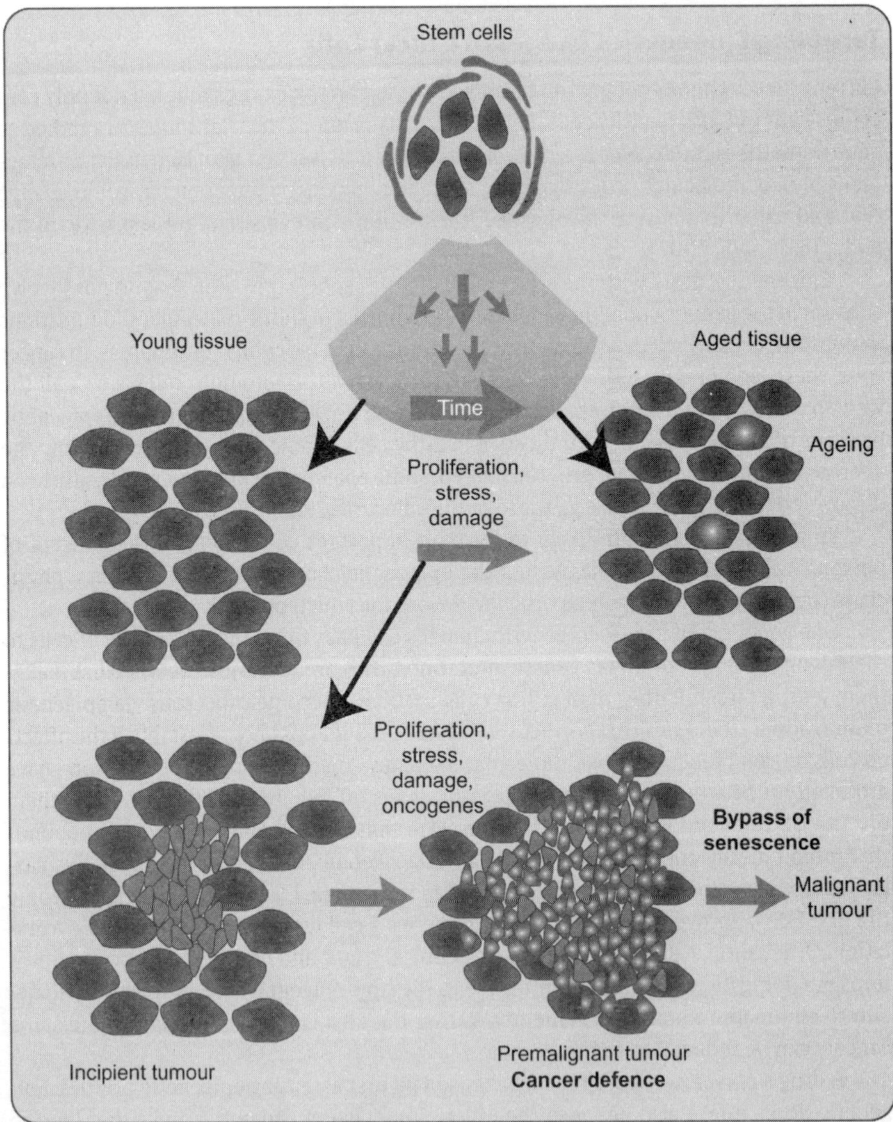

Fig. 4.2 POTENTIAL INTERACTION BETWEEN STEM CELLS, STRESS, AGEING AND CANCER: During normal ageing, stem cells accumulate damage and subsequent stress-dependent changes (for example, de-repression of the *CDKN2a* (*INK4a*/*ARF*) locus or telomere shortening). This leads to the increasing abundance of senescent cells within differentiated tissues. Incipient tumours, arising directly from stem cells or from more committed cells, proliferate rapidly. These pre-malignant tumour cells rapidly accumulate damage, partly owing to the presence of oncogenes, leading to a higher proportion of tumour cells becoming senescent. Tumour progression to full malignancy is favoured when tumour cells acquire certain mutations that impair the senescence program (after Finkel et al., 2007).

of mitochondrial metabolism and energetic-dependent signal transduction in both processes. All these findings collectively point to a distinct possibility that both cancer and ageing represent complex biological processes that are often—but not always—woven by similar molecular connections (Finkel et al., 2007).

The relevance of senescence for cancer protection makes sense if we consider senescence as a stress-induced barrier that limits the proliferative potential of damaged cells. In accordance with this view, recent data show that there are abundant senescent cells within tumours (Collado and Serrano, 2006) (Fig. 4.2). This intra-tumoural senescence is probably triggered by oncogenic signals that can function in part by de-repressing the *CDKN2a* (cyclin dependent kinase inhibitor 2a) locus. Oncogene-induced senescence may also be mediated by the activation of the DNA damage response (DDR) pathway, presumably by the hyper-replication so characteristic of cancer cells (Di Micco et al., 2006).

Figure 4.2 also illustrates the potential interactions among stem cells (see Chapter 5), stress, ageing, and cancer. Considerable amount of recent human genetic data indicate that single nucleotide polymorphisms (SNPs) near *CDKN2a* might be associated with ageing and age-related pathologies (see Melzer et al., 2007). There is also evidence for a connection between p16INK4a and stem cell biology. This link was surmised on the basis of the analysis of mice deficient in certain Polycomb genes, which normally repress p16INK4a. These Polycomb-deficient animals suffer from defects in stem cell self-renewal (Valk-Lingbeck et al., 2004). Age-induced expression of *p16INK4a* in adult stem cells appears to be associated with widespread impairment in tissue regeneration (Krishnamurthy et al., 2006). Also, mice that lack *p16INK4a* have increased regenerative potential in diverse niches including the nervous system, the pancreas and the haematopoietic system. These observations point to *p16INK4a* both serving as a break for the proliferation of cancer cells as well as limiting the long term renewal of stem cells. This means that excessive inhibition of pathways linked to cancer might reduce the robustness of various stem cell niches. In essence, cancer may be prevented but at the expense of an accelerated decline in tissue regeneration and repair (Finkel et al., 2007).

Genomic Instability links Cancer and Ageing

How to maintain DNA is a major challenge to every cell. Several distinct pathways can sense and repair damaged DNA, depending on the nature of the damage and on the phase of the cell cycle in which the damage occurs. In view of the fact that genomic instability is a hallmark of most cancers, it is not surprising that many of the factors implicated in sensing and responding to DNA damage are altered in human tumours. A less well known fact is that genomic instability is also a hallmark of ageing. An age-dependent increase in chromosomal instability occurs in mammals (see Curtis, 1963). There are indications that the age-dependent accumulation of somatic mutations might vary significantly between different tissues of the same organism and that these genetic alterations may possibly contribute to the stochastic variation in gene expression often seen in mammalian ageing (Bahar et al., 2006).

Molecular analyses of human inherited cancer syndromes such as Li-Fraumeni syndrome, ataxia-telangiectasia (AT) and some forms of familial breast and ovarian cancers have reinforced the connection between the maintenance of genome integrity and cancer susceptibility. These conditions are sometimes caused by germline mutations in the genes for *p53*, the ataxia-telangiectasia mutated (ATM) kinase and breast cancer 1

(*BRCA1*), respectively—three proteins that are essential in the surveillance of DNA damage. Interestingly, these three proteins have also been linked to cellular or organismal ageing (Finkel et al., 2007).

The work of Bahar et al. (2006) on the analysis of mice with targeted deletions or humans with inherited deficiencies in several factors involved in sensing or repairing DNA damage has strengthened the correlation between DNA damage and the rate of ageing. Reducing the level of various mitotic checkpoint genes leads to chromosomal instability, augmented aneuploidy, and the phenotypic appearance of progeroid mice. These and other recent observations indicate that severe deficiencies in proteins involved in DNA damage sensing and DNA repair probably accelerate ageing, while milder mutations in these same pathways tend to predispose individuals to cancer. While the mechanism for ageing in the absence of faithful DNA repair is not very clear, it seems to be secondary to the induction of senescence or apoptosis of crucial stem and progenitor cells.

Telomeres and Telomerase

Telomeres are specialized structures at the ends of chromosomes. These protect natural chromosome ends from fusions and are essential for chromosomal stability. However, soon after the discovery of the structure of DNA, James Watson and Alexey Olovnikov realized that the replication of the very ends of chromosomes (telomeres) would probably be impaired because conventional DNA polymerases needed a primer to initiate DNA synthesis. This problem has been termed the 'end-replication problem'. Its solution—or lack thereof—provides yet another link between cancer and ageing (Finkel et al., 2007).

Most adult cells have small amounts of telomerase which cannot prevent telomere loss, resulting in the shortening of telomeres with age (Harley et al., 1990). Since telomeres are indispensable for chromosomal stability, their progressive loss has been proposed to be the basis of cellular senescence and ageing in the 'telomere hypothesis'. Telomere length can predict the replicative capacity of human cells and the appearance of certain age-associated pathologies in humans (Cawthon et al., 2003). Telomerase-deficient mice with short telomeres show reduced function of several stem cell compartments such as those in the bone marrow and skin (Lee et al., 1998). Human patients who have inherited or acquired genetic defects that limit telomere maintenance also face increased risk of various disorders such as aplastic anaemia and idiopathic pulmonary fibrosis (see Armanios et al., 2007).

Most human cancers activate telomerase at some point during tumourigenesis, while this activity is largely absent in most normal tissues (Kim et al., 1994). Also, by activating a program of telomere maintenance, tumour cells can escape from replicative senescence. Conversely, mice with short telomeres are usually resistant to tumours (Blanco et al., 2007). This suggests that telomere shortening is a potent in vivo tumour suppressor mechanism.

Autophagy

The manner in which cellular waste is managed or disposed off is another area in which the biologies of cancer and ageing converge. One overlap area involves autophagy. In this process, old and damaged proteins and organelles, including mitochondria, are sequestered into double-membraned structures known as autophagosomes which can then

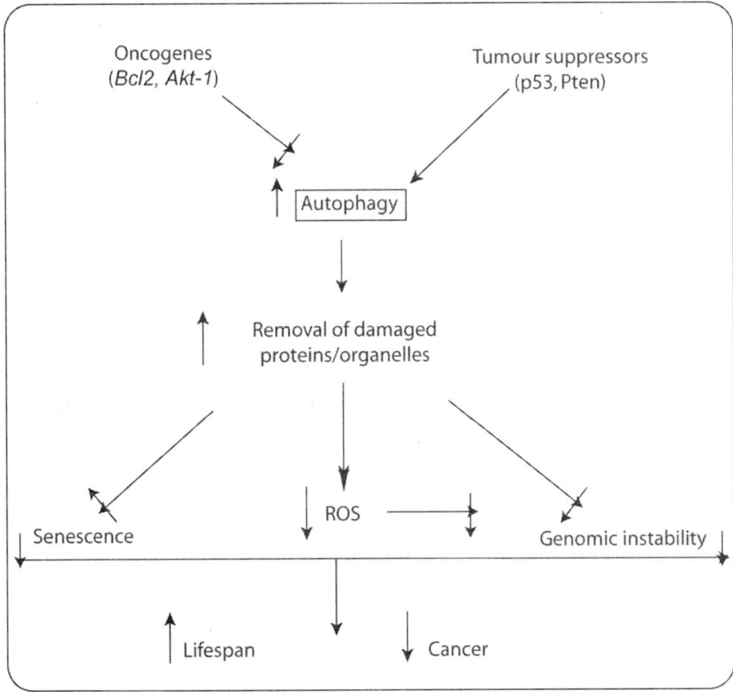

Fig. 4.3 The potential role of autophagy in cancer and ageing.

fuse with the lysosome in mammalian cells to further degrade the used cargo back to reusable building blocks (see Ohsumi, 2001).

The first link between autophagy and cancer emerged from the observation that the product of the mammalian gene *beclin 1* (*Becn1*), bound to the human oncogene B-cell [CLL/lymphoma 2 (BCL2)] (Liang et al., 1999). The binding of BCL2 to *beclin* seems to inhibit autophagy. This pointed to the possibility that, in tumours characterized by increased BCL2 expression, the oncogene may be working at least in part by suppressing autophagy. This notion was supported from mice engineered to have lost one copy of the *Becn1* gene—the haloinsufficient mice developed tumours, indicating that autophagy probably acts as an *in vivo* tumour suppressor (Qu et al., 2003). However, although it appears that oncogenes can inhibit autophagy and tumour suppressors can stimulate it, the precise link between cancer and autophagy is not clear (Fig. 4.3). Conceivably, interfering with the normal degradation of organelles leads to the retention of older, damaged mitochondria that serve as a source for damaging reactive oxygen species. Such a mechanism suggests a robust connection between common insults that could both contribute to cancer and accelerate ageing (Finkel et al., 2007).

Autophagy is a regulated process for the removal of damaged proteins and organelles. Autophagy occurs under basal conditions and is stimulated by environmental factors such as starvation. Proteins linked to tumourigenesis may regulate the rate of autophagy, with oncogenes in general blocking and tumour suppressors stimulating the process. The removal of damaged cellular components, especially damaged mitochondria, might decrease the level of reactive oxygen species (ROS), which in turn may reduce genomic instability or forestall cellular senescence. Such mechanisms might allow moderate increases in autophagy to reduce the incidence of cancer and prolong lifespan (after Finkel et al., 2007).

Metabolism links Cancer and Ageing

In lower organisms such as the nematode worm *Caenorhabditis elegans*, mutations that prolong lifespan are usually intimately connected with the organism's ability to withstand oxidative, metabolic and other stresses. This same stress resistance could also well be crucial to a rapidly growing tumour cell, where the supply and availability of nutrients and oxygen is critical. This strategic metabolic overlap has been reinforced by observations of specific genes that interconnect the triad of lifespan, cancer and energetics (Finkel et al., 2007). One such gene, *Trp53*, encodes *p53*. This tumour suppressor is a most frequently mutated gene in human cancers and its increased activity can accelerate ageing.

Also, there is a strong link between *p53* and cellular metabolism, which is strengthened even more firmly by reports that *p53* regulates the transcription of two proteins, TP53-induced glycolosis and apoptosis regulator (TIGAR) and the SCO cytochrome oxidase deficient homologue 2 (SCO2), which are crucial in the utilization of glucose and mitochondrial respiration, respectively (Bensaad et al., 2006; Matoba et al., 2006). Another pathway that allows cells and organisms to adapt to changes in nutrient availability is the TOR (target of rapamycin) signalling network, on which much work has been published. TOR is activated in the presence of abundant nutrients, and inactivated under starvation. Some upstream regulators of TOR, e.g., PTEN are usually altered in human tumours. The use of the TOR inhibitor rapamycin is currently being actively explored as a possible treatment for human malignancies. In mammalian cells, mammalian TOR (mTOR) may be an important regulator of overall mitochondrial metabolism (Schieke et al., 2006).

5 Stem Cells and Cancer

Introduction

Genes and genomes represent one of the two pillars of 21st century progress in biomedicine, while the second is stem-cell biology. Yet, while everyone knows of Watson and Crick, hardly anyone has heard of Leroy Stevens and other early stem-cell pioneers. In fact, many scientists are still unaware of the advances that occurred before the 1998 isolation of human embryonic stem cells. Parson (2004) has filled this gap. She has traced the birth of modern stem-cell research from 1953—the year of the double helix debut. Although the means for composing and reproducing life's genetic recipes were a fundamental secret of life, they were certainly not the only one. Equally mysterious was the process by which a microscopic embryo developed into a fully functional mammal. It was known that development occurred through the controlled growth, division and specialization of individual cells, but how developmental control was asserted was not known. The assumption was that a permanent loss of biological components or capabilities narrowed cellular potential; by implication, a postembryonic mammalian cell should never be able to reverse course and return to an embryonic state. The exceptions were the germ cells (eggs and sperm), which did have the potential to retrace normal development only after combining with each other (Silver, 2004).

Even in recent times, some believe that from the zygote stage onwards, the major development of a human embryo's growth is controlled and directed from within, by the organism itself. Consequently, human zygotes and blastocysts (newly fertilized embryos that have just started to divide) are already living beings and need to be protected from being killed by researchers.

In 1953, Leroy Stevens was looking for morphological differences among inbred mice at the Jackson Laboratory in Bar Harbor, Maine, when he incidentally observed an enlarged testicle in about 1 per cent of adult males of the 129 strain. The enlargements were caused by an independently growing mass of a type previously found only in human patients. It attracted the term teratoma in view of its monster-like characteristics. Human teratomas are typically covered with skin and hair, and contain a bizarre diversity of tissues and organs that are normally found in other parts of the body, including synaptically connected neurons, muscle, beating heart tissue, bone, teeth, occasionally eye-like structures or whole limbs.

Stevens realized that this strain's predisposition to develop teratomas offers a unique means for tackling the mystery of their origin, which could provide insight into normal developmental processes. Two years and several thousand animals later, Stevens had dissected his way back through younger and younger mice, and ultimately foetuses, to discover that random genital-ridge cells occasionally developed like the early embryos before exploding into teratomas. In some other strains, females were similarly predisposed to teratoma formation. Ovarian cells morphed, by themselves, into an organism that at first appeared just like a normal embryo, but later would get mixed up, becoming disorganized and forming a tumour instead of a baby mouse. When normally fertilized embryos were placed into unusual environments, such as the kidney capsule, they also became teratomas instead of mice.

Teratomas are not ordinary tumours. Like their adult tissues, some have cells that grow and divide for years without becoming specialized. When dispersed and injected into mouse abdomens, these cells developed into thousands of small structures resembling 5- or 6-day mouse embryos floating freely. Such 'embryonic carcinoma' (EC) cells could settle down and participate in completely normal tissue and organ development, if given a chance in a normal embryonic environment. Others could produce chimaeric mice derived from a mixture of normal embryo cells and EC cells.

In 1981, Evans and M Kaufman of Cambridge University, and G. Martin of the University of California, San Francisco, independently extracted embryonic stem cells directly from mouse embryos and made them grow in culture indefinitely without differentiating. In 1998, the same process was developed for use with human embryos, heralding the age of regenerative medicine. The goal today is to discover the factors and conditions that will transform embryonic-like cells into whatever tissue is required to treat a particular disease (Silver, 2004).

Parson also offers a balanced assessment of the therapeutic potential of stem cells in both the short and long term, disease by disease and organ by organ.

Stem Cells

Most tissues in higher animals (vertebrates) are complex mixtures of cell types that are subject to periodical, continual turnover. Almost every tissue is an intricate mixture of several different cell types that must remain different from one another while they coexist in the same environment. In most adult tissues, cells are continually dying and are replaced. Through all these happenings, the integrity of the tissue has to be preserved. This is achieved through three chief processes, viz., cell communication, selective cell-cell adhesions, and cell memory. Whereas the selectivity of adhesion prevents the different cell types in a tissue from becoming chaotically mixed, cell memory also plays a crucial role—specialized patterns of gene expression elicited by signals that operated during embryonic development, tend to be maintained stably thereafter. This enables cells to autonomously preserve their distinctive identity or traits and transmit it to their progeny. This is why the endothelial cell divides to produce more endothelial cells or the fibroblast likewise produces more fibroblasts. The diversity of cell types in the tissue is preserved in this way.

Many of the differentiated cells that need to be continually replaced by themselves cannot divide: some examples are red blood cells, surface epidermal cells and some cells of the gut lining. Cells of these examples are referred to as terminally differentiated as they lie at the dead end of their developmental pathway (see Alberts et al., 1998).

More such cells are produced from a stock of precursor cells called stem cells, which tend to be retained in the corresponding tissues along with the differentiated cells. As they are not terminally differentiated, stem cells can go on dividing for the lifetime of

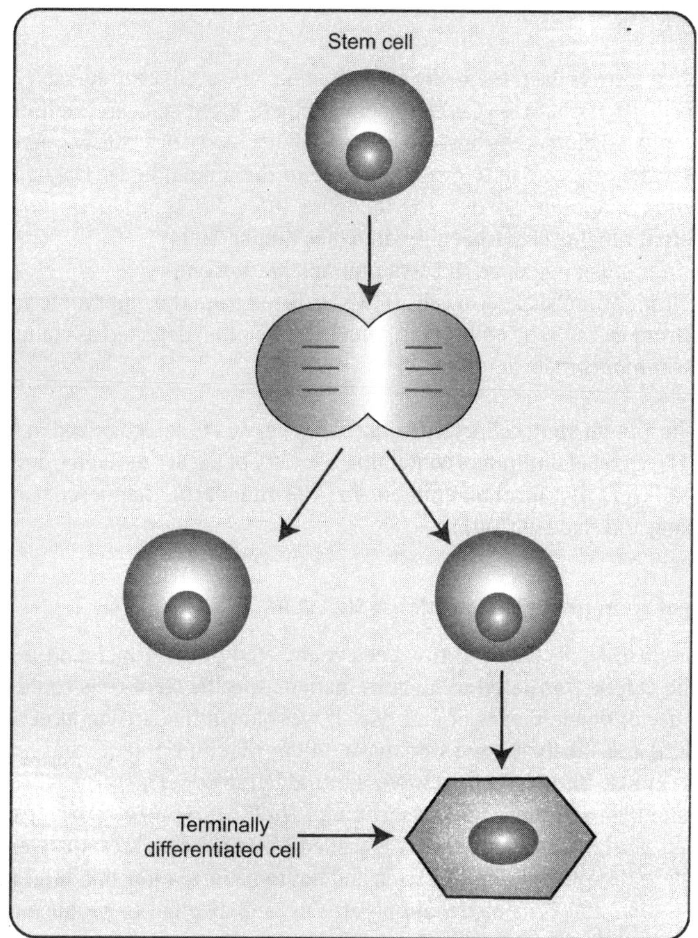

Fig. 5.1 DIVISION OF A STEM CELL: Each daughter can either remain a stem cell or may become terminally differentiated (after Alberts et al., 1998).

the individual. But when a stem cell does divide, each daughter has a choice—either it may continue to be a stem cell, or it can take a route that leads irreversibly to terminal differentiation (Fig. 5.1).

Stem cells that are not terminally differentiated are nevertheless quite determined—they stably express sets of gene regulatory proteins which make sure that their differentiated descendants will be of the appropriate types.

Quite often, a single type of stem cell can give rise to several types of differentiated progeny—the process of blood cell formation is an extreme example. All the different cell types in the blood, e.g., the red cells that carry oxygen and the different types of white blood cells engaged in fighting infection, ultimately come from a shared haematopoietic stem cell which is normally found in the bone marrow.

Stem cells can proliferate as well as produce differentiated progeny. This property facilitates growth and tissue repair, as well as normal maintenance.

Pluripotent Stem Cells

Spermatogonial stem cells in the testis are unipotent, i.e., produce only one type of differentiated cell (a spermatozon), while haematopoietic stem cells are multipotent and produce not only red blood cells but also various white blood cells. Pluripotent stem cells have the potential to give rise to every cell type in the animal body. They are derived from embryonic (not adult) tissues. The following three different types of mammalian pluripotent stem cell lines have been isolated (see Kumar, 2004):

1. ES cells, from inner cell mass (ICM) of preimplantation embryo.
2. EG cells, from primordial germ cells (PGCs) isolated from the embryonic gonad; and
3. EC cells, from PGCs in the embryonic gonad but are often detected as components of testicular tumours in an adult.

In fact, the pluripotent stem cell, as a distinct cell type, was first recognized in teratocarcinomas—bizarre gonadal tumours containing a variety of tissues derived from the three primary germ layers that form an embryo, viz., the endoderm, the mesoderm, and the ectoderm (Jiang and Nadeau, 2001).

Engineering of Stem-like Cells from Mouse Skin Cells

Embryonic stem-like cells have recently been engineered from normal mouse skin cells. If this method can be translated to humans, patient-specific stem cells could be made without the use of donated eggs or embryos. It was shown by Cartwright et al. (2005), Lie et al. (2005) and Takahashi and Yamanaka (2006) that pluripotent stem cells can be induced from mouse fibroblasts by retroviral introduction of *Oct3/4* (also called *Pou5f1*), *Sox2*, *c-Myc* and *Klf4*, and subsequent selection for *Fbx15* (also called *Fbxo15*) expression. These induced pluripotent stem (iPS) cells (called *Fbx15* iPS cells) resemble embryonic stem (ES) cells in morphology, proliferation and teratoma formation, but differ in respect of gene expression and DNA methylation patterns, and also fail to produce adult chimaeras (Okita et al., 2007). Owing to the possibility that the incomplete reprogramming might be due to the selection for *Fbx15* expression, and that by using better selection markers, it might be possible to generate more ES-cell-like iPS cells, Okita et al. decided to use *Nanog* as a candidate of such markers. Okita et al. have now shown that selection for *Nanog* expression results in germline-competent iPS cells with increased ES-cell-like gene expression and DNA methylation patterns compared with *Fbx15* iPS cells. The four transgenes (*Oct3/4, Sox2, c-Myc* and *Klf4*) are strongly silenced in *Nanog* iPS cells. Adult chimaeras were obtained from seven *Nanog* iPS cell clones; one clone could be transmitted through the germline to the next generation. Approximately 20 per cent offspring developed tumours attributable to reactivation of the *c-Myc* transgene. So, iPS cells competent for germline chimaeras can be obtained from fibroblasts. But retroviral introduction of *c-Myc* needs to be avoided for clinical application (Okita et al., 2007).

The apparently simple method can change differentiated adult cells into pluripotent stem cells (Okita et al., 2007; Wernig et al., 2007; Maherali et al., 2007). The 'acid' test for pluripotency is the ability of a cell to contribute extensively to all adult cell types, including the germline. The cells generated by these authors certainly pass this test. Four gene-transcription factors could be introduced into fibroblast cells originating from mouse skin; and specifically those cells were selected that, in response to these factors, expressed genes indicative of a pluripotent state. The research teams managed to isolate cell lines that resembled mouse embryonic stem (ES) cells. Upon being injected into early embryos, the cells differentiated into all normal adult cell types.

Unfortunately, some iPS-cell derived chimaeras developed tumours. Furthermore, it is not known whether the same set of factors can reprogramme other, more specialized cell types. Clearly, the current methodology represents only a proof-of-principle and much further work is required. From proof-of-principle in mice to application in humans is also a big jump. The pluripotent nature of human ES cells holds enormous potential for future cell-based therapies for degenerative diseases. Use of human embryos to derive such cells is very controversial. The possibility of making cell lines with all of the properties of ES cells directly from non-controversial adult sources such as skin is therefore appealing. It could be a powerful way of creating patient-specific stem cells to provide tissue-matched cells for therapy, and a source of cells for research into the pathogenesis of complex diseases (Rossant, 2007).

Nanog selection allows the generation of high-quality iPS cells comparable to ES cells in morphology, proliferation, teratoma formation, gene expression and competency for adult chimaeras. Nearly all Nanog iPS clones manifested these properties, indicating that Nanog is a major determinant of quality in cellular pluripotency. However, germline competence varied among Nanog iPS clones, pointing to the existence of other important determinants of germline competency besides Nanog. The high quality of Nanog iPS cells highlights the potential of using this technology to generate patient-specific pluripotent stem cells. In another study, Okita et al. also found that germline-competent iPS cells can be obtained from adult mouse somatic cells (T Aoi and SY, unpublished data).

Considering the fact that reactivation of *c-Myc* retrovirus may result in tumour formation, there is need to find ways to address this problem. Strong silencing of the four retroviruses in Nanog iPS cells indicates that they are only required for the induction and not the maintenance of pluripotency. Hence, the retrovirus-mediated system might be eventually replaced by transient expression, such as the adenovirus-mediated system. Alternatively, high-throughput screening of chemical libraries may facilitate identification of small molecules that can replace the four genes.

We do not know whether the same magic brew of molecular factors will work to generate iPS cells in humans. Critical tests may provide the answer. Translation from proof-of-principle to any therapy poses formidable challenges. First, human cells would have to be given a built-in drug-selectable pluripotent marker by some efficient means. Second, potentially cancer-causing factors such as *c-Myc* must be avoided. Third, factors would need to be introduced by some technique other than retroviral transfection because retroviruses can activate cancer-causing genes. Transient gene expression by direct introduction of membrane-permeable transcription factors into cells could possibly help in achieving this, and screens for small molecules which can replace the gene products can prove useful. Despite these challenges, however, direct reprogramming of adult cells potentially promises to open up new frontiers not only in human biology but also future therapy (Rossant, 2007).

Chemotherapy and Stem Cells

Higher doses of chemotherapy drugs and radiation therapy being used during cancer treatment occasionally also cause some damage to normal cells besides destroying the cancer cells. The normal cells that are most sensitive to destruction by high-dose therapy are the stem cells in the bone marrow.

It is important to collect stem cells prior to treatment with high-dose chemotherapy so that these cells may then be infused to 'rescue' bone marrow and hasten blood cell production and immune system recovery.

The stem cells may not only be taken from the bone marrow, but also from peripheral blood or umbilical cord. Stem cells may be sourced from the patient (autologous), an identical twin (syngeneic), or someone other than the patient (allogeneic).

Stem Cells and Brain Tumours

Stem cells have been increasingly implicated in maintaining or supporting certain cancers. Studies of an intractable type of brain tumour provide some clues as to why such cells could possibly determine the tumours' resistance to therapy (Dirks, 2006).

Rare populations of cancer stem cells have been found in solid tumours (Al-Hajj et al., 2003, Singh et al., 2004). Papers published by Bao et al. (2006) and Piccirillo et al. (2006) discussed the stem-cell nature of human glioblastoma, an especially serious type of brain cancer. Glioblastomas are heterogeneous tumours that contain a few tumour-initiating $CD133^+$ stem cells among other, more differentiated, $CD133^-$ cells, including glioblastoma progenitor cells. Both teams were inspired by the identification of a tumour-initiating subpopulation of cells that express a cell-surface marker, CD133, which is a hallmark of neural precursor cells (see Singh et al., 2004).

Bao et al. found that glioblastoma cells expressing CD133 ($CD133^+$ cells) are resistant to ionizing radiation because they are more efficient at inducing the repair of damaged DNA than are the bulk of the tumour cells. While radiation therapy for glioblastoma treatment is transiently effective, it provides no lasting cure. It fails in the long run because it cannot kill the subpopulation of $CD133^+$ tumour-initiating cells (Dirks, 2006).

Piccirillo et al. worked on bone morphogenetic proteins (BMPs); soluble factors that normally induce neural precursor cells to differentiate into mature astrocytes—a subtype of brain cells called glial cells. They showed that BMPs can also induce the differentiation of $CD133^+$ brain tumour cells and weaken their tumour-forming ability. These results imply that tumour populations partially retain a developmental hierarchy based on stem cells, and continue to be able to respond to the normal signals that induce them to mature. These findings generate considerable interest in devising therapies that can promote the differentiation of cancer cells (Dirks, 2006). The knowledge that a tumour retains a developmental hierarchy suggests that targeting different cell populations is a promising therapeutic strategy.

Stem Cell Malignancy

Stem cells can potentially turn malignant, leading to some cancers. One among thousands of tumour cells may be a cancer stem cell responsible for driving the disease. Eliminating the disease could depend on tracking down and destroying the elusive killer stem cells.

In some cases, it proves very difficult to eradicate cancer. One reason for this may be that tumour cells behave like stem cells. Several years ago, John Dick and his associates at the University of Toronto noticed that only a very small population of leukaemia cells could transmit the cancer from one experimental animal to another, and that these cells had a property previously seen only in stem cells: the ability to produce an exact copy of themselves each time they divide, thereby maintaining the ability to reproduce repeatedly. It is these cancer stem cells which might make cancer difficult to treat with radiation or chemotherapy.

Such cancer stem cells have been reported from many other cancers also, including those of the breast, brain, colon, head and neck, the prostate, lung, pancreas, and the deadly skin cancer, i.e., melanoma. This suggests that therapies that target cancer stem cells may be more effective than current treatments. Radiation and many chemotherapeutic drugs only wipe out dividing cells; as stem cells are quiescent most of the time, they may survive these treatments.

Cancer stem cells lead to the formation of new blood vessels needed to feed tumour growth. Better understanding of how normal and cancer stem cells differ could facilitate formulating a new class of less toxic drugs (see Marx, 2007).

Cancer stem cells seem to stimulate the formation of new blood vessels that support tumour growth. Glioma stem cells in culture produce much more of the angiogenesis-promoting protein VEGF than do other glioma cells. The drug bevacizumab (Avastin) is an antibody designed to block VEGF action; it is already used for cancer therapy. When human glioma stem cells are transplanted into mice and the animals treated with the antibody, the tumours from cancer stem cells shrink greatly. This points to the possibility that bevacizumab may be a kind of anticancer-stem cell therapy.

Cancer stem cells may also have another dangerous property: the ability to promote the spread of tumours in the body. It appears that oncogenic mutations arising either in normal tissue stem cells or in the more developmentally advanced progenitor cells can produce cancer stem cells. When these cells divide, one daughter is a true exact copy of the original; it not only retains the ability to divide but can also initiate additional tumours—whereas the other target differentiates to produce nontumourigenic cells (see Marx, 2007).

Chronic myelogenous leukaemia (CML) can be treated with Gleevec which has benefited many patients but it appears that they are not truly cured, because a reservoir of malignant cells responsible for maintaining the disease has not been eradicated.

Any tumour cell remaining in the body can potentially re-ignite the disease. Current treatments focus on killing the greatest number of cancer cells—a hit-or-miss affair.

In CML and a few other cancers, only a tiny percentage of tumour cells can produce new cancerous tissue, and targeting these specific cells for destruction is a far more effective way to eliminate the disease. Being the engines driving the growth of new cancer cells and also probably initiating the malignancy itself, these cells are termed cancer stem cells. They were once normal stem cells or their immature offspring that have undergone a malignant transformation.

Today, the study of stem cells is shedding light on cancer research (see Parson, 2004; Bissell and LaBarge, 2005). Scientists have provided considerable details over the past 50 years about mechanisms regulating the behaviour of normal stem cells and their cellular progeny. Recent insights have led to the discovery of hierarchies among cancer cells within a tumour, supporting the theory that rogue stem-like cells are at the root of many cancers. Successfully eradicating these cancer stem cells requires a better understanding of how a good stem cell could turn bad (Clarke and Becker, 2006).

The human body is a highly compartmentalized system made up of discrete organs and tissues, each performing an essential function. But individual cells that make up these tissues are often short-lived. A constant population of working cells is maintained in such tissues by a mechanism that centers on small pools of long-lived stem cells that serve as factories for replenishing functional cells. This manufacturing process follows tightly regulated and organized steps wherein each generation of a stem cell's offspring becomes more and more specialized, exemplified by the haematopoietic family of blood and immune cells.

All the functional cells found in the blood and lymph arise from a single common parent, the haematopoietic stem cell (HSC), found in bone marrow. Although the HSC pool represents less than 0.01 per cent of bone marrow cells in adults, each of these rare cells gives rise to a larger, intermediately differentiated population of progenitor cells which in turn divide and differentiate through several stages into mature cells responsible for specific tasks. When a cell has reached that final functional stage, it cannot proliferate or alter its destiny—it is terminally differentiated.

The stem cells themselves meanwhile remain undifferentiated, a state maintained through their unique capacity for self-renewal. To begin producing new tissues, a stem cell divides in two, but only one of the daughter cells might proceed down a path toward increasing specificity. The other daughter often retains the stem cell identity. Numbers in the overall stem cell pool can thus remain constant, whereas the proliferation of intermediate progenitors allows populations of specific haematopoietic cell types to expand rapidly in response to changing needs.

The most important defining property of stem cells is their capacity to re-create themselves through self-renewal. It alone gives them the potential for unlimited life span and future proliferation. In contrast, with increasing differentiation, the ability of the progenitors' offspring to multiply declines steadily.

Cellular hierarchies similar to those of HSCs have been identified in brain, breast, prostate, intestines and skin. Principles of regulated stem cell behaviour are shared across these tissues, including mechanisms for controlling stem cell numbers and for directing decisions about the fates of individual cells.

There are many similarities between stem cells and cancer cells. The classical definition of malignancy itself includes cancer cell's apparent capacity to survive and multiply indefinitely and ability to invade neighbouring tissues and to migrate (metastasize) to distant sites in the body. The usual constraints that tightly control cellular proliferation and identity seem to have been lifted from cancer cells (see Clarke and Fuller, 2006).

Normal stem cells' ability to self-renew exempts them from the rules which limit life span and proliferation for most cells. Stem cells' ability to differentiate into a broad range of cell types allows them to form all the different elements of an organ or tissue system. A core trait of tumours is the heterogeneity of cell types they contain, as though the tumours were a very disorderly version of a whole organ. HSCs migrate to distant parts of the body in response to injuries, as do cancer cells.

In healthy stem cells, strict genetic regulation restrains their potential for unlimited growth and diversification. If those control mechanisms are removed, malignancy can result. It seems that failures in stem cell regulation are how many cancers initiate and perpetuate (Clarke and Becker, 2006).

Malignancies seem to arise when an accumulation of 'oncogenic' changes in key genes within a cell leads to the abnormal growth and transformation of that cell. Gene mutations typically happen through some direct insult, such as exposure to radiation or chemicals, or simply through random error when the gene is improperly copied before cell division. The rare stem cells are the only long-lived cells in the organs where most cancers develop; they can be a small potential reservoir for cumulative genetic damage. But because they are very long-lived, they become the most likely repository for such damage. In fact, this longevity probably also accounts for why many cancers develop decades after tissues are subjected to radiation—the initial injury may be only the first in a series of mutations that turn a healthy cell into a malignant one. Also, a stem cell's huge proliferative capacity makes it an ideal target for malignancy. Nature strictly regulates self-renewal—a cell population already having that ability needs fewer additional mutations for malignant transformation than do cells lacking that capacity.

There may be several possible routes to malignancy. One could involve mutations in the stem cells themselves, with their resulting loss of control over self-renewal decisions producing a pool of stem cells predisposed to malignancy. Additional oncogenic events that start proliferation of the malignant cells into a tumour might take place in the stem cells or in their descendants, the committed progenitor cell population. Another possibility is that oncogenic mutations initially occur in stem cells but the final steps in transformation to cancer occur only in the committed progenitors which somehow reactivate their lost self-renewal power.

Recent evidence that stem cells could become malignant and that only certain cancer cells share a variety of traits with stem cells has supported the view that the driving force underlying tumour growth might be a subpopulation of stem-like cancer cells. This hypothesis can now be tested experimentally by modern techniques. One crucial technique is based on a flow cytometer, which can automatically sort different living cell populations based on the unique surface markers they bear. Another landmark event has been the advent of conclusive tests for self-renewal. Assays to establish self-renewal in human cells could be made by following development of methods that allow normal human stem cells to grow in mice. Using flow cytometry and this new mouse model, JE Dick (Toronto University) has published reports identifying cancer stem cells in leukaemia.

In 2003, R Jones (Johns Hopkins University) similarly identified a cancer stem cell population in multiple myeloma. The same year Clarke et al. (University of Michigan, Ann Arbor) showed cancer stem cells in solid tumours. By transplanting sorted populations of cells from human breast tumours into mice, they confirmed that not all human breast cancer cells have the same capacity to generate new tumour tissue. Only one subpopulation of the cells could re-create the original tumour in the new environment, suggesting that the transplanted tumourigenic cells could both self-renew and give rise to all the different cell populations present in the original tumour, including the non-tumourigenic cells (see Clarke and Becker, 2006). This points to the presence of a hierarchy of cells within a breast cancer similar to those identified in blood malignancies. Since then, many labs have found similar subpopulations of tumourigenic cells in other forms of cancer.

Further support for the cancer stem cell model comes from a related area. The signalling environment (niche) in which tumours reside, seems to strongly influence the initiation and maintenance of malignancy. Studies of normal body cells as well as of stem cells have established the crucial role of signals emanating from surrounding tissue and the supportive extra-cellular matrix in sustaining a given cell's identity and in directing its behaviour. When normal cells are removed from their usual context in the body and placed in a dish, they lose some of their differentiated functional characteristics. Stem cells, in contrast, must be cultured on a medium that provides signals informing them to remain undifferentiated, or they will quickly begin proliferating and differentiating—seemingly as though that is their default programmemed behaviour, and only the niche signals hold it in check (see Clarke and Becker, 2006).

Within the body, stem cell niches are enclaves surrounded by specific cell types, such as stromal cells that form connective tissue in the bone marrow. With a few exceptions, stem cells always remain in their niche, sometimes are physically attached to it by adhesion molecules. In contrast, progenitor cells move away from the niche as they become increasingly differentiated.

Niche signalling, thus, maintains stem cells' undifferentiated state and keeps them quiescent until they are called on to produce new cells, suggesting that these local environmental signals might exert similar regulatory control over cancer stem cells. Experiments have shown, for example, that when transplanted into a new niche, stem cells predisposed to malignancy because of oncogenic mutations will nonetheless fail to produce a tumour. Conversely, normal stem cells transplanted into a tissue environment that has been previously damaged by radiation do give rise to tumours (Clarke and Becker, 2006).

The therapeutic implications of a stem cell model of cancer are dramatic. Current therapies aim against all tumour cells when, in fact, only a small fraction of cancer cells can reconstitute and perpetuate the malignancy. If traditional therapies shrink a tumour but miss these cells, the cancer can return. Treatments that specifically target the cancer stem cells are designed to destroy the engine driving the disease, which leaves any remaining non-tumourigenic cells to eventually die off on their own.

The intriguing hypothesis that tumour growth may be sustained by a rare subpopulation of cancer stem cells is supported by the heterogeneous cellular composition of certain tumours and the observation that only a very small proportion of the cells ($\sim 1/10^6$) in some human acute myeloid leukaemia (AML) samples can seed tumour growth when transplanted into sub-lethally irradiated nonobese diabetic (NOD) severe combined immunodeficient (*scid*) mice (Hope et al., 2004). Such a low frequency of human AML cells producing tumours in NOD/scid mice probably reflects, in part, the rarity of human tumour cells that can readily adapt to growth in a foreign milieu. According to Kelly et al. (2007), the frequency of cells that can sustain tumour growth, and hence the generality of the cancer stem cell hypothesis, is best tested by transfer of titrated numbers of mouse tumour cells into non-irradiated histocompatible recipient mice. The researches of Kelly et al. challenge the idea that growth of AML is always sustained by a rare cancer stem cell. While cancer stem cells may drive the growth of many cancers, especially those that are extensively differentiated, observations of mouse lymphomas and leukaemia suggest that at least certain malignancies (particularly those with substantial homogeneity) can be maintained by a fairly large proportion (>10 per cent) of tumour cells. Of course, mouse and human tumours differ notably, but the significant disparity with results from human AML cells indicate that xenotransplantation probably underestimates the percentage of tumour sustaining cells. With common human solid tumours (for example, brain, colon, and breast), transplantation places the tumour growth-sustaining cells within subpopulations (for example $CD133^+$) that make up to 20 per cent of the cells (Singh et al., 2004, O'Brien et al. 2007); and most of the remaining cells are probably at differentiation stages that cannot be supported by the mouse microenvironment. Cancer stem cells in AML and colon cancer being rare, might reflect the need to co-transfer an essential human accessory cell. It is very important to determine whether the growth of various tumours is sustained by most of the tumour cells or by a rare subpopulation, as this can have crucial implications for designing novel therapies. The need to focus research on testing the cancer stem cell hypothesis critically is urgent.

Rogue Stem-like Cells

Over 75 per cent survival rates for some potentially fatal childhood cancers can now be achieved. In other malignancies, new drugs can reduce the severity of the disease to a condition with which a patient can live. In 2001, Gleevec was approved for the treatment of chronic myelogenous leukaemia (CML) and has recorded great clinical success with many patients now in remission after treatment with Gleevec. But strong evidence points to the possibility that these patients are not truly cured—a reservoir of malignant cells responsible for maintaining the disease is not completely eradicated (Clarke and Becker, 2006).

Since any tumour cell remaining in the body can potentially re-ignite the disease, current treatments are aimed at killing the largest number of cancer cells. But this strategy involves considerable trial and error, and some cancer cells can still escape and survive. Further, in CML as well as some other cancers, only a very small percentage of tumour cells can produce new cancerous tissue, and hitting these specific cells may be a much more effective way to eliminate the disease. Being the engines driving the growth of new cancer cells and very probably the source of the malignancy itself, these cells are called cancer stem cells. They were once normal stem cells or their immature offspring that later became malignant.

It is now believed that rogue stem-like cells lie at the root of many cancers. For successful eradication of these cancer stem cells, we need a much better understanding of how a good stem cell turns bad. Contrary to a popular belief that all cancer cells have the same potential to proliferate and expand the disease, in many types of cancer only a small subset of tumour cells have that power. The tumour-generating cells share some important traits with stem cells, including an unlimited life span and the ability to generate a diverse range of other cell types. This is why they are described as cancer stem cells. It is believed that these malignant progenitors arise from regulatory failures in damaged stem cells or their immediate offspring. This highlights the need for cancer treatments to target cancer stem cells to eradicate the disease (Clarke and Becker, 2006).

The most important defining property of stem cells is their capacity to re-create themselves through self-renewal. It alone gives them the potential for unlimited life span and proliferation.

There are many similarities between stem cells and cancer cells. The traditional definition of malignancy is based on the apparent capacity of cancer cells to survive and multiply indefinitely, ability to invade neighbouring tissues, and spread to distant sites in the body. Indeed, the usual constraints which strongly control cellular proliferation and identity appear to have been lifted from cancer cells. The ability of normal stem cells to self-renew exempts them from the rules limiting life span and proliferation for most cells. Stem cells' ability to differentiate into a wide range of cell types enables them to form the various elements of an organ or tissue system. A core trait of tumours too is the heterogeneity of cell types they contain, as if the tumour were a highly disorderly version of a whole organ. Strict genetic regulation limits or checks the potential of healthy stem cells for unlimited growth and diversification. But if those control mechanisms are lost or compromised, malignancy may result. It is these commonalities that suggest that failures in stem cell regulation are how many cancers initiate, how they perpetuate themselves, and possibly how malignancies metastasize (see Huntly and Gilliland, 2005; Clarke and Fuller, 2006).

Malignancies seem to arise when certain 'oncogenic' changes in key genes within a cell have accumulated and lead to the abnormal growth and transformation of that cell. Gene mutations can appear through a direct insult, such as exposure of the cell to radiation or mutagenic chemicals, or simply through random error when the gene is improperly copied before cell division. The rare stem cells being the only long-lived cells in the organs where most cancers develop, represent a much smaller potential reservoir for cumulative genetic damage that sometimes eventually causes cancer. The crucial point here is the long life of stem cells—they become the most likely repository for such damage (Clarke and Becker, 2006). This is how stem cells' longevity explains why some cancers can develop even decades after tissues are exposed to radiation—the initial injury may be only the first in a series of mutations needed to transform a healthy cell into a malignant one. Besides collecting and preserving these oncogenic scars, a stem cell's high proliferative capacity renders it a particularly suitable target for malignancy.

There can be several different routes to malignancy. Mutations may take place in the stem cells themselves, and their resulting loss of control over self-renewal decision, which thereafter creates a pool of stem cells predisposed to malignancy. Subsequent additional oncogenic events that can trigger proliferation of the malignant cells into a tumour can take place in the stem cells or in their descendants (the committed progenitor cell population). Another scenario is that oncogenic mutations at first occur in stem cells but the final steps in transformation to cancer take place only in the committed progenitors. This model would require the lost self-renewal capacity of the progenitors to be somehow reactivated. Current evidence supports both models in different cancers (see Clarke and Becker, 2006 for specific examples).

One currently hot area of research supports the cancer stem cell model. The signalling environment, or niche, in which tumours are found, influences the initiation and maintenance of malignancy. Studies of normal body cells as well as of stem cells have established the crucial importance of signals originating from surrounding tissue and the supportive extra-cellular matrix not only in sustaining a given cell's identity but also in guiding its behaviour. Normal cells removed from their usual context in the body and placed in a Petri dish tend to lose some of their differentiated functional properties. Stem cells, in contrast, need to be cultured on a medium that signals them to remain undifferentiated, or they will quickly begin proliferating and differentiating—seemingly as though that is their default programmemed behaviour, and only the niche signals hold it in check (Clarke and Becker, 2006).

Within our body, stem cell niches are like enclaves surrounded by such specific cell types as stromal cells that form connective tissue in the bone marrow. With some exceptions, stem cells always reside in their niche, sometimes even physically attached to it by adhesion molecules. In contrast, progenitor cells migrate away from the niche, often escorted by guardian cells, as they become increasingly differentiated.

The crucial role of niche signalling in maintaining stem cells' undifferentiated state and in keeping them quiescent until they are needed to produce new cells points to the strong possibility that these local environmental signals also exercise a similar regulatory control over cancer stem cells. This idea is supported by experiments that, when transplanted into a new niche, stem cells predisposed to malignancy because of oncogenic mutations are not able to produce a tumour. Conversely, normal stem cells transplanted into a tissue environment that has suffered some damage by radiation do produce tumours.

Most current therapies are targeted against all tumour cells. It is now emerging that only a minor fraction of cancer cells carry the power to reconstitute and perpetuate the malignancy. If conventional therapies shrink a tumour but miss these cells, the cancer can return. On the other hand, treatments that are specially aimed at the cancer stem cells can destroy the engine driving the disease, leaving any remaining non-tumourigenic cells to eventually die off on their own (Bissell and LaBarge, 2005; Clarke and Becker, 2006).

Sources of Cancer Stem Cells

Certain tumours have been reported to be sustained by a rare population of cancer stem cells that show one defining property of normal stem cells, the ability to renew themselves. In fact, it is self-renewal that allows stem cells to persist during the lifetime of the organism and to generate new cells for tissue repair, maintenance and regeneration after some stress or injury. Importantly, it is these characteristics that cancer stem cells show not only in initiating and maintaining malignant growth but also in regenerating a tumour when the cancer stem cells escape treatment (Passegue, 2006). This prompts the question whether cancer stem cells are always derived from normal stem cells that run amok, producing cancer cells instead of normal cells (Fig. 5.2A, B). This view seems quite plausible because many cancer stem cell populations indeed express cell-surface proteins that are also present on normal stem cells. However, stem cells may not be the only source of cancer stem cells. Krivtsov et al. (2006) reported the formation of cancer stem cells by a leukaemia-associated protein that can somehow befool non-stem cells to acquire stem-cell-like behaviour and support tumour formation (Fig. 5.2C).

Human leukaemias usually contain recurrent chromosome translocations where segments of the chromosomes have shifted around. For example, the 'mixed lineage leukaemia' gene (*MLL*) is repeatedly found fused to different partners, including the *AF9* gene used by Krivtsov et al. *MLL* is the vertebrate homologue of the fruit fly *trithorax* gene which regulates many developmental programmes by maintaining expression of the *Hox* family of genes (Ernst et al., 2002). *Hox* genes act as master regulators of development. As shown by Daser and Rabbitts (2004), *MLL* fusion genes are associated with the development of acute-type myeloid leukaemias; in mice, they can produce leukaemia upon expression either in the blood-forming stem cells or in myeloid progenitors only (So et al., 2003). As discussed by Akashi et al. (2000) myeloid progenitors are produced by the blood-forming stem cells and have begun to specialize, so that they do not self-renew and are typically destined only to form mature white blood cells or myeloid cells. Krivtsov et al. showed that *MLL-AF9* induces the aberrant expression of a specific set of 'stem cell genes' in myeloid progenitor cells; this induces the cells to self-renew, turning them into cancer stem cells that initiate, maintain and propagate the leukaemia (Passegue, 2006).

While self-renewal is not well understood at the molecular level, it is possible to track it by means of micro-arrays to profile the expression levels of many genes (Forsberg et al., 2005). Hence it is possible to sum up stem-cell identity as a gene-expression signature which differs from the signature of non-stem-cell populations. Some of these differences could possibly underpin self-renewal and other stem-cell-specific proper-

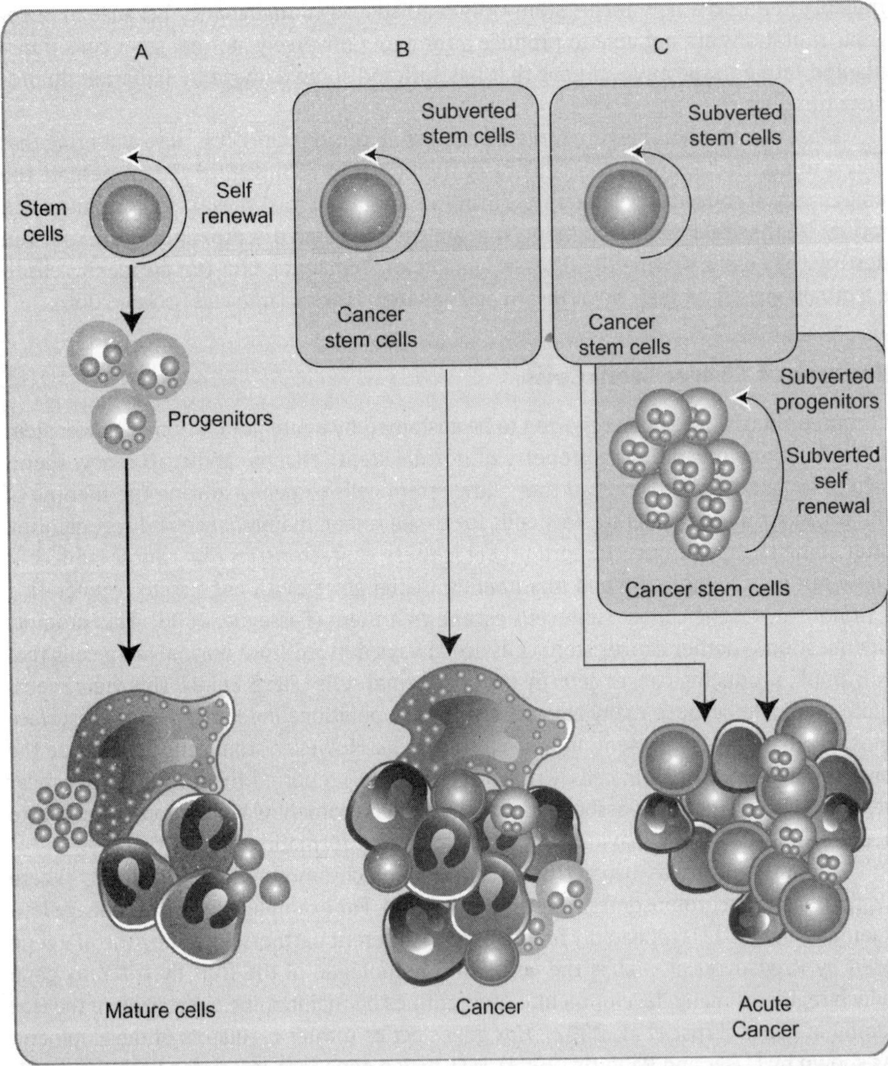

Fig. 5.2 SOURCES OF CANCER STEM CELLS: A. The only cells that self-renew for the lifetime of the organism are normal stem cells. They give rise to the progenitor and mature cell populations required for tissue function and maintenance (here, the blood system). B. Subversion of the stem-cell population by cancer genes to turn it into cancer stem cells, which then produce cancer cells instead of normal cells. Some cancer genes involved in acute myeloid leukaemia can also turn progenitor cells into cancer stem cells by inducing expression of a specific set of stem-cell genes. This expression subverts the progenitor cells to self-renew and to support tumour formation (after Passegue, 2006).

ties. Krivtsov et al. showed that transformed myeloid progenitors abnormally express a small number (363) of stem-cell genes while still displaying the overall gene-expression profile of myeloid progenitor cells—the transformed progenitors do not become stem cells; they only acquire stem-cell-like behaviour. The acquired stem-cell signature is lost when cancer stem cells are forced to abandon their self-renewal properties. This points to the strong possibility that the stem-cell genes identified indeed mediate the erratic self-renewal of the myeloid progenitor cells (Passegue, 2006).

It seems that the stem-cell self-renewal programme is hierarchical, with a specific set of genes activated as an early response to *MLL-AF9* expression. This early programme includes known regulators of stem-cell self-renewal activity, such as members of the *Hox* gene family. Krivtsov et al. examined one of these early-response genes, *Mef2c*, and showed that it modulates stem cell behaviour *in vitro* and *in vivo*. The overall architecture of the self-renewal programme is not clear. This also applies to the specific genes and/or pathways that are crucial for its establishment both in normal- and cancer-stem-cell populations. However, there is hope that interfering with such deregulated self-renewal genes may prevent or reverse the formation of cancer stem cells (Passegue, 2006).

Stem-Cell Divisions and Cancer

Immature cells and stem cells are more likely to go ahead and divide if their chromosomes are entangled. This makes them naturally more prone to becoming cancerous.

Bestor et al. (2005) studied multipotent progenitor cells—which divide to give rise to more specialized cells—in humans and mice. They used a drug to block the action of an enzyme that normally disentangles chromosomes, and observed that a greater proportion of progenitor cells went on with cell division, compared with similarly treated specialized cells.

Cells that divide produce daughters with damaged and abnormal chromosomes. Conceivably, such aberrations could help to give rise to cancer stem cells, a subset of tumour cells thought to be involved in cancer development.

The cancer stem cell hypothesis postulates that tumour cell growth is driven by a small population of malignant cells that are able to self-renew and differentiate—a capacity that is shared with normal tissue stem cells. This attractive idea suggests that drugs could be designed to target cancer stem cells selectively, if and when these cells are identified. Although the stem cell origin of leukaemias is now widely acknowledged, the role of stem cells in solid tumours is not so clear. Shipitsin et al. (2007) made a thorough molecular characterization of two classes of cells purified from human breast cancer: one class expressed a cell surface marker (CD44) previously associated with high tumourigenicity and stem cell-like properties, and the second class expressed a marker (CD24) previously associated with low tumourigenicity and a more differentiated state. $CD44^+$ breast cancer cells expressed many genes in common with progenitor cells in normal breast tissue. The abundance of these cells in the tumour correlated with decreased patient survival. However, the CD44+ and $CD24^+$ cells within individual breast tumours showed genetic differences; this observation is not consistent with the simplest version of the cancer stem cell hypothesis. An alternative model is that many cancer cells retain the capacity to adapt to changing conditions, whether this means reverting to a more primitive, stem-like state or evolving into a more differentiated state.

Stem cells can make more stem cells (i.e., have a 'self-renewal') and they are able to produce cells that differentiate (Fig. 5.3A). Asymmetric cell division enables stem cells to accomplish these two tasks: each stem cell divides to generate one daughter with a stem-cell fate (self-renewal) and one daughter that differentiates (Clevers, 2005) (Fig. 5.3B). Asymmetric division manages both tasks with a single division, but a disadvantage is that stem cells are unable to increase in number. This clear disadvantage argues

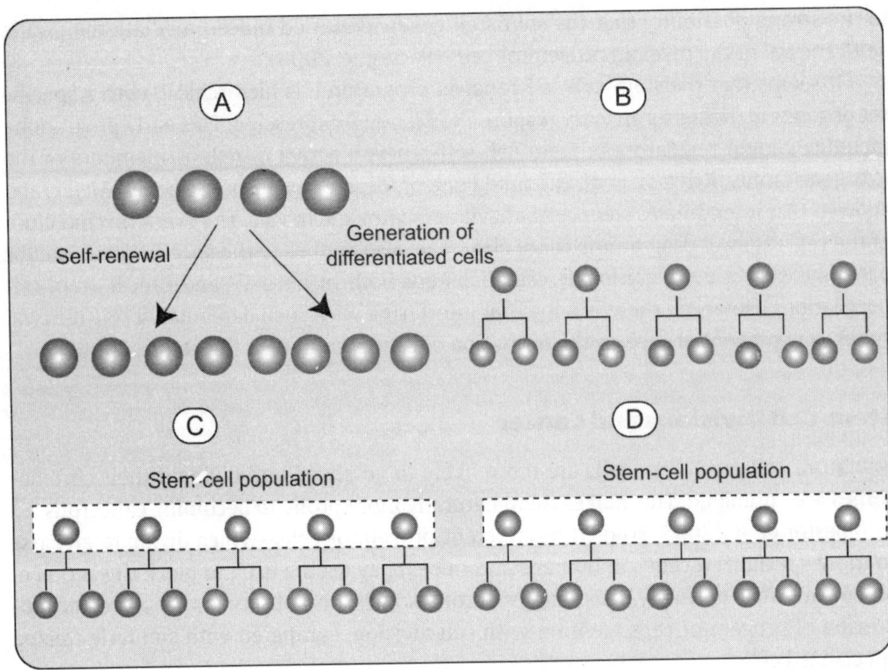

Fig. 5.3 STEM-CELL STRATEGIES: A. Stem cells must accomplish the dual task of self-renewal and generation of differentiated cells. B–D. Possible stem-cell strategies that maintain a balance of stem cells and differentiated progeny. B. Asymmetric cell division: each stem cell generates one daughter stem cell and one daughter destined to differentiate. C and D. Population strategies. A population strategy provides dynamic control over the balance between stem cells and differentiated cells; this ability is necessary for repair after injury or disease. In this scheme, stem cells are defined by their 'potential' to generate both stem cells and differentiated daughters, rather than their actual production of a stem cell and a differentiated cell at each division. C. Symmetric cell division: each stem cell can divide symmetrically to generate either two daughter stem cells or two differentiated cells. D. Combination of cell divisions: each stem cell can divide either symmetrically or asymmetrically (after Morrison and Kimble, 2006).

against the general belief that asymmetric cell division is a defining characteristic of stem cells that enables them to simultaneously perpetuate themselves (self-renew) and generate differentiated progeny—in fact, many stem cells can divide asymmetrically, particularly when they are increasing in number during development or after injury. Thus, asymmetric division is not necessary for stem-cell identity but rather is a tool that stem cells use to maintain appropriate numbers of progeny (Morrison and Kimble, 2006). The facultative use of symmetric or asymmetric divisions by stem cells may be a key adaptation that is crucial for adult regenerative capacity.

Stem cells can also use symmetric divisions to self-renew and to produce differentiated progeny. Symmetric divisions mean the generation of daughter cells destined to acquire the same fate. The notable point is that stem cells are defined by their 'potential' to generate more stem cells and differentiated daughters, rather than by their production of a stem cell and a differentiated daughter at each division. When considered as a population, a pool of stem cells with equivalent developmental potential may produce only stem-cell daughters in some divisions and only differentiated daughters in others.

In principle, stem cells can rely either completely on symmetric divisions (Fig. 5.3C) or on a combination of symmetric and asymmetric divisions (Fig. 5.3D). Symmetric stem-cell divisions have been reported not only in model organisms such as *Caenorhabditis elegans* and *Drosophila*, but also vertebrates.

Morrison and Kimble explored the idea that most stem cells can divide by either asymmetric or symmetric modes of division, and that the balance between these two modes is controlled by developmental and environmental signals to produce appropriate numbers of stem cells and differentiated daughters. Most stem cells possess the ability to switch between asymmetric and symmetric modes of division. The balance between these two modes of division becomes disturbed in some disease states.

Available data on the modes of division used by adult mammalian stem cells *in vivo* are limited. Adult mammalian stem cells are quiescent most of the time (Cheshier et al., 1999). The rarity of adult stem-cell divisions make them technically difficult to image. Although some adult stem cells appear to divide asymmetrically, they do retain the capacity to divide symmetrically to restore stem-cell pools depleted by injury or disease, e.g., in the nervous and haematopoietic systems. In general, stem cells seem to adopt a symmetric mode of division to regenerate depleted stem-cell pools after injury. In mammals, symmetric divisions also increase in number after physiological injuries (Morrison and Kimble, 2006).

The capacity for symmetric stem-cell self-renewal seems to confer some developmental plasticity, increased growth and enhanced regenerative capacity; however, it may also create some risk of cancer. Even in the fruit fly (*Drosophila*), neuroblasts normally divide asymmetrically (Doe and Bowerman, 2001) as a result of the asymmetric localization of cortical cell polarity determinants (e.g., Partner of Inscuteable, PINS) and cell fate determinants, and regulated alignment of the mitotic spindle. But when the machinery that regulates asymmetric divisions is disrupted, these neuroblasts begin dividing symmetrically and form tumours (Caussinus and Gonzalez, 2005).

Cell clones lacking PINS are tumourigenic (Caussinus and Gonzalez, 2005) and double mutant cells lacking both PINS and Lethal giant larvae (LGL) generate a brain composed largely of symmetrically dividing and self-renewing neuroblasts (Lee et al., 2006). Cell clones lacking the cell fate determinants Numb or Prospero are tumourigenic and can be propagated after transplantation into new hosts (Caussinus and Gonzalez, 2005). These tumour cells become aneuploid within 40 days of adopting a symmetric mode of division, indicating that invertebrate cells can undergo rapid neoplastic transformation. Conceivably, the capacity to divide symmetrically may be a prerequisite for neoplastic transformation and that cancer may reflect, at least in part, the capacity to adopt a symmetric mode of cell division (Morrison and Kimble, 2006).

According to Clevers (2005), the machinery that promotes asymmetric cell divisions has an evolutionarily conserved role in tumour suppression. The *adenomatous polyposis coli* (*APC*) gene is required for the asymmetric division of *Drosophila* spermatogonial stem cells and is an important tumour suppressor in the mammalian intestinal epithelium (Kinzler et al., 1991). Loss of Numb could possibly be involved in the hyperactivation of Notch pathway signalling observed in breast cancers (Stylianou et al., 2006). Although these gene products could inhibit tumourigenesis through several different mechanisms that are independent of their effects on cell polarity, the fact that these genes consistently function as tumour suppressors suggests that asymmetric division itself may protect against cancer.

The connection between symmetric cell divisions and cancer derives support from the observation that some gene products can both induce symmetric cell divisions and also function as oncogenes in mammalian cells. Possibly, asymmetric division suppresses carcinogenesis, besides its role in maintaining a balance between stem cells and differentiated progeny (Morrison and Kimble, 2006).

Symmetric modes of division probably promote the expansion of stem-cell numbers and also allow for secondary events leading to aneuploidy. Consistent with this possibility, the machinery that controls asymmetric division is known also to regulate the orientation of mitotic spindles (Lee et al., 2006). One potential source of aneuploidy in symmetrically dividing fly neuroblasts is a defective centrosome—either duplicated or abnormal in shape—that presumably leads to errors in chromosome segregation. This means that regulation of centrosome function by tumour suppressors is also crucial to avoid genomic instability in mammalian cells. Notably, centrosomes and mitotic spindles are tightly regulated in asymmetrically dividing cells—this ensures that daughter cells adopt different fates. Conceivably, tightly regulated centrosomes might also protect chromosomes from errors in segregation. If so, symmetric divisions might increase stem-cell numbers and also increase the probability of aneuploidy and other secondary mutations by loosening the controls on mitotic spindles (Morrison and Kimble, 2006).

Protein Wip1

A new way has been found to trick cancer cells into self-destructing via a protein. Researchers are aiming to potentially inhibit cancer. The focus is on a protein called Wip1 found in stem cells—that is where many cancers originate. Stem cells are able to develop into any type of cell in the body. Cells must have the ability to multiply to produce new daughter cells, but the multiplication also needs to be controlled. This is where Wip1 comes in: it provides the checks and balances that control cell multiplication. If there is too much Wip1, the cell goes into overdrive and goes on multiplying, so causing cancer. 'More Wip1, more cancer'. This prompted the idea that by reducing the amount of Wip1, cancer might potentially be inhibited. In mice, knocking off this protein out of their cells made them cancer-resistant. Now plans are afoot to start Phase I clinical trials soon.

Loss of Heterozygosity (LOH) Mutations

Cancers are thought to originate in pluripotential stem cells. When clinically detected, these cells contain several mutations. Cancer cell genomes are frequently aneuploid, epigenetically altered, and rich in mutations (Feinberg et al., 2006). Some of these mutations result in a loss of heterozygosity (LOH). The mutations in cancer cells include random events that damage DNA, such as attack by environmental carcinogens and reactive cellular metabolites. Mutations in oncogenes (e.g., *K-ras* and *myc*) and tumour-suppressor genes (e.g., *RB* and *APC*) confer growth advantages to malignant cells and can be clonally selected (Weinberg, 2006).

Other non-clonal mutations appear randomly throughout the genome and contribute to the characteristic heterogeneity of malignant cells within a tumour (Bielas et al., 2006). Bielas and Loeb (2005) discussed the quantification of clonal mutations, including LOH in tumours. In contrast, the detection of random mutations requires an analysis of single cells or single DNA molecules.

Donahue et al. (2006) demonstrated that exposure of mouse embryonic stem cells to nontoxic amounts of mutagens triggers a marked increase in the frequency of LOH. Thus, mutagen induction of LOH in embryonic stem cells points to a new pathway to account for the multiple homozygous mutations in human tumours. This induction appears to mimic early mutagenic events that generate cancers in human tissue stem cells (Bielas et al., 2007).

The high frequency of LOH induced by chemical carcinogens throughout the mouse ES genome provides a good protocol for the production of double-knockouts in cultured cells. Homozygous mutants can be recovered directly from genetic screens of mouse ES cells. Even more importantly, nonviable homozygous mutations can be induced in heterozygous mouse ES cells by chemical carcinogens. The need of the hour is to determine whether the high frequency of induction of LOH at retrovirally induced loci in mouse ES cells is also observed at endogenous loci in human ES cells and whether tissue stem cells—the precursors for malignant transformation—also show a high frequency of LOH in response to chemical carcinogens (Bielas et al., 2007).

6 Nucleic Acids and Cancer

Dynamic DNA

The DNA double helix is not a static structure but the molecule gyrates like a seasoned dancer and can perform endless acrobatics. DNA enjoys a fascinating life not in three dimensions but four, the fourth dimension being of time—that makes it far more than a simple string of code. The molecule coils in the cell's nucleus and structural biologists believe that it is sometimes unfaithful to its famous structure—the double helix—it regularly assumes alternative shapes and weaves itself into knots (Pearson, 2003).

The behaviour of the molecule after it crumples up into chromosomes is markedly dynamic. Chromosomes form short-lived liaisons with proteins, move around and spread out exploratory arms. The nucleus, like DNA, once believed to be fairly static, is actually a very lively place. Conceivably, these mysterious movements might be just as important as the genetic sequence itself in determining which genes are switched on or off. A failure to coordinate this sub-cellular waltz may underlie some human diseases. Although half a century has elapsed since the double helix made its debut, scientists have only just begun to understand this wonder molecule as it twirls in time and space.

That the double helix is by no means the alpha and omega of genetics is indicated partly by the discovery of DNA in other peculiar and wonderful shapes. One such variant is called Z-DNA (Wang et al., 1979). Although still a double helix, this Z-DNA swirls in the opposite orientation to Watson and Crick's right-handed coil. But because it was identified in test-tube conditions, the Z-DNA wasn't considered an important player in cellular life. Only recently it has emerged that Z-DNA might be important in controlling gene activity.

Liu et al. (2001) showed that part of the regulatory sequence of an immune-system gene must flip into Z-DNA before the gene can be activated. Similar stretches of transiently existing Z-DNA, of which there are perhaps 100,000 in the human genome, may help to switch on genes by enhancing their access to proteins, such as transcription factors, that stimulate gene activity. Indeed, there is indication that the vaccinia virus, which is related to smallpox, may specifically hijack vulnerable Z-DNA, thereby crippling human cells. In mice, preventing a viral protein from binding to Z-DNA weakens an infection (see Siddiqui-Jain et al., 2002).

Parkinson et al. (2002) reported another unusual form that is adopted at the ragged ends (telomeres) of chromosomes, where the two sister strands give way to a lone string. X-ray crystallography revealed that this single strand can weave itself into a tidy propeller-like loop, which may prevent the molecule from fraying away. This propeller-like structure of DNA is known as 'G-quadruplexes'; they occur in guanine-rich sequences.

Another member of the class seems to prevent genes from being switched on. L. Hurley of the University of Arizona (Tucson) has showed (see Pearson, 2003) that one type of G-quadruplex forms next to the potent cancer-causing gene *c-Myc*. Affecting this structure by mutating its genetic sequence boosts the gene's activity (Phair and Misteli, 2000; Misteli et al., 2000). The shape change seems to ward off gene-activating proteins and drugs are being sought that might stabilize G-quadruplexes and thereby serve as anti-cancer agents.

Improved cellular imaging and other modern techniques to watch living cells in real time have revealed an unexpected brisk activity of proteins buzzing around DNA. Almost all nuclear proteins scuttle constantly back and forth, moving at speeds that would allow them to traverse the nucleus in as little as five seconds. Even histone H1, a protein that was thought to rest in the arms of DNA, now appears to actively attach and detach itself rapidly (Phair and Misteli, 2000; Misteli et al., 2000). Possibly, this swirl of proteins helps in regulating gene activity.

Chromosomes, which seem to be carefully arranged in the nucleus, may be positioned so that those that are most important to the cell gain preferential placement. Human chromosome 18, which carries only a handful of active genes, is spotted to the edge of the nucleus, whereas the gene-packed chromosome 19 is positioned near the middle (see Croft et al., 1999; Tanabe et al., 2002).

Some scientists feel that pushing a chromosome to the edge of the nucleus may help to hive it off from gene-activating machinery thereby keeping unwanted genes gagged. Others suspect that peripheral chromosomes may have a defensive role, shielding genomic DNA from mutagenic chemicals. Chromosomes are constantly in motion. In cells of most organisms, they move rapidly within their confined territories. The shuddering motion probably enables scudding proteins to find their targets in the vast genome.

Brown et al. (1999) showed that chromatin's wanderings may help to lock unwanted genes in an 'off' configuration. In developing immune cells, chromatin carrying genes that are no longer needed move close to regions of inactive DNA (heterochromatin) which suppresses neighbouring genes. If this relocation does not occur, the genes reactivate.

In view of the observations that chromosomal and chromatin movements may spark or silence gene activity, it is being asked whether disruptions in location could trigger disease. Parada et al. (2002), for example, found that in mouse lymphoma cells, chromosomes 12, 14 and 15 huddle closer together than normal. Their proximity might predispose the cells to become cancerous by facilitating the abnormal exchange of chromosome regions that trigger uncontrolled cell division. It is hoped that patients with a susceptibility to cancer might be diagnosed on the basis of the positions of their chromosomes within the nucleus.

Odd (Alternative) DNA Structures

The DNA double helix sometimes contains some unruly bases which get out of line, affecting its function and integrity. This can cause disease. DNA can actually have a left-handed twist. When the double helix untwists so that a gene's code can be read, it sometimes flips into this reverse twirl, a form called Z-DNA because the DNA backbone has a zigzag (Z-shaped) appearance. DNA's strands can also split, kink, or loop back over themselves and form hairpins, crosses and other structures. About a dozen of these abnormal forms have been found at repetitive or symmetrical sequences along chromosomes; these alternative DNA structures have usually been dismissed as transient and biologically unimportant (Pennisi, 2006).

In fact, these forms of DNA deserve critical scrutiny—they can affect transcription and either strengthen the activity of a gene or silence it. In some cases, the formation of these structures affects genetic activity and disrupts the health of cells, ultimately causing mental retardation or cancer. Alternative structures have also been implicated in chromosomal weak spots called fragile sites that play a role in several disorders.

Researchers who have established links between these altered DNA states and diseases such as viral infections and cancer hope to develop drugs that target these unusual forms of DNA.

Alexander Rich of the Massachusetts Institute of Technology, Cambridge (USA) unveiled the structure of Z-DNA in 1979 by using X-ray crystallography. In 2003, he noticed that a poxvirus virulence factor, E3L, mimicked a mammalian protein that binds Z-DNA. After infecting animals with mutated poxviruses, attaching to Z-DNA was crucial to E3L's then-unknown function. If the protein lacked the Z-DNA binding region, then mice infected by an otherwise lethal poxvirus survived. More recently, Rich and his associates

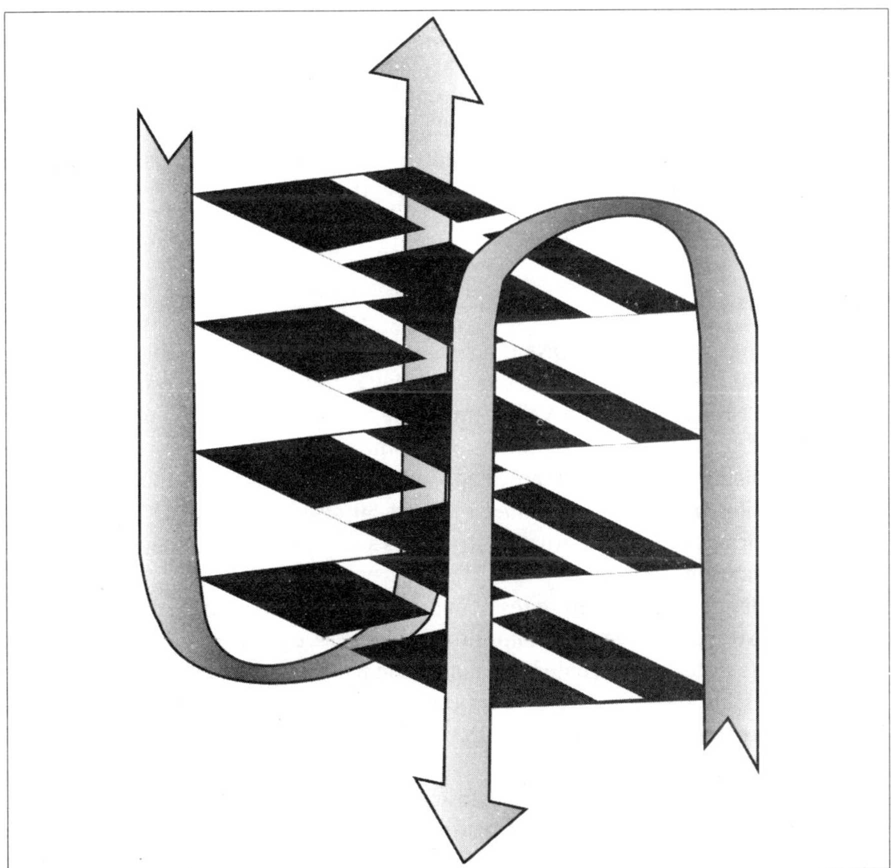

Fig. 6.1 The DNA quadruplex which forms when repetitive bases, in this case guanine (G), align the two strands of the DNA double helix in an unusual configuration (after Pennisi, 2006).

have elucidated the function of E3L. When expressed in human cells, E3L greatly increases the production of several genes that block a cell's ability to self-destruct in response to infection. Once E3L binds to the Z-DNA in the regulatory regions of these genes and stops apoptosis, the poxvirus converts infected cells into viral production factories (Pennisi, 2006). The Z-DNA may be necessary for transcription and E3L stabilizes the Z-DNA, prolonging expression of the anti-apoptotic genes. Conceivably, a small molecule that interferes with the E3L binding to Z-DNA could thwart the activation of these genes and help protect people from pox infections (see Pennisi, 2006).

Some researchers are targeting alternative DNA structures with drugs that might fight cancer. A particular quadruplex DNA structure (Fig. 6.1) has been discovered. It arises naturally from the regulatory sequence that controls the expression of the oncogene *c-Myc*. This quadruplex looks like a chair. Cells produce proteins that stabilize *c-Myc*'s regulatory sequence into a quadruplex, preventing transcription. The gene silencing depends on this alternative structure. Cancer cells often have an overactive *c-Myc*. L. Hurley (University of Arizona, Tucson, USA) showed that if the regulatory sequence's bases are changed, the quadruplex becomes unstable and *c-Myc* expression goes awry, stimulating uncontrolled cell growth. In 2002, Hurley and his associates had reported that such an over-expressed *c-Myc* could be blocked with a small molecule that stabilizes the quadruplex. And without *c-Myc*'s constant prodding, cancer cells self-destructed.

Cylene Pharmaceuticals Inc. (San Diego, California), instead of aiming to silence *c-Myc*, has developed drugs to inhibit a quadruplex that promotes the production of ribosomal RNA, which is needed to make the cell's ribosomes. Their quadruplex is still a sensible anti-cancer target: To have enough protein to fuel their growth, cancer cells need more ribosomes than other cells do. Safety trials of the company's candidate quadruplex inhibitor are underway.

DNA Breakage

One interesting question about DNA is how alternative DNA structures might disrupt the genome. These unusual DNA features are probably central to certain "fragile sites" (i.e., sites where DNA readily breaks while being copied). During replication of DNA at these sites, parts of genes can drop out, pieces of chromosomes can translocate, or repetitive DNA gets copied many times; all these happenings make the site even more vulnerable.

Fragile sites have been implicated in about 50 diseases, including Fragile X syndrome and various cancers. Alternative structures such as cruciforms may possibly have a role in chromosome fragility.

The tendency of cruciforms to result in broken chromosomes may also explain why DNA is often swapped between certain chromosomes (as, e.g., 11 and 22 in humans). The breaks tend to occur at the center of palindromic patterns of A's and T's on these two chromosomes; this creates a window for translocations to occur. The bigger the palindrome, the greater the likelihood that DNA translocation will occur, see *Science*, 17 Feb. 2006 (p. 971).

DNA sequences with repeating cytosine and guanine bases, which are prone to twisting counterclockwise into Z-DNA, also take a toll on the genome, especially in mammalian cells.

It has also been seen that the chromosomal breaks in mammalian cells may not appear just at the point where Z-DNA is inserted but even in remote regions several hundred bases away, resulting in larger-scale deletions and translocations that are so typical in leukaemias and lymphomas. It appears that this breakage is not the result of stalled DNA replication but probably occurs as repair enzymes try to fix the Z-DNA (Pennisi, 2006).

P. Shing Ho of Oregon State University (Corvallis) found that 70 per cent of the regulatory regions for human genes contain sequences that could convert to Z-DNA. Hurley has found thousands of potential quadruplexes in a quick scan of the human genome for the appropriate DNA sequence. Others have identified over 800 regions in the human genome with the DNA signature for triplexes, an alternative DNA structure in which an extra strand latches onto the double helix. These widespread abundances clearly suggest that alternative DNA structures probably perform crucial roles in genome function, such as fine-tuning gene expression. Even though these structures are sources of disease-causing alterations, the genome may like to keep them around because these mutational hotspots generate the genetic diversity so crucial for evolution.

Sanger DNA Sequencing

The Sanger method of DNA sequencing helps in generating long and accurate sequence reads. Some alternative low-cost methodologies aimed at displacing Sanger sequencing currently produce shorter and less accurate sequence reads, which can limit their usefulness in *de novo* sequencing of complex genomes and in the detection of structural variations (Blazej et al., 2006). Comparative analysis of mammalian genomes focuses attention on the importance of such structural variations as insertions, inversions, deletions and duplications in speciation, evolution, disease and cancer (Check, 2005). This underscores the necessity to critically evaluate modern technologies for low-cost genome sequencing and eventual ultra-low-cost sequencing technologies (see NIH, 2004) in terms of their ability to generate accurate short-range as well as long-range genome assemblies. Some such emerging technologies include two cyclic array methods that produce highly parallel, short-read data. Shendure et al. (2005) used DNA ligation to generate 26-base reads that were confidently aligned to 70.5 per cent of the 3.3-Mb *Escherichia coli* genome. Using a pyrophosphate-based approach, Margulies et al. (2005) generated read-lengths of approximately 110 bases for sequencing and *de novo* assembly of 90.4 per cent of the 2.1-Mb *Streptococcus pneumoniae* genome. They took precautions to exclude repetitive DNA sequences from the assembly. Such repeat sequences are vital to genome structure and regulation, in view of the fact that over half of the human genome is composed of repetitive DNA. Repetitive sequences are also ubiquitous and functionally important in prokaryotic and eukaryotic genomes; and gene duplications are involved in disease, speciation and cancer (Lengauer et al., 1998; Gonzalez et al., 2005). Longer, more accurate read-lengths increase sequence coverage and improve *de novo* genome assemblies, but extending cyclic sequencing reads is difficult because the process is serial and requires many enzymatic steps. So, genomes sequenced thus far by using cyclic methods are much smaller than the human genome.

Since Sanger sequencing is the only proven technology for complete sequencing of plant and animal genomes (Lander et al., 2001), some pertinent questions are: what are the ultimate limits of Sanger sequencing and how to achieve these? Paegel et al. (2003) discussed the possible application of nanotechnology, performing completely integrated, nanoliter-scale Sanger sequencing from a femtomole of template. The difficulty in creating such a system is the integration of diverse biochemical processes and high-performance electrophoretic separation onto a single micro-device. Sequencing separations alone were shown on a single-channel glass micro-device in 1995 and later scaled to 96 and 384 channels (Paegel et al., 2002). But in these cases, sample production and purification was done by using conventional microliter-scale processing that generates a 1000-fold more product than is required for analysis. A significant cost in Sanger sequencing is associated with reagent consumption, equipment expense and labour. Conversion to an integrated lab-on-a-chip technology (Dittrich and Manz, 2005) can potentially revolutionize Sanger sequencing by efficiently linking miniaturized analysis to ultra-low-volume sample generation and purification (Blazej et al., 2006). In this context, Blazej et al. have developed an efficient, nanoliter-scale micro-fabricated bioprocessor (see Fig. 6.2) by integrating all three Sanger sequencing steps (thermal cycling, sample purification and capillary electrophoresis). Hybrid glass-polydimethylsiloxane (PDMS) wafer-scale construction is used to combine 250-nl reactors, affinity-capture purification chambers,

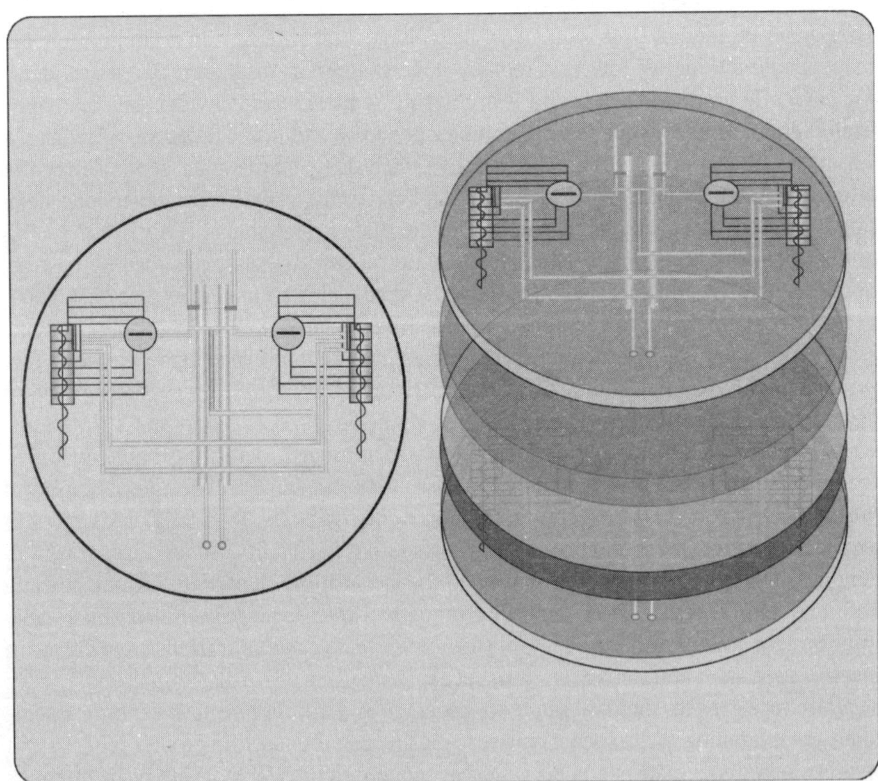

Fig. 6.2 INTEGRATED NANOLITRE-SCALE NUCLEIC ACID BIOPROCESSOR FOR SANGER DNA SEQUENCING: A. Top view of the assembled bioprocessor containing two sets of thermal cycling reactors, purification/concentration chambers, CE channels, RTDs, microvalves/pumps, pneumatic manifold channels and surface heaters. B. Enlarged view, showing micro-device layers. The top two glass wafers are thermally bonded and then assembled with a featureless PDMS membrane and manifold wafer (after Blazej et al., 2006). (NB: CE, capillary electrophoresis; PDMS, polydimethylsiloxane; RTD, resistive temperature detector).

high-performance capillary electrophoresis channels and pneumatic valves and pumps onto a single micro-fabricated device. Lab-on-a-chip-level integration enables complete Sanger sequencing from only 1 fmol of DNA template. Over 550 continuous bases could be sequenced accurately, demonstrating read lengths required for *de novo* sequencing of human and other complex genomes. The performance of this miniaturized DNA sequencer may be a benchmark for predicting the ultimate cost and efficiency limits of Sanger sequencing (Blazej et al., 2006).

DNA Damage and Repair

Cancer arises from a normal cell that changes into a tumour cell through a multistage process involving typical change of a precancerous lesion to a malignant tumour. Multi-stage accumulation of genetic alterations in a single cell changes expression of genes that modulate growth and apoptosis pathways. The disregulation of these critical cellular pathways leads to the uncontrolled growth of cancer. Sustained cancer growth also requires alterations in pathways that control formation of new blood vessels (angiogenesis).

Many types of genetic alterations can initiate cancer. Cancer-related mutations may arise from changes in single bases within the DNA sequence, DNA replication errors (RER) that add or delete bases within mononucleotide or dinucleotide repeat sequences, malfunction of the DNA mismatch repair genes that change the length of simple repetitive sequences (micro-satellite instability), or deletion or amplification of sequences ranging from short to large portions of chromosomal arms. Further, various chromosomal changes, including increased or decreased number of chromosomes and chromosomal rearrangements have been identified in cancer cells.

All these gene alterations can impair the ability of the cell to repair DNA damage resulting in additional mutations and accelerated tumour progression. Somatic cell mutations in individual cells during cancer development account for most cancers. Some cancers are hereditary and appear in individuals with specific germline mutations that convey a much higher risk of developing cancer. Two good examples of hereditary cancers are breast-ovarian cancer associated with mutations in the *BRCA1/2* genes and colorectal cancer associated with mutations in the *HNPCC* or *FAP* genes.

The aesthetic appeal of the DNA double helix initially hindered notions of DNA mutation and repair. But it later emerged that DNA is subject to continuous damage and the cell has many ways of responding to such injury. Mutations or deficiencies in repair can have catastrophic consequences, causing a range of human diseases.

Work on three 'R's' of DNA metabolism—replication, recombination and repair—clearly brought out the dynamic state of DNA. DNA in all living organisms continually suffers diverse types of damage and cells have devised elegant mechanisms for tolerating and repairing the damage. Failure of these mechanisms can cause serious disease, best illustrated in the human hereditary diseases xeroderma pigmentosum (XP), hereditary non-polyposis colon cancer (HNPCC) and some forms of breast cancer. XP is characterized by about a 10,000-fold increased risk of skin cancer associated with sunlight exposure; individuals with HNPCC manifest an increased hereditary predisposition to colon (and other) cancer (Friedberg, 2003).

The early work on DNA damage and repair in the 1930s preceded the elucidation of the double helical structure of DNA (see Pontecorvo, 1958; Friedberg, 2002, 2003). There was strong cooperation and collaboration involving integration of physics and biology in pre-war Germany between German physicists Karl Zimmer and Max Delbrück with the Russian geneticist Nikolai Timoféeff-Ressovsky (Timofeeff-Ressovsky et al., 1935). This effort was greatly stimulated by the work of Muller (1927) on the fruit fly *Drosophila*; Muller first proved that ionizing radiation causes mutations in living organisms.

Whereas Timoféeff-Ressovsky and Zimmer were intrigued primarily by the fact of how small amounts of energy in the form of ionizing radiation could have such marked biological effects, Delbruck and Muller wished to find out whether such mutations could shed light on the physical nature of the gene.

Their efforts to explain these confounding observations led to the discovery of the phenomenon now known as photoreactivation, whereby the DNA damage incurred by exposure to UV light is repaired by a light-dependent enzyme reaction (Friedberg et al., 1995). Photoreactivation reverses DNA damage. DNA exposed to ultraviolet (UV) radiation results in covalent dimerization of adjacent pyrimidines, typically thymine residues (thymine dimers). These lesions are recognized by a photoreactivating enzyme which absorbs light at wavelengths less than 3,000 nm (such as fluorescent light or sunlight) and facilitates a series of photochemical reactions that monomerize the dimerized pyrimidines, restoring them to their native conformation (Friedberg, 2003).

Tautomerism allows a compound to exist in two interconvertible chemical states; in the case of DNA bases, as either keto or enol forms. Watson and Crick had initially overlooked tautomerism and were grappling in vain to construct their DNA model with the rare enol form of bases. It was only after Jerry Donohue suggested to Watson to use the more common keto form that the problem of how bases could stably pair was solved (see Watson, 1968). But it was not realized at that time that the chemical liability of DNA implicit in tautomerism could have wider implications for the stability of genes. Indeed, the field gave little thought to the precise nature of DNA damage and its possible biological consequences. In those days; or even after the DNA double helix was unveiled, its 'pathology' attracted little interest—much higher priority was given to deciphering the genetic code or understanding DNA replication. This is indeed strange considering that the repair phenomenon of photoreactivation was known before the elucidation of the structure of DNA.

DNA replicates in a semi-conservative fashion, whereby each strand of the double helix pairs with a new strand generated by replication. This allows any errors introduced during DNA replication to be corrected by excision repair, which relies on the redundancy inherent in having two complementary strands of the genetic code. If the nucleotides on one strand are damaged; they can be excised and the intact opposite strand used as a template to direct repair synthesis of DNA (Hanawalt and Haynes, 1967).

DNA repair now embraces the direct reversal of some types of damage (such as the enzymatic photoreactivation of thymine dimers) and also multiple distinct mechanisms for excising damaged bases, termed nucleotide excision repair (NER), base excision repair (BER) and mismatch repair (MMR). The underlying principle in all three mechanisms is splicing out the damaged region and inserting new bases to fill the gap, followed by ligation of the pieces (Friedberg et al., 1995; Friedberg, 2003).

Double-strand breaks (DSBs) in DNA can result from exposure to ionizing radiation, oxidative damage and the spontaneous cleavage of the sugar-phosphate backbone of the DNA molecule. They can be repaired by either rejoining the broken ends or by homologous recombination with a sister DNA molecule. Both processes involve different multiprotein complexes (Friedberg, 2003).

Cell Suicide

Biological responsiveness to genetic insult covers more than the repair and tolerance of DNA damage. The exposure of cells to many DNA-damaging agents leads to the transcriptional upregulation of many genes, the precise function(s) of some of which is not known. Also cells have evolved complex signalling pathways to arrest the progression of the cell cycle in the presence of DNA damage, thereby providing more time for repair and tolerance mechanisms to operate (Zhou and Elledge, 2000). Lastly, if the burden of genomic insult is simply too heavy to be effectively handled, cells can initiate programmed cell death (apoptosis), thereby eliminating themselves from a population that otherwise might suffer serious pathological consequences (Cory and Adams, 2002).

Somatic Mutation Hypothesis

The 'somatic mutation hypothesis' of cancer was prompted by the idea that neoplastic transformation arises from mutations that change the function of specific genes (now termed oncogenes and tumour-suppressor genes) that are critical for cell division. The genetic basis of many cancers is abnormal recombination events, such as chromosomal translocations, where a region of one chromosome is juxtaposed to another chromosome; also mutagenesis is a fundamental cornerstone of the molecular basis of all forms of cancer (Vogelstein and Kinzler, 1998).

Validation of the somatic mutation hypothesis came from the discovery that defective responses to DNA damage and the accumulation of mutations underlie two distinct types of hereditary cancer: skin cancer associated with defective NER and colorectal cancer associated with defective MMR. In both instances, researchers of DNA repair contributed greatly to our understanding.

Elucidation of the genes defective in XP patients and their role in NER of damaged bases in human cells (De Weerd-Kastelein et al., 1972; Wood, 1996) attests to the triumph of modern genetics and its application to molecular biology. Another finding that the process of NER in eukaryotes requires elements of the basic transcription apparatus has illuminated the complex relationships between deficient DNA repair, defective transcription and hereditary human diseases (Friedberg et al., 1995).

According to Friedberg (2003), biological responsiveness to DNA damage includes DNA repair, mutagenesis, damage tolerance, cell-cycle checkpoint control, programmed cell death and other cellular processes concerned with tackling genomic insult. This whole field is now unravelling the regulatory pathways transduced by signalling mechanisms that detect DNA damage and/or arrested DNA replication. Parallel technological gains in gene therapy and therapeutic intervention by rational drug design are likely to generate new strategies for blocking the unwanted consequences of DNA damage, especially cancer.

Base-excision Repair and Colorectal Cancer

Living organisms constantly face the challenge of how to maintain the chemical integrity of DNA when exposed to oxidizing agents. Base-excision repair (BER) plays a crucial role in preventing mutations associated with a common product of oxidative damage to DNA, 8-oxoguanine (8-oxoG). Recent structural studies have shown that 8-oxoG DNA glycosylases use an intricate series of steps to find and excise 8-oxoguanine lesions efficiently against a high background of undamaged bases (David et al., 2007). The importance of preventing mutations associated with 8-oxoguanine is borne out by a direct association between defects in the DNA glycosylase MUTYH and colorectal cancer. The properties of other guanine oxidation products and the associated DNA glycosylases that remove them are now becoming clear.

The importance of preventing mutations associated with 8-oxoG was appreciated with the discovery of a direct link between colorectal cancer and mutations in the gene encoding the human MutY homologue (MUTYH) (Al-Tassan et al., 2002). This work established the first link between inherited defects in BER and cancer.

In 2001, Fearnhead et al. had shown that in familial adenomatous polyposis, the colon of afflicted patients littered with adenomatous polyps as a result of mutations in the adenomatous polyposis coli gene (*APC*). The APC protein controls the proliferation of colon cells and suffers mutation in most colorectal tumours. Although the familial nature of familial adenomatous polyposis is usually a consequence of inherited mutations in APC, this was not the case in one British family, N Work done on this family prompted the hypothesis that certain MUTYH variants show reduced capacity to initiate the repair of 8-oxoGA mismatches, leading to increased numbers of G-to-T transversions in APC and eventually resulting in inactivation of the APC protein (David et al., 2007). This is an elegant mechanism by which inherited defects in a gene encoding a BER enzyme (*MUTYH*) lead to mutations in a gene associated with predisposition to cancer (*APC*). This mechanism of predisposition to colorectal cancer is referred to as MUTYH-associated polyposis (Sampson et al., 2005; Cheadle and Sampson, 2007).

Since the discoverv of family N, much subsequent work has supported the relationship between mutations in MUTYH and colorectal adenomas and carcinomas and this disorder is now referred to as MUTYH-associated polyposis (see Tenesa et al., 2006). MUTYH-associated polyposis appears to be an autosomal recessive disorder (requiring mutations in both alleles).

Current estimates of the frequency indicate that MUTYH-associated polyposis accounts for –1 per cent of all colorectal cancer. This contribution to colorectal cancer is lower than the present estimate of 1–6 per cent for hereditary non-polyposis colorectal cancer (HNPCC) (Jo and Chung, 2005; Strate and Syngal, 2005). HNPCC, like MUTYH-associated polyposis, arises from an inherited DNA-repair defect, particularly in genes involved in mismatch repair (MMR). But HNPCC differs from MUTYH-associated polyposis in being an autosomal dominant disorder and it results from a different type of DNA-repair defect.

Alternative Splicing and RNA Therapy

Alternative splicing edits the information stored in the genes of complex organisms in such a way that a single gene can specify two or more distinct proteins. Alternative splicing accounts for much of the diversity among organisms with relatively similar gene sets. Within a single organism, alternative splicing allows different tissue types to perform diverse functions working from the same small gene assortment (Ast, 2005).

The prevalence of alternative splicing increases with an organism's complexity; as many as three quarters of all human genes can undergo alternative editing. In the shorter term, scientists are learning how faulty gene splicing leads to several cancers and congenital diseases and how the splicing mechanism can be used therapeutically (Ast, 2005). Indeed, life and death depend on alternative editing—at least when a damaged cell must determine whether to go on living or die. Each cell constantly senses the conditions inside and outside itself, so that it can decide whether to maintain growth or to self-destruct by apoptosis. Cells that cannot repair DNA activate their apoptotic program. B. Thompson (University of Pennsylvania) has shown that a gene called *Bcl-x*, which is a regulator of apoptosis, is alternatively spliced to produce either of two distinct proteins, Bcl-x(L) and Bcl-x(S). The former suppresses apoptosis, while the latter promotes it.

Genome comparisons have revealed that the process whereby cells give rise to different forms of protein from a single gene is both common and crucial. It strongly changes the classical view of how information stored in a gene is translated into a protein. Most of the well-known facts still hold true: the instructions for making and maintaining an organism are encoded in the four-letter language of DNA nucleotides. When the gene's instructions are to be expressed, the double-stranded zipper of DNA opens just long enough for a single-stranded copy of the gene's sequence to be manufactured from RNA. Each sequence of DNA bases that is transcribed into an RNA version in this way is termed a gene. Some of the resulting RNA molecules are never translated into proteins but perform housekeeping and regulatory functions within the cell. The RNA transcripts of genes that do code for a protein will ultimately be read by the ribosomes and translated into a corresponding sequence of amino acids. But first the preliminary transcript must be edited.

These initial or primary RNA transcripts contain many non-meaningful codons inserted at intervals. These codons, called introns, must be excised and the protein-coding ones connected together for the RNA to tell a coherent story. The cutting-and-ligation process is termed splicing. In this, the introns are snipped out of the primary transcript and discarded. Segments of the transcript containing functional protein-coding sequences, called exons, are joined together to create a final version of the transcript, known as messenger RNA (mRNA).

By 1980 it had emerged that the above basic view of pre-mRNA splicing, in which all introns are always discarded and all exons are always included in the mRNA, does not always hold true. In fact, the cellular machinery can "decide" to splice out an exon or to leave an intron, or pieces of it, in the final mRNA transcript. This ability to alternatively edit pre-mRNA transcripts increases any gene's versatility and gives the splicing mechanism great power to determine how much of one type of protein a cell will produce over the other possible types encoded by the same gene (Ast, 2005).

Splicing Machine

The basal machinery is found in all organisms whose genomes contain introns. It consists of five small nuclear RNA (snRNA) molecules, called U1, U2, U4, U5 and U6. These molecules associate with as many as 150 proteins to form a complex called the spliceosome that recognizes the sites where introns begin and end, cutting the introns out of the pre-mRNA transcript and joining the exons to form the mRNA.

Four short base sequences within introns act as signals that guide the spliceosome where to cut. One of these splicing signals lies at the beginning of the intron and is called the 5' splice site; the others, sitting at the end of the intron, constitute the branch site, the polypyrimidine tract and, finally, the 3' splice site (Ast, 2005).

A separate regulatory system regulates the splicing by directing the basal machinery to these splice sites. Over 10 different splicing regulatory (SR) proteins are known. Their forms may vary in different tissues or stages of development in the same tissue. SR proteins bind to short base sequences within the exons of the pre-mRNA transcript. These binding sites are termed exonic splicing enhancers (ESE) because the binding of the appropriate SR protein to an ESE directs the basal machinery's snRNAs to the splice sites adjacent to either end of the exon. However, an SR protein can also bind to an exonic splicing suppressor (ESS) sequence within the exon—this suppresses the basal machinery's ability to bind to the ends of that exon and results in it being spliced out of the final mRNA (Ast, 2004, 2005).

Skipping just one exon can produce a dramatic effect on an organism. Exon skipping is the commonest type of alternative splicing reported in mammals, besides several other uncommon kinds, including one that causes introns to be retained in mature mRNA, which is most prevalent in plants and lower multi-cellular organisms. Intron retention may be the earliest version of alternative splicing to have evolved. Even today the splicing apparatus of yeast operates by recognizing introns, in contrast with the SR protein system of higher organisms, which defines exons for the basal machinery (Ast, 2005).

In the unicellular system, the splicing machinery can recognize only intronic sequences of less than 500 nucleotides; this is okay for yeast because it has very few introns, averaging just 270 bases long. But with genomes expanding during evolution, their intronic stretches multiplied and grew and cellular splicing machinery had to switch from a system that recognized short intronic sequences within exons to one recognizing short exons amid a lot of introns. The average human protein-coding gene, for instance, is 28,000 nucleotides long, with 8.8 exons separated by 7.8 introns. While the exons are relatively short (usually about 120 nucleotides), the introns can range from 100 to 100,000 nucleotides long.

Humans have the highest number of introns per gene of any organism. The size and quantity of these introns raises an interesting issue. Introns are an expensive habit to maintain. A large fraction of the energy we consume daily helps in the maintenance and repair of introns in their DNA form, transcribing the pre-mRNA and deleting the introns and even causing the break-down of introns at the end of the splicing reaction. This system can also make costly mistakes. Each miscut and ligation of pre-mRNA can change the gene transcript's protein-coding sequence and possibly lead to the synthesis of a defective protein (Ast, 2004, 2005).

By creating more than one type of mRNA molecule and, hence more than one protein per gene, alternative splicing enables humans to manufacture more than 90,000 proteins without having to maintain 90,000 genes. On average, each of our genes generates about three alternatively spliced mRNAs. Yet, this number does not account for our need for so many introns and why exonic sequences are left to make up only 1 to 2 per cent of the human genome (Ast, 2005).

RNA Therapy

Many scientists are trying to understand the complex reactions involved in alternative splicing. There are pointers toward future therapeutic applications, such as new gene therapy strategies that exploit the splicing mechanism to treat both inherited and acquired disorders, e.g., cancer.

A short stretch of synthetic RNA or DNA nucleotides, called antisense oligonucleotides (oligos) may possibly be directed to bind to a specific target on the patient's DNA or RNA. Antisense oligos could be delivered into cells to mask either a specific splice site or some other regulatory sequence, which would shift the splicing activity to another site. This approach has been applied to human cancer cells grown in culture. By masking a 5' splice site of the *Bcl-x* apoptosis-regulating gene transcript, splicing activity could be shifted to generate the Bcl-x(S) form of mRNA rather than the Bcl-x(L) form, decreasing the cancer cells' synthesis of the antiapoptotic protein and enhancing synthesis of the proapoptotic protein. In some cancer cells, this change activates the apoptotic program; in others, it enhances the apoptotic effects of chemotherapeutic drugs administered along with the oligos (Ast, 2005).

Another possibility to exploit the alternative splicing mechanism for therapy is to induce cells to splice in an exon that would otherwise be skipped. A synthetic molecule has been created and can be programmed to bind to any piece of RNA according to its sequence and then attached to the RNA-binding part of an SR protein. This chimeric molecule can not only bind to a specified sequence on the pre-mRNA but also recruit the basal machinery to the appropriate splice signal.

A third approach exploits the ability of the spliceosome to join two different pre-mRNA molecules from the same gene to form a composite mRNA. This trans-splicing event is common in worms but is rare in human cells. Forcing the spliceosome to trans-splice could allow a mutated region of pre-mRNA responsible for disease to be precisely excised and replaced with a normal protein-coding sequence.

Alternative splicing is indeed the pivotal process that permits a small number of genes to generate the much larger assortment of proteins needed to produce the complex human body and mind while precisely orchestrating their manufacture in different tissues at different times. Splicing also explains how the tremendous diversity among humans and presumably all mammals, could originate in such similar genomes.

Gene Mutations and Human Cancers

An accumulation of mutations and other heritable changes causes cancer in susceptible cells. Abnormalities in about 350 genes have been implicated in human cancers, but the true number of 'cancer genes' is not known. Stephens et al. (2004) and Greenman et al. (2007) did extensive work on breast, lung and brain tumours by identifying mutations in the genes encoding all known protein kinases across various types of cancer. These enzymes regulate other proteins through the addition of a phosphate residue. A whole-genome resequencing analysis of a smaller number of breast and colorectal cancers done by Sjöblom et al. (2006) provides an informative overview of the spectrum of mutations involved in human cancers (Haber and Settleman, 2007).

Greenman et al. sequenced 518 protein-kinase-encoding genes in 210 cancers. Kinases have not only been implicated in tumourigenesis but several have also been validated as targets for drug therapy. The spectacular success of the drug imatinib (Gleevec) in treating chronic myeloid leukaemia is attributed to its suppression of a kinase known as BCR-ABL, which is the product of a gene located within a cancer-specific, translocated chromosome (Kantarjian et al., 2002). In their analysis of the 'kinome', the collection of cellular kinases, Greenman et al. identified 1000 mutations. These were common in cancers of the lung, stomach, ovary, colon and kidney, but rare in those of the testis, breast and in carcinoid tumours, which usually appear in the gastrointestinal tract. Tumours with defects in DNA-mismatch repair contained many mutations, whereas other types of tumour revealed no detectable mutations. Specific patterns of nucleotide substitution differed among cancers from various tissue types and probably mirrored the effects of external mutagens or defects in DNA repair.

By the time a cancer is diagnosed as such, it already contains billions of cells carrying the DNA abnormalities that initiated malignant proliferation and many additional genetic lesions acquired later. Some of these secondary mutations arise due to selective pressure during tumourigenesis (drivers) whereas others may be incidental (passengers) and result from mutational exposures, genome instability or merely the numerous cell doublings that lead from a single transformed cell to a clinically detectable cancer (Haber and Settleman, 2007). To distinguish driver from passenger mutations, Greenman et al. used a statistical model comparing the observed-to-expected ratio of synonymous (no amino-acid change) mutations with that of non-synonymous (altered amino acid) mutations. An increased proportion of non-synonymous mutations indicate selection pressure during tumourigenesis. Overall, 158 predicted driver mutations could be identified in 120 genes encoding kinases. Unlike the recurrent mutations in the gene encoding a kinase known as BRAF identified by Davies et al. (2002) in malignant melanomas, most kinase mutations identified by Greenman et al. across different tumour types represented 'single hits'. Sjöblom et al. (2006) also reached generally similar conclusions. Both these teams emphasized the requirement for a very large number of samples to catch the full spectrum of genetic heterogeneity in cancer (Haber and Settleman, 2007).

The US National Cancer Institute and the National Human Genome Research Institute have proposed the Human Cancer Genome Project (see von Eschenbach and Collins, 2005). It is sequencing 12500 tumour samples (250 specimens from 50 different cancers) and focusing on about 2000 genes implicated in tumourigenesis. The large scale analysis is expected to reveal recurrent mutations in subsets of cancer, an important clue to identifying truly significant drivers. However, small nucleotide changes within genes that can be detected by sequencing make up only a small group of abnormalities underlying human cancer; gene amplification or deletion, inactivation of genes through epigenetic silencing and chromosomal translocations which also contribute substantially to alterations in cancer genes (Fig. 6.3); cannot be detected by sequence analysis of known genes (Haber and Settleman, 2007). The figure illustrates the various defects that can lead to cancer.

The initial sequencing studies published by Greenman et al. and Sjöblom et al. throw light on mutational profiles in various cancers that might help in identifying the molecular mechanisms responsible for tumour initiation and progression. But, it should be remembered that each cancer genome carries several unique abnormalities and not all mutations identified contribute equally to the manifestation of the associated cancers. A choice of appropriate genetic and functional approaches is essential to correctly identify true drivers from the many passengers on the road to tumourigenesis (Haber and Settleman, 2007).

DNA-sequencing strategies described by Greenman et al. and Sjöblom et al., allow detecting small nucleotide changes within genes (intragenic mutations) and identify these genes as the target of a mutational event. Various abnormalities can be transmitted from a cancer cell to its progeny, some of which activate specific genes (gain-of-function mutations), whereas others inactivate them (loss-of-function mutations). Comparative

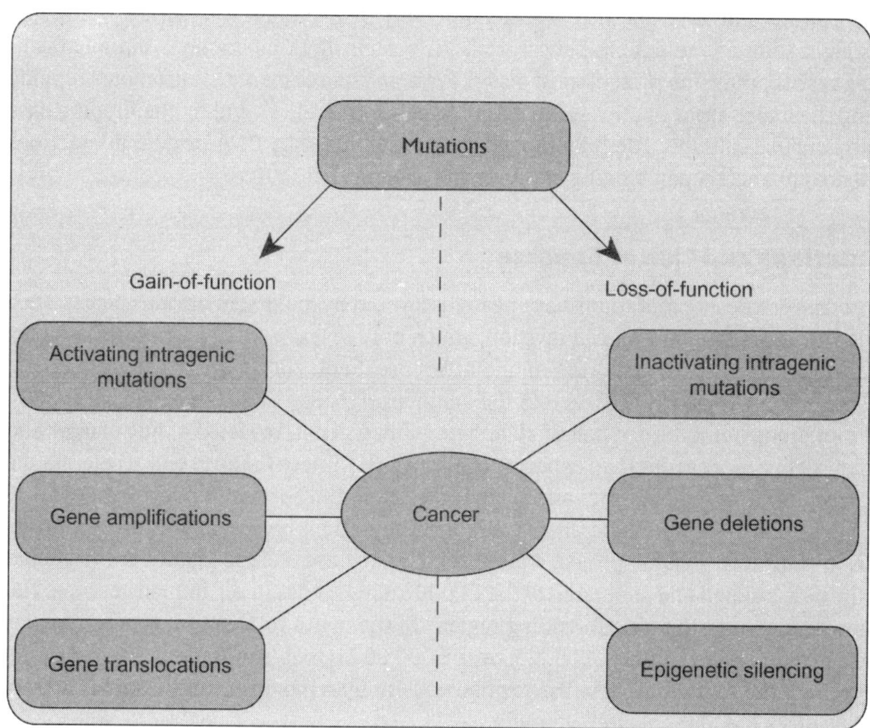

Fig. 6.3 The various defects that underlie human cancer (after Haber and Settleman, 2007).

genomic hybridization is needed to scan for deletion or amplification of chromosome fragments, which often contain many genes, making it very difficult to identify the specific gene(s) targeted by these events. Epigenetic silencing involves heritable modifications of nucleotides and histones in regulatory regions of genes, leading to suppression of gene expression in the absence of DNA mutations. Translocations lead to the fusion of DNA fragments from different chromosomal regions, either creating an abnormal fusion protein or leading to aberrant expression of a normal gene (Haber and Settleman, 2007).

Base Flipping and Cancer Etiology

DNA methylation plays an important role in gene regulation of eukaryotes and in protection of "self" DNA in prokaryotes. It is involved in the etiology of some cancers. For methylation of the target base, as catalyzed by methyltransferases, the base has to be flipped out of the DNA double helix and into the enzyme's active site (Roberts and Cheng, 1998). Base flipping is also important for other enzymes that chemically modify DNA, including DNA-mismatch repair enzymes, such as uracil glycosylase and endonucleases (Huang et al., 2003). Base flipping is also probably linked to early events in the opening and unwinding of DNA for transcription and replication processes. Enzyme-mediated base flipping is therefore a crucial first step in elucidating the more complex enzyme-catalyzed DNA processing involved in transcription and replication (Huang et al., 2003). Flipping occurs via the major groove of the DNA. Structural analysis suggests that it is facilitated by destabilization of the DNA double-helical structure and substitution of DNA base-pairing and base-stacking interactions with DNA-protein interactions. Although destabilization of the double-helical state via protein-DNA interactions initially facilitates base flipping, the protein must also provide an environment that promotes flipping along the major groove pathway. This can happen by merely excluding the flipping base from aqueous solution. The fully flipped state is stabilized by DNA-protein interactions that are enhanced upon binding of coenzyme (Huang et al., 2003).

Mutations and Cancer Genome

Most cancer-causing mutations have been discovered by looking in obvious places, such as in the genes that control cell division, which only reveal a small part of the complex picture. A recent search reported online in *Science* (Sept. 2006) (www.sciencemag.org/cgi/content/abstract/1133427) across the genomes of breast and colorectal cancer cells, for mutations in more than half of all known human genes, revealed a much larger and richer set of cancer genes than expected (Kaiser, 2006). These findings will accelerate the race for new drugs, diagnostics and a better understanding of tumour development.

Even this first effort at describing all cancer mutations reveals daunting complexity. This mini-cancer-genome project started with a database of 13023 genes is considered as the best-studied and annotated of the 21,000 known genes in the human genome. The team resequenced the protein-coding regions of the genes in 11 breast cancer samples and 11 colon cancer samples, yielding over 8,000,000 possible mutations. More than 99 per cent of the mutations were then winnowed out by removing errors, normal variants and changes that did not alter a protein.

It was found that the average breast or colon tumour has 93 mutated genes and at least 11 appear to be cancer-promoting. This yielded a total of 189 'candidate' cancer genes. Although some are familiar—the tumour-suppressor gene *p53*, for example—most had never been found to be mutated in cancer before. The abundance of certain genes, such as those involved in cell adhesion and transcription, points to the possibility that these processes have a strong role in cancer. Of course, it will not be easy to verify that each candidate gene is important to cancer. The cancer genes differed between colon and breast cancers and each tumour had a different pattern of mutations. The number of genes indicates that there may be more steps to cancer than believed hitherto.

The mutation differences from tumour to tumour may account for why 90 per cent of drugs fail in patients.

The advent of several high-throughput technologies and their application in many gene expression profiling studies have focused interest in tumour signatures that can discriminate cancer patients with good vs. poor outcomes (van't Veer et al., 2002; Sotiriou et al., 2003). Unfortunately, understanding the biological basis of why these signatures are predictive and how the identified risk groups relate to activation of oncogenic pathways and sensitivity to molecularly targeted therapies are no easy tasks. It appears that optimal efficacy of targeted therapies can be possible only when the appropriate subgroups of patients with target and/or pathway-activated tumours can be identified and used to guide treatment (Shaw and Cantley, 2006; Bild et al., 2006).

There seems little doubt that in the coming years, pathway-specific therapy will gain importance and be helpful in cancer management. The oncogenic phosphatidylinositol 3-kinase (PI3K) pathway is frequently activated in solid tumours; however, no reliable test for PI3K pathway activation has yet been designed for human tumours.

Prompted by the observation that loss of PTEN, the negative regulator of PI3K, results in robust activation of this pathway, Saal et al. (2007) developed and validated a microarray gene expression signature for immunohistochemistry (IHC)-detectable PTEN loss in breast cancer (BC). The most significant signature gene was *PTEN* itself; pointing to *PTEN* mRNA levels as the primary determinant of PTEN protein levels in BC. Some PTEN IHC-positive BCs showed the signature of PTEN loss, which was associated to moderately reduced *PTEN* mRNA levels cooperating with specific types of *PIK3CA* mutations and/or amplification of *HER-2*. This shows that the signature is more sensitive than PTEN IHC for identifying tumours with pathway activation. In independent data sets of breast, prostate and bladder carcinoma, prediction of pathway activity by the signature correlated significantly to poor patient outcome. Stathmin, encoded by the signature gene *STMN1*, turned out to be an accurate IHC marker of the signature and had prognostic significance in BC. Stathmin was also pathway-pharmacodynamic *in vitro* and *in vivo*. Thus, the signature or its components such as stathmin may be clinically useful tests for stratification of patients for anti-PI3K pathway therapy and monitoring therapeutic efficacy. Aberrant PI3K pathway signalling is strongly associated with metastasis and poor survival across carcinoma types, highlighting the huge potential impact on patient survival achievable through pathway inhibition.

Recent Nucleic Acid Technologies

Innovations in biotechnology that integrate molecular biology, micro-fabrication and bioinformatics have moved nucleic acid technologies from futuristic possibilities into common laboratory and clinical procedures.

Screening-based approaches are changing the way hypothesis-driven research is conducted. Genome-sequencing efforts are giving place to 'post-genome' efforts so as to coordinate and interpret the wealth of information generated. In clinical practice, for nucleic acid diagnostics to become routinely used, these procedures will need to be adapted to high-throughput situations, with greater reproducibility and reduced expense.

The explosive growth of molecular technology has brought it to the stage of commercialization without basic standard reference materials. The acceptance of molecular diagnostics will be enhanced by adopting industry standards, similar to those in other fields.

The work of Cheng et al. (1998) on the so-called gene-chip has been a major breakthrough—every site on their chips, currently up to 400 per chip, is an electrode that can be selectively handled. This allows substances to be moved around the chip by electrical charge. Nanogen (San Diego, California) is trying to create a less-expensive, more flexible gene-chip system that could be used for varied research goals (see Freeman and Gioia, 1999).

An alternate route to multiplex analysis by combining some aspects of chip technologies with mass spectrometry is being taken by Sequenom (San Diego) in view of the fact that mass spectrometry offers greater accuracy and precision than some gel- and hybridization-based sequencing methods. This technology can be used for long sequences and is especially suited to determining micro-satellite repeats and polymorphisms (see Freeman and Gioia, 1999).

P. Kleyn (Millennium Predictive Medicine, Cambridge, MA) has suggested a new approach to therapeutics called 'diagnomics'. The bioinformatic combination of a patient's individual gene-expression profile with nucleic acid and protein databases can be used for diagnostic, prognostic, screening and monitoring purposes during drug discovery, clinical trials and patient care. This is expected to improve medicine and also reduce the costs of pharmaceutical development and health care.

Molecular-structure information from possible therapeutic compounds can be added to the bioinformatic mix to find new targets of action and new anti-cancer drugs (see Weinstein et al., 1997). Membrane-bound DNA probes are being used to find differences in gene-expression profiles between drug-resistant and drug-sensitive tumour-cell lines. This technology is already commercially available and, although it contains fewer genes than some 'gene chips', many molecular biologists can use it.

One serious problem with *in situ* hybridization has been how to amplify the signal of rare gene messages easily at the level of tissue slices and individual cells. V.P. Antao (Chiron Diagnostics, Emeryville, CA) has described the use of branched DNA, a non-isotopic approach that utilizes signal rather than nucleic acid amplification. The desired nucleic acid is bound by a target-specific probe; this in turn is bound by a preamplifier and amplifiers so as to generate a detectable signal.

Y Li (Advanced Bioscience Laboratories, Fredrick, MD) has worked on a nucleic-acid-sequence-based amplification (NASBA) method to quantify HIV-1. This seems to be a good alternative to PCR that would apply linear amplification to detect mRNA without the concern of DNA contamination. Another merit of NASBA is that reverse transcription is incorporated into the amplification process, thereby reducing the potential for contaminations. However, the long established nature of PCR casts some doubt on whether this method will achieve wide usage.

Wittwer et al. (1997) have worked on the 'Light Cycler' which combines rapid PCR cycling with simultaneous detection and quantification through fluorescence and melting-curve analysis. Systems such as this help the researcher to maximize both throughput and result quality and ease the confirmation of results from multiplex gene-expression arrays.

Linking Genes, Drugs and Diseases

Systematically linking gene expression profiles with compounds and phenotypes can greatly advance basic and applied biomedical research. New combinations of genomic, proteomic and bioinformatic research can provide deeper insights into disease mechanisms, novel markers for diagnostics and new molecular targets for therapeutic intervention. DNA and protein micro-arrays and high-throughput molecular profiling have revealed information on a human organism as having 20,000–25,000 genes, less than 100,000 transcript splice variants of those genes and about 10^6 protein states of possible functional significance. However, the tremendous scope and anticipated potential of 'omic' science has not so far overflowed drug pipelines. Several chemical genetic strategies have linked gene profile signatures to drug activity patterns and mechanisms of action, yet none proved universally useful. But now, Lamb et al. (2006) have proposed a large-scale chemical genetic approach which can potentially connect genes and drug action with human diseases.

Lamb et al. described a 'connectivity map', which uses gene-expression signatures to link small molecules to each other and to disease. They point to the discovery of novel inhibitors of known drug targets (histone deacetylases and heat-shock protein 90 (HSP90) and the discovery of new small molecules that correlate negatively with the gene expression profiles of complex diseases such as diet-induced obesity and Alzheimer's disease -

Weinstein and Pommier, 2006). The other two groups have applied the same approach to identify gedunin, a plant folk medicine and HSP90 inhibitor with antiandrogenic activity, as a new lead for treatment of prostate cancer and rapamycin as a potentially useful drug for treatment of acute lymphocytic leukaemia resistant to dexamethasone.

Lamb et al. made use of photolithographically synthesized oligonucleotide chips and calculated the change in each transcript's expression as a result of various perturbations to generate a 'reference database' of ~22000 gene up- or down-regulation values for 164 agents. They used the nonparametric Kolmogorov-Smirnov statistical algorithm, embodied in a 'Gene Set Enrichment Analysis', to rank the drugs according to how well their patterns in the reference database correlate (positively or negatively) with a binary 'query signature'. The query signature consists of a list of genes whose expression is correlated with a biological state of interest. That state might, for example, correspond to relative gene expression values in a drug-resistant, as opposed to a drug-sensitive, cancer (Wei et al., 2006).

Both parametric and nonparametric statistics are used in the analyses to identify gene-drug relationships (Weinstein and Pommier, 2006). The issues addressed in recent studies relate to: 'What baseline molecular characteristics predict sensitivity or resistance to the compound tested' and 'What the molecular effects of the treatment are?' These two approaches provide complementary information on mechanism and they are not mutually exclusive. The former is somewhat like an epidemiological study, finding themes in the molecular and pharmacological diversity of different cell types (from the same or different tissues); the latter then focuses basically at the level of a single cell type and asks about molecular differences between pre- and post-treatment states of the cells. This latter mode treats each cell as its own control, rather than searching for patterns across cell lines with different phenotypic backgrounds; however, much larger numbers of molecular profiles—proportional to the number of compounds in the reference data-base—have to be generated.

Of course, it will be important to make careful choices among the many free variables in a perturbation protocol. A one-size will not fit all or be optimal across all drugs, diseases and cell lineages. The authors focused on transcript expression as a molecular signature, but other possibilities exist.

An expanded Connectivity Map should be generated in the context of large drug libraries and would require large numbers of micro-arrays, which would be expensive and should be preceded by additional pilot studies to test the experimental design dimensions, particularly cell type, dose and time. An initial goal is to profile all approved drugs and inhibitory RNAs targeting a large collection of genes in a few diverse cell lines. The resulting database would be useful for researchers in biology, molecular pharmacology and pharmaceutics.

Cancer Gene Therapy

Antisense Therapy

Much recent work has led to identifying, cloning, sequencing and characterizing some genes involved in cancer development. Genetic therapy involves two general approaches: one, termed gene therapy, means the introduction of a vector that can insert a gene into the patient's genome to restore normal function or to correct an abnormal function;

Table 6.1 Antisense anti-cancer drugs in clinical trials since 1995 (Source: *Progress in Drug Research, Advances in Targeted Cancer Therapy*, vol. 63, p. 229).

Drug	Target	Chemical modification(s)	Company
Affinitakl/ISIS3521/ Aprinocarsen	PKC-alpha	PS	Lilly/ISIS
Oblimersen, G3139	Bcl-2	PS	Aventis/Genta
ISIS2503	H-ras	PS	ISIS
GTI-2040	RR R2 subunit	PS	Lorus Therapeutics
GTI-2501	RR R1 subunit	PS	Lorus Therapeutics
GEM-231	PKA	MBO (PS/2/-O-Me)	Hybridon
MG98	DNA methyl-transferase	MBO (PS/2/-O-Me)	MethyGene, MGI Pharma, British Biotech
Oncomyc-NGI/AVI 4126	*c-Myc*	Morpholino	AVI BioPharma
AVI 4557	Cyp3A4	Phosphorodiamidate Morpholino	AVI BioPharma
AP12009	TGF-B2	PS	Antisense Pharma
ISIS5132	c-raf	PS	ISIS
LErafAON	c-raf	PS (liposome)	NeoPharm
OGX-011	Clusterin	MBO (PS/2/-O-Me)	Oncogenix ISIS
LR-3001	c-Myb	PS	Lynx Therapeutics/ Inex/Temple Univ.
OL(1)p531/EL-625	p53	PS	Lynx Therapeutics/ Elos Inc.

the second, termed RNA-based therapy, which includes antisense technology. It delivers RNA silencing molecules that hybridize with and inhibit the expression of pathogenic genes in target cells.

In general, antisense nucleic acids (DNA, RNA and DNA/RNA chimeras) are single-stranded oligonucleotides (oligos) complementary to the sequence of a target RNA or DNA. Antisense RNA is really a natural mode of regulation of gene expression in most living cells. Recent advances in automated oligo synthesis and better understanding of gene regulation have greatly stimulated work on developing antisense techniques. Antisense technology as an RNA silencing approach is useful in many areas such as: (i) identification of gene function and of novel targets for therapy; (ii) pharmacogenetics and pharmacogenomics; and (iii) novel therapeutic agents.

Vitravene, the first antisense drug has already been approved for the treatment of patients with cytomegalovirus-induced retinitis. Several other antisense oligos are undergoing clinical trials as anti-cancer agents (Table 6.1) and several are in preclinical development.

Gene Therapy

Scientists today can alter genetic material of patients to fight or prevent disease by introducing DNA or RNA into a patient's cells. It is undergoing clinical trials for many different types of cancers, but no gene therapy has yet been approved for routine clinical use. Some approaches to treat cancer by using gene therapy include:

- Replacing missing or altered genes with healthy genes. Some of the missing or altered genes (e.g., *p53*) can lead to cancer.
- Stimulating the body's immune response.
- Injecting cancer cells with genes that make them more sensitive to chemotherapy, radiation therapy, or other treatments.
- Placing genes into healthy blood-forming stem cells to make them more resistant to the side effects of high doses of anti-cancer drugs.
- Injecting cancer cells with genes ("suicide genes") that destroy the cells. This is followed by administering a pro-drug (an inactive form of a toxic drug) to the patient. The pro-drug is activated in cancer cells containing these "suicide genes." This leads to the destruction of those cancer cells.
- Preventing cancer cells from developing new blood vessels (angiogenesis).

Cancer therapies aim at eliminating both primary tumours and metastases. The objective of gene therapy for the treatment of cancer is to kill tumour cells but not normal tissue. An ideal gene therapy agent would be one that is targeted for specific transduction of tumour cells and shows highly specific cytotoxic action (Palmer et al., 2006). The latter tend to escape detection by conventional methods and hence have to be treated by systemic agents—a treatment that is usually associated with significant systemic toxicity; this may be overcome by using targeted approaches, including gene therapy.

Vectors

It has become possible to create enzyme—pro-drug activating systems, correct genetic mutations that contribute to the malignant phenotype and stimulate a T-cell-mediated anti-tumour immune response. Crucial to the success of all these strategies is an effective vector that can direct appropriate expression of the therapeutic gene. A vector is needed to deliver the therapeutic agent specifically to tumour cells or the supporting vasculature. An ideal vector would be one that is easy to produce, possesses an unlimited capacity for transgene inserts, be non-immunogenic and can mediate transgene expression efficiently and specifically in target cells. Table 6.2 lists some available vectors that are a compromise of these features.

Weak gene transfer and the lack of ability to administer systemically, strongly limit cancer gene-therapy by using the available vectors. However, this situation might improve if and when selectively replicating viruses are developed (Palmer et al., 2006). Viruses have many properties that can be adapted to achieve this therapeutic endpoint. They can be engineered to replicate selectively in cancer cells and lyse them. The current challenge is to translate these features into effective therapies that can supplement or supplant existing treatments (Palmer et al., 2006).

Immunogene Therapy

Some human tumours express tumour-associated antigens (TAAs) that distinguish them from normal cells, but clinically effective anti-tumour immune responses are not only restricted by the low level and low avidity of TAA-specific cytotoxic T-lymphocytes

Table 6.2 Commonly used gene therapy vectors employed in cancer gene-therapy clinical trials (after Palmer et al., 2006).

Vector	Advantages	Disadvantages
Non-viral		
Naked DNA	Production is easy.	Transduction efficiency low.
DNA complexed with lipids or polymer	Gene insert size is unlimited. Nonimmunogenic.	
Viral		
Retrovirus	Integration into host genome. Long-term gene expression.	Risk of insertional mutagenesis. ; Infects dividing cells only. Low viral titre.
Lentivirus	Infects dividing and non-dividing cells. Long-term gene expression.	Risk of insertional mutagenesis. Low viral titre.
Adenovirus	Wide tissue tropism. Facilitates infection of a variety of tumours but infection of non-target tissue can increase unwanted toxicity. Infects dividing and non-dividing cells. High titre.	Transient transgene expression (might be advantageous in limiting unwanted toxicity).
Adeno-associated virus	Wide tissue tropism. Non-pathogenic.	Immunogenicity. Limited gene-insert capacity.

(CTLs) but also by immune evasion strategies, such as down-regulation of MHC and local production of inhibitory cytokines.

Some gene therapy approaches (e.g., pro-inflammatory cytokines, such as IL-2, IL-4 and IL-12 and co-stimulatory molecules, such as HLA-B7) to stimulate anti-cancer immune responses are undergoing clinical trials. The therapeutic gene is usually administered by intratumoural injection and has the potential to stimulate anti-tumour responses in the injected lesion as well as distant non-injected lesions; it can also induce long-lasting protective immunity.

Recombinant vaccines expressing TAA are also used. Viruses (such as poxviruses) present antigens efficiently and induce both humoral and cell-mediated responses. An alternative is to deliver TAAs and co-stimulatory molecules to antigen-presenting cells such as dendritic cells *in vitro*, before returning these to the patient as an autologous vaccine; this avoids the difficulties of *in vivo* gene delivery (Collins and Cerundolo, 2004; Banchereau and Palucka, 2005).

Clinical trials have generally confirmed the ability to stimulate immune responses but these have not translated into objective clinical responses. Immunogene therapy probably fails as the result of inefficient gene transfer, tumour mechanisms to evade immune responses (e.g., selective down-regulation of TAA) and the complex regulation of immune responses against self-antigens. This failure also points to the limitations of conventional clinical trial design in which efficacy must first be shown against advanced disease, whereas immunogene therapy might be more effective in an adjuvant setting in patients with normal immune function as compared with the relative immunosuppression in patients with advanced cancer (Palmer et al., 2006).

Mutant Gene Correction

Although an understanding of cancer at a molecular level points to the rationale for gene correction as a cancer therapy, the multi-step nature of the malignant process appears to limit this strategy. Another problem is that this approach depends on highly efficient gene transfer at the tumour site, which cannot yet be attained with current vector technology (Palmer et al., 2006).

***p53* tumour-suppressor gene over-expression** *p53*, the most frequently mutated gene in human cancers, is expressed in response to DNA damage. It mediates a G1 cell-cycle arrest to enable DNA repair. If repair is not possible, it mediates apoptosis, stopping the replication of damaged DNA.

Expression of wild-type *p53* induces apoptosis, enhances chemo-sensitivity, inhibits angiogenesis and prolongs survival in *p53*-deficient animal models. Clinical trials using replication-defective adenovirus vectors (Ad-*p53*), administered by intratumoural, intravesical and intravascular routes, have led to *p53* gene expression in tumours but no up-regulation of *p53*-dependent genes (e.g., *p21*, *bax*) and no significant anti-tumour effects (Pagliaro et al., 2003).

In contrast, intraperitoneal administration of Ad-*p53* to women with ovarian cancer resulted in transgene expression and up-regulation of *p53*-dependent genes in most patients. Although it has been safely administered in combination with systemic chemotherapy, no significant therapeutic benefit was seen, perhaps owing to dominant mutant *p53*, which is frequently expressed in ovarian cancers, forming inhibitory heterodimers with the wild-type *p53*.

Phase II and Phase III trials may determine the effect of *p53* gene therapy on survival endpoints. According to Palmer et al., future study of *p53* replacement should focus on the synergy between *p53* correction and conventional therapies, as observed in preclinical studies (Roth et al., 1999).

Antisense and RNA interference. Mutation of oncogenes being crucial to the development of human malignancies makes the inhibition of the expression of mutant oncogenes a sensible therapeutic target. Synthetic oligonucleotides which hybridize to specific mRNAs can block the expression of protein; anti-sense therapy could possibly provide a safe, non-toxic treatment (Sakakura et al., 1995).

Short inhibitory RNAs (siRNA) are synthetic sequences of 21–22 nucleotides which, unlike long dsRNA, do not induce non-specific interferon-γ responses. This makes them an effective and simple means of silencing specific genes. This approach may be even better than antisense-based silencing (Aoki et al., 2003).

Transcribed RNA is single stranded in human cells but the use of a palindromic sequence that folds to form a hairpin results in the same specific degradation of homologous mRNA and it is possible to incorporate these constructs into viral vectors. siRNA sequences against oncogenes (e.g., *ras*), oncogenic viral proteins (e.g., hepatitis B HBx), cell cycle-regulatory genes (e.g., *cyclin E*) or anti-apoptotic genes also show growth-inhibitory effects against tumour cell lines (Brummelkamp et al., 2002; Li et al., 2003; Crnkovic-Mertens et al., 2003; Chen et al., 2003). In fact, siRNA might also prove useful in targeting multi-drug resistance genes to overcome resistance to conventional anticancer therapies (Nieth et al., 2003). Paroo and Corey (2004) have pointed out certain challenges facing the successful application of this technology.

Pro-drug Activation

Pro-drug activation therapy aims at expressing an activating enzyme within the tumour, which can activate a systemically delivered, inactive pro-drug at the target site only. One widely studied enzyme-pro-drug combination has been the combination of phosphorylated ganciclovir (GCV) which, by competing with dGTP, inhibits DNA synthesis and herpes simplex virus thymidine kinase (HSV-TK), which catalyses GCV phosphorylation much more efficiently than the human enzyme.

In a large phase III trial, 248 patients with primary brain tumours were randomized to receive surgery and adjuvant radiotherapy with or without HSV-TK. The enzyme-encoding gene was delivered by retrovirus-producing vector producer cells (VPCs) injected into the resection site and followed by systemic administration of GCV. No clinical benefit manifested (Rainov, 2000). The failure was probably because of the non-migratory nature of retrovirus VPCs resulting in gene expression being confined to the immediate vicinity of the needle track. Another study investigated the use of adenovirus-delivered HSV-TK (Ad-HSV-TK) and subsequent GCV administration, as an adjuvant to surgery for patients in similar circumstances. Patients were randomized to either Ad-HSV-TK by direct injection into the resection plus intravenous GCV or to conventional therapy: in this case, the gene therapy was associated with improved median survival from 37.7 to 62.4 weeks (Immonen et al., 2004).

Genetically Modified Oncolytic Virus Therapy

Some viruses show oncolytic and anti-tumour effects *in vivo*. This points to the rationale of modifying a viral gene that is normally required for virus replication and whose function might be complemented by the cellular mutations in cancer cells.

Oncolytic virus replication in normal cells can be abrogated either by the mutation of crucial viral replicative genes or through normal cellular antiviral responses. Abolition of cell cycle regulatory checkpoints such as *p53*, *pRb* or antiviral responses in cancer cells promotes virus replication and cell lysis (Palmer et al., 2006).

Conditionally replicating viruses, modified to code for such therapeutic transgenes as cytokines or pro-drug-activating enzymes could possibly increase transgene expression as compared with non-replicating vectors. Some oncolytic viruses that have been genetically modified are Adenovirus (e.g., dl1520), Herpes simplex virus (HSV), Reovirus, Vesicular stomatitis virus (VSV) and Newcastle disease virus (NDV).

Some improvement in the low level of transgene expression observed in the clinical trials of enzyme-pro-drug gene therapy might be achieved by using replicating viruses to deliver the gene encoding the enzyme. Pre-clinical studies of a replication-competent HSV vector encoding the *TK* gene have shown that GCV reduces cytotoxicity, probably because of an anti-viral effect of the activated pro-drug (Carroll et al., 1997).

Gene Therapy for Manipulating Apoptotic Pathways

Cell death in drug-resistant tumour cells can be enhanced, *in vitro*, through a combination of conventional chemotherapeutic drugs with ligation to surface death-receptors by tumour necrosis factor (TNF) or other ligands of the TNF receptor superfamily, such as CD95L, TRAIL, or CD40L (Knox et al., 2003). To cross the hurdles associated with large-scale production of soluble trimeric TNF-receptor ligands, their low *in vivo* stability and to provide specific tumour targeting, replication-defective adenoviruses encoding these ligands have proved effective (Griffith and Broghammer, 2001). It may be possible to further enhance such a therapeutic potential by the combination of selectively replicating adenovirus vectors with death-receptor ligands (Sova et al., 2004).

Other Options for Cancer Gene-therapy

Tumour development beyond a critical size requires a new blood supply which can make the tumour susceptible to anti-angiogenic therapies. Replication-defective adenoviruses delivering angiostatin or endostatin by inhibiting endothelial cell proliferation, *in vitro*, also inhibit tumour growth *in vivo*.

Chemotherapy is limited by its toxicity to normal tissues, particularly the bone marrow. Transfer of a drug-resistant gene to hematopoietic progenitor cells could possibly improve the therapeutic index of chemotherapeutic drugs. According to Schiedlmeier et al. (2002), multidrug resistance 1 gene transfer confers chemoprotection to human peripheral blood progenitor cells engrafted in immunodeficient mice. There may be scope for more progress through improvements in vector technology and stem cell isolation from peripheral blood.

Gene Therapy Targeting of Cancer

Most cancer gene-therapy trials have used direct intratumoural injection of the vector which secures tumour targeting but limits its use to solitary tumours. Systemic gene-delivery requires mechanisms to ensure tumour selectivity which might be achieved by targeting the vector specifically to tumour cells (transductional targeting) or by restricting transgene expression to the tumour (transcriptional targeting). In the former case, vectors may be re-targeted to specific tumour receptors, enabling systemic delivery. For instance, adenovirus fibre can be such modified as to block its interaction with its natural receptor (CAR) and to target novel tumour-specific receptors (Douglas et al., 1996).

Another approach is to coat adenovirus with an inert polymer to block virus infection. The incorporation of specific ligands or monoclonal antibodies against tumour-specific receptors or antigens into the polymer then facilitates tumour retargeting (Fisher et al., 2001). Coating adenovirus with polyethylene glycol (PEG) incorporating fibroblast growth factor (FGF) increases transgene expression in the tumour and reduces infection of normal tissue as compared to unmodified virus in an ovarian-cancer animal-model (Lanciotti et al., 2003).

Indeed, polymer coatings also tend to reduce the anti-adenovirus immune responses. Bartosch and Cosset (2004) have described strategies for retargeted gene delivery by employing vectors derived from lentiviruses.

For transcriptional targeting, tumour or tissue-specific promoters can be used to limit specific gene expression (Miller and Whelan, 1997). Specific anti-tumour effects may also be generated on the basis of biological differences in the activity of enzymes, such as ribonucleotide reductase, between normal cells and cancer cells (Yoon et al., 2000).

One possibility is to place the expression of a key viral gene under the control of a tumour-specific promoter so as to restrict viral replication to tumour cells. Adenoviruses have been constructed with T-cell factor (TCF)-binding sites in early promoters so that virus replication could be confined to cancer cells with dysregulated WNT and/or β-catenin signalling (Fuerer and Iggo, 2002).

De Weese et al. (2001) have used a replication competent PSA selective oncolytic adenovirus for the treatment of locally recurrent prostate cancer following radiation therapy. This work is undergoing Phase I/II trials. According to Palmer et al., cancer gene-therapies may have the greatest impact as adjuvants and in combination with conventional therapies.

7 DNA, Immunology and Cancer

Introduction

Till hitherto, cancer research has been mostly based on an understanding of genetic changes as the underlying cause of the disease. It now appears that a better understanding of chronic inflammation may be crucial to revealing the mysteries of cancer. It has emerged that the developing tumour can commandeer the immune system's inflammatory component—normally part of the wound-healing process—to foster carcinogenesis (Stix, 2007).

The hallmark of innate immunity is inflammation, which is a significant contributor not only to cancer but also to many other chronic ailments (see Weinberg, 2006). Tumour development in some cancers progresses through the effects of a 'smoldering' inflammation, in which the tumour recruits immune cells that linger in its surroundings and within the malignant mass (Balkwill et al., 2006).

The immune system consists of: (a) innate cells that constitute a first line of defense against pathogens and (b) members of the adaptive system, which target invaders with greater specificity. The former category includes macrophages which engulf and consume pathogen invaders (see Lewis and Pollard, 2006); mast cells (which release histamine and other chemicals that promote inflammation); granulocytes (include three cell-types with tiny granules in their interior—the neutrophil, eosinophil and basophil and participate in the inflammatory response); dendritic cells (present antigens—fragments of protein or other molecules from pathogens or cancer cells—to adaptive immune cells, inducing the cells to attack bearers of the displayed antigens); and natural killer (NK) cells (which destroy the body's own cells that have become infected with pathogens; NK cells also go after cancer cells).

Second Category (Adaptive Cells) Involves B Cells and T Cells

Immunology exemplifies a field that was completely transformed during the past five decades by the discovery of the structure of DNA and the emergence of various DNA technologies. The short history of research in lymphocyte receptors attests to the power of DNA technology not only to explain known biological phenomena, but also to contribute to the discovery of new biological systems.

Indeed, the immune system can recognize and produce antibodies to virtually any molecule in the Universe. This enormous diversity stems from the ingenious reshuffling of DNA sequences encoding components of the immune system. The secret of genetic processes that control the vast variety of synthetic potential within an immune system

Table 7.1 Approximate percentage (per cent) of lymphocytes in various organs of humans*.

	T Cells	B Cells
Thymus	90	<5
Bone marrow	5	90
Lymph node	70	25
Spleen	45	45
Thoracic duct lymph	90	5
Blood	75	20

*NK and K cells appear as either large granular lymphocytes or small lymphocytes. These cells account for most of those not included in the T and B cell categories listed. Accordingly, 5-10 per cent of the lymphocytes from various tissue sources do not qualify as either T or B cells.

capable of reacting specifically to virtually any microbe or foreign molecule lies in unique DNA processing that occurs during the development of lymphocyte cells that are responsible for the specific immune response to a foreign agent (antigen). B lymphocytes produce antibodies (on their surface as well as secreted) and T lymphocytes mount cellular attacks on pathogenic infiltrators (Nossal, 2003). Table 7.1 shows the relative abundance of T and B lymphocytes in humans. Figure 7.1 is a diagrammatic sketch of cross section through a lymph node to show location of T cells and B cells.

B and T lymphocytes are the two types of cells involved in antibody formation. B cells are derived from bone marrow whereas T cells are produced by the thymus gland. B cells keep circulating in the blood serum and generate humoral immunity. They secrete immunoglobulins. T cells are specialized cells having surface receptors capable of recognizing specific antigens. These cells attack and destroy the antigens and are responsible for cell-mediated immunity. They can act as killer cells that attack virus infected or cancerous cells (Cooper, 1982; Hood et al., 1983).

There are five classes of immunoglobulins called IgG, IgA, IgM, IgD and IgE (Table 7.2). Each type has a distinct chemical structure and specific biological role, IgG is the most prevalent antibody population. A mother transmits this antibody to the developing foetus, as IgG can pass through the placenta. IgA is produced by the lymphoid tissues lining the respiratory, gastrointestinal and other secretory systems and helps stop organisms from penetrating the body through mucus membranes. IgM is the first antibody formed and is important during the first few days of the primary immune response. IgD occurs on the surface of lymphocytes of newborn infants but its role is uncertain. IgE attaches to certain cells which release histamine and is responsible for the major symptoms of allergy.

Immunoglobulin molecules contain four polypeptide chains: two identical light chains (L), each comprising about 220 amino acids and two identical heavy chains (H), each having about 400 amino acids. Each chain has an amino terminal protein, which is the variable region and a carboxy terminal portion, which is the constant region. The four chains are held together by noncovalent interactions and are stabilized by the existence of several disulphide bridges. The general shape of immunoglobulin molecules is like a Y. The antigen binding sites are at the two tips of the Y arms. The constant region of the Y is responsible for the effector functions of the antibody molecule such as cytotoxicity. All antibodies tend to have at least two antigen binding sites of identical specificity. Differ-

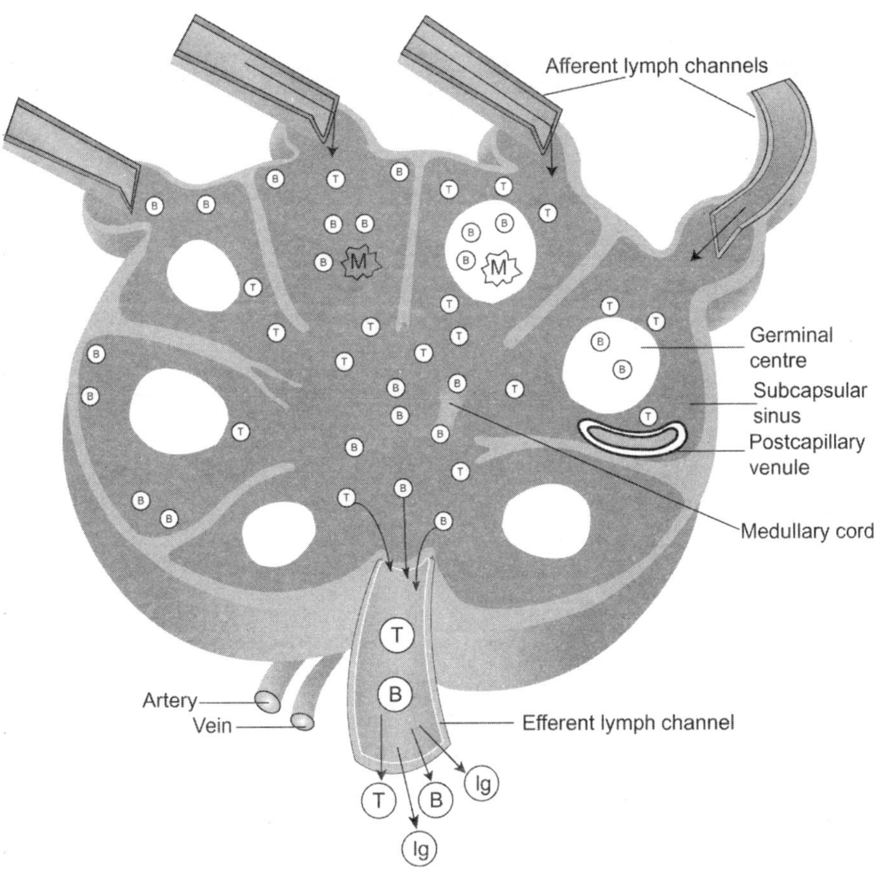

Fig. 7.1 Diagrammatic cross-section through lymph node showing localization of T cells and B cells. M, macrophages (after Hildemann, 1984).

ent H chains impart different conformations and biological properties to the Ig molecule (Kumar, 1998).

As lymphocytes develop, an array of short genes become rearranged and assembles together and their products recognize distinct antigens. This process is usually random, so each lymphocyte makes different choices with the result that a large repertoire of lymphocytes reactive to different antigens is created. This process has implications for antibody formation, cell-mediated immunity and malignancies of the immune system (Nossal, 2003).

One B cell produces one antibody (Nossal and Lederberg, 1958). Jerne (1955) postulated the random synthesis of a million or more different sorts of antibodies. Upon entering the body, an antigen unites with an antibody that just happens to fit it; the antigen-antibody complex is taken up by a cell and the antibody acts as the template for the formation of more of itself. Burnet (1957) stated that this theory would make more sense if the postulated natural antibodies were located on the surface of what are now called B lymphocytes. If each cell had only one sort of antibody specificity, then the antigen could select one lymphocyte out of a repertoire, induce its clonal division and stimulate anti-

Table 7.2 Characteristics of the five antibody classes.

Characteristics	IgM	IgG	IgA	IgE	IgD
per cent of total Ig in normal human serum	8	74	17	<1	1
Form:	Pentamer	Monomer	Dimer	Monomer	Monomer
Mainly found in:	Blood stream	Tissue	Seromucous secretions	Blood	Blood
Activities:	Agglutination, Cytolysis, Opsonization	Neutralization, Opsonization, Cytolysis	Prevention of bacterial adherence	Rejection of metazoan parasites (gut); Degranulation of mast cells (allergy)	Influence of lymphocytes
Complement fixation:	Yes	Yes	Alternative pathway	No	No
Remarks:		Predominant	Locally produced		Found on surface of B lymphocytes

body production and secretion (Fig. 7.2). Nossal and Lederberg (1958) proved the clonal selection theory,i.e., one B cell always produces only one antibody.

While a single B cell produces antibody of a single antigen-binding specificity, a person must be able to make 10^7 to 10^8 different specificities of antibodies. The implication is that 10^7 or more clones of B cells must differentiate to create the needed library of potential responses (Hildemann, 1984). Figure 7.2 illustrates the clonal selection model of antibody diversity.

Malignancies usually develop in three stages, viz., initiation (hereditary mutations or exposure to chemicals or radioactivity produce genetic changes in one or more cells); promotion (cells in premalignant tissue proliferate, usually in the presence of an inflammatory stimulus and become markedly abnormal); and progression (tumour cells invade surrounding tissue and spread to the blood and lymph nodes; full malignancy develops). Metastases tend to establish themselves at distant sites (see de Visser et al., 2006).

Antibody Formation

Antibodies are multichain proteins of different forms. The most abundant, immunoglobulin-γ (IgG), consists of two identical light (L) chains and two identical heavy (H) chains (Fig. 7.3). Whereas the carboxy-terminal halves of the two light chains are identical to each other, the amino-terminal halves differ in over 50 residues, called the 'variable' region. The heavy chains, too, consist of a variable (V) part and a constant (C) part.

Dreyer and Bennett (1965) floated the idea that the carboxy-terminal C region of the L chain was always encoded by a single gene, but that the amino-terminal V half could be encoded by many different genes. This meant that a chosen V gene must then somehow become associated with a C gene by a DNA rearrangement event in each lymphocyte,

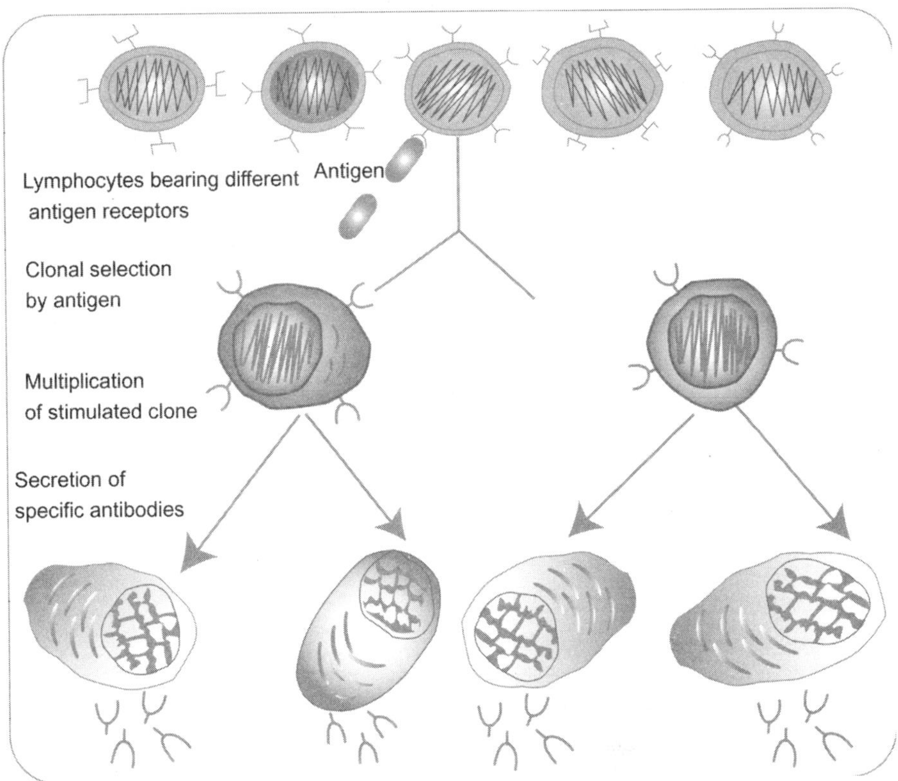

Fig. 7.2 CLONAL SELECTION MODEL OF ANTIBODY DIVERSITY: Antigen interacts with the appropriate cell by combining specifically with the membrane-bound receptor, thus stimulating the cell to undergo rapid division, leading to a clone of daughter cells synthesizing and secreting the specific antibody (after Hildemann, 1984).

because only when the V-C regions were spliced together could a functional protein be expressed (Nossal, 2003).

In 1976, Hozumi and Tonegawa performed a landmark experiment by using a restriction endonuclease to digest the DNA extracted from a mouse embryo and from an antibody-secreting tumour. The resulting DNA fragments were separated on the basis of size and were treated with radioactive probes, one corresponding to the whole L chain, the other to just the C portion.

In the tumour, both probes lit up the identical fragment, whereas in the embryonic extract, two different fragments hybridized to the full-length probe, but only one hybridized to the C-region probe. Both fragments from the embryo sample differed in size from the hybridizing fragment in the tumour sample. This suggested that the V and C genes were located some distance away from each other in the embryo, but became reshuffled and assembled during development of antibody-forming cells in adults, so forming a continuous DNA sequence of the full L-chain gene.

Later work of Bernard et al. (1978) showed that V-region genes in the germline were significantly shorter than what is needed to encode the V region of the L chain. It turned out that there is a series of 'minigenes' known as 'joining' (J) genes, which code for about

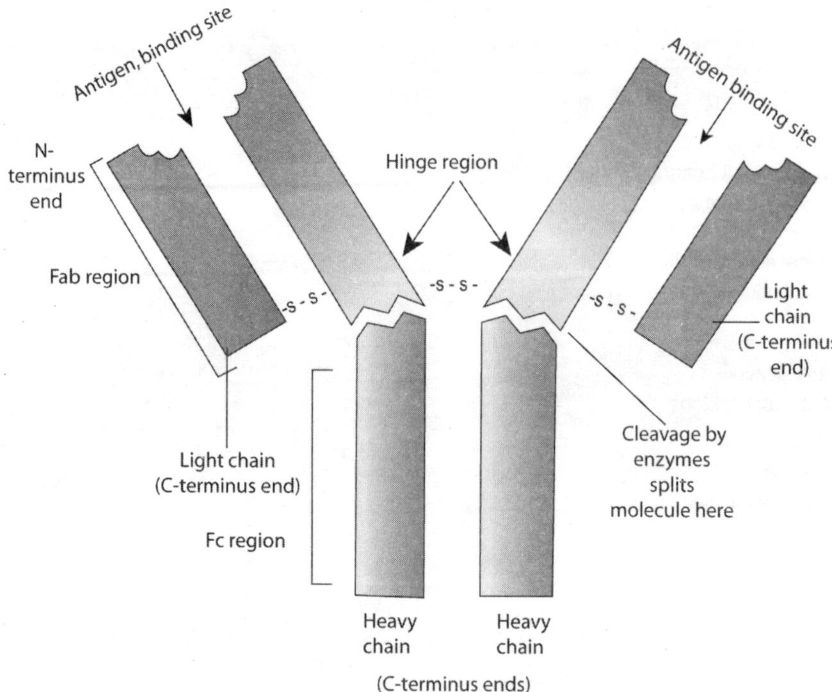

Fig. 7.3 The basic structure of an antibody molecule, showing the points at which the heavy chains can be cleaved by certain proteolytic enzymes. Two identical heavy chains are connected by disulphide linkages. The antigen-recognizing site is composed of the variable regions of the heavy and light chains, whereas the effector site (which determines its function) is determined by the amino-acid sequence of the heavy chain constant region (after Davey, 1994).

13 amino acids of the L chain. Thus, the full L chain is actually encoded by V, J and C genes (Fig. 7.3). For the H chain, it is even more complicated, because some 'diversity' (D) genes encode up to eight amino acids lying between the V and J regions. So, the H chain is encoded by V, D, J and C genes (Fig. 7.3). A complete H-chain V region is assembled in two steps: first, one of the D regions joins with one of the J regions and then one of several V regions joins with that DJ assembly. After the joining, the intervening DNA is deleted between the chosen minigenes. This constitutes the first example of a somatic cell having a different genome from its fellow cells (Nossal, 2003).

The minigene assembly process can generate tremendous antibody diversity. In humans, Nossal (2003) estimated potentially 2,478,600 different types of germline-encoded antibodies. But still greater diversity can be generated by mutations of DNA in dividing B cells; the latter which express newly assembled immunoglobulin genes, each with its own unique specificity, make up the 'primary repertoire'. When an antigen stimulates a chosen B cell to divide, a part of the progeny move near antigen-capturing follicular dendritic cells (FDGs), forming a 'germinal centre'. FDCs retain antigen on their surface for long periods and stimulate further series of division. Within the germinal centre the B cells show very high rate of somatic mutation in V genes, estimated at 10^{-3} per nucleotide per division (Kocks and Rajewski, 1989). With production of more antibodies, only those

B cells with stronger affinity for the antigen find access to FDC-bound antigen and so become further stimulated to divide. In this way, B-cell clones secreting higher affinity antibody get selected.

The 'memory' B cells emerging from the germinal centre make up the 'secondary repertoire', which is even more diverse than the primary one—twenty mutations per chain are not uncommon, nor are thousand-fold increases in affinity. Thus rearrangement of germline genes gives the naïve B-cell repertoire, while somatic mutation ensures further diversification during memory B-cell development (Nossal, 2003).

Switching Function

Several different classes of antibodies have distinct roles arising from DNA rearrangements. Eight different genes for the C region of the H chain specify different antibody functions. Each B cell first links the chosen VDJ assembly to a C gene known as □, creating an antibody class called IgM. If that cell is thrust into a pathway favouring the production of an antibody prominent in mucus secretions (such as in the gastrointestinal tract), the VDJ section is switched over to a C region encoded by C gene □ and the cell produces IgA. If, on the other hand, the antigen is of parasite origin, or an allergen such as a pollen grain, the cell forms IgE, in which case the VDJ region associates with the product of the C gene. All this happens without any change in the specificity of the antibody being secreted. The class switching again involves sequential excision of portions of the genetic material. Cytidine deaminase induced by B-cell-specific activation appears to be involved in both the processes of class switching and somatic hypermutation (Nossal, 2003).

Assembly of T-cell Receptors

Whereas B cells generate antibodies against antigens, the thymus-derived or T cells also respond to foreign agents but specialize in a more localized battle. Cytotoxic T cells can kill virus-infected cells or cells displaying cancer-specific antigens. Other T cells secrete potent stimulatory and inflammatory molecules, which usually function in a strictly localized context. T cells also help to guide B cells along appropriate pathways of differentiation.

Like B cells, T cells have one-receptor specificity as exemplified by the $\alpha\beta$ T-cell receptor (TCR), a heterodimer consisting of two subunits, the α- and β-chains, joined by disulphide bonds. The manner of generating T cells with different receptors is very similar to the strategy used by B cells to form different antibodies. The β-chain of the TCR is assembled in somatic cells form V, D, J and C genes; the α-chain from V, J and C genes. There are additions of N-region nucleotides between V and D, as well as between D and J on the β-chain; and between V and J on the α-chain.

A peculiarity about T-cell recognition was discussed by Hengartner (2001)—cytotoxic T cells could recognize viral antigens only if a specific 'self' molecule was also present on the target cell. The T-cell recognition puzzle was solved by the discovery that the TCR recognized short antigenic peptides bound to the groove of a self molecule known as the major histocompatibility complex (MHC), as well as surrounding portions of the MHC molecule itself. Cells can fragment proteins into peptides of 8-24 amino acids in length, attach these to MHC molecules and take the entire complex to the cell surface. TCRs then 'see' these short linear portions of antigens, be these of viral, bacterial or parasitic origin, or even portions of normal intracellular components. Such a system helps in controlling infections where the pathogen remains hidden inside a cell and can also eliminate cells with mutated self antigens, such as cancer cells (Nossal, 2003).

Immunotherapy

Immunotherapy potentially promises not only the development of new approaches to cancer and other diseases, but also throws valuable light on the human immune response. In order for this potential to be realized, however, biomedical researchers need to overcome challenges which reflect the difficulties inherent in conducting investigations in human patients (Steinman and Mellman, 2004).

Cancer immunotherapy aims to harness the power and specificity of the immune system for the treatment of malignancy. Although cancer cells are less immunogenic than pathogens, the immune system can recognize and eliminate tumour cells. Unfortunately, as tumours frequently interfere with the development and function of immune responses, it is difficult to use advances in cellular and molecular immunology for developing strategies that effectively and safely augment antitumour responses (Blattman and Greenberg, 2004).

Unlike the situation in conventional cancer therapy, the immune system has evolved strategies, largely in response to infections, to efficiently seek, search and specifically destroy diseased targets. As discussed by Shankaran et al. (2001), strong evidence suggests that immune cells play a crucial role in the control of malignancy, as borne out by both occasional spontaneous regressions of cancers in immunocompetent hosts and increased cancer incidence in immunocompromised individuals.

Also, tumour immunity can be shown in experimental animal models, such as mice. In fact, modern technologies have enabled direct detection of antitumour immune responses from many patients (Blattman and Greenberg, 2004). There is considerable therapeutic interest in strategies by which the immune system might be harnessed for therapy of established malignancies.

Figure 7.4 illustrates one such strategy and shows how the innate immune response may be gainfully manipulated. One well known but old strategy to enhance immune responses to cancer was the administration of adjuvants directly into solid tumours to stimulate inflammation and recruit immune effector cells. This approach is even currently used for treatment of superficial bladder carcinomas and has previously been used to treat melanoma and neurological tumours. Many of these adjuvants contain bacterial products such as lipopolysaccharide (LPS) or CpG-containing oligodeoxynucleotides recognized by toll-like receptors (TLRs) on innate immune cells, leading to the production of pro-inflammatory cytokines and facilitating productive interactions between the innate and adaptive immune responses (Takeda et al., 2003). But many tumours make this strategy ineffective by producing proteins such as transforming growth factor (TGF)-β to prevent activation of the immune response (Gorelik and Flavell, 2001).

Recent researches have indicated that obstacles present at tumour sites might be bypassed and tumour immunity initiated by providing pro-inflammatory cytokines and/or chemokines at sites of solid tumours (Homey et al., 2002). Expression of secondary lymphoid-tissue chemokine or the TNF superfamily member LIGHT in tumour sites has successfully converted these microenvironments into highly immunogenic structures. This makes the approach potentially useful.

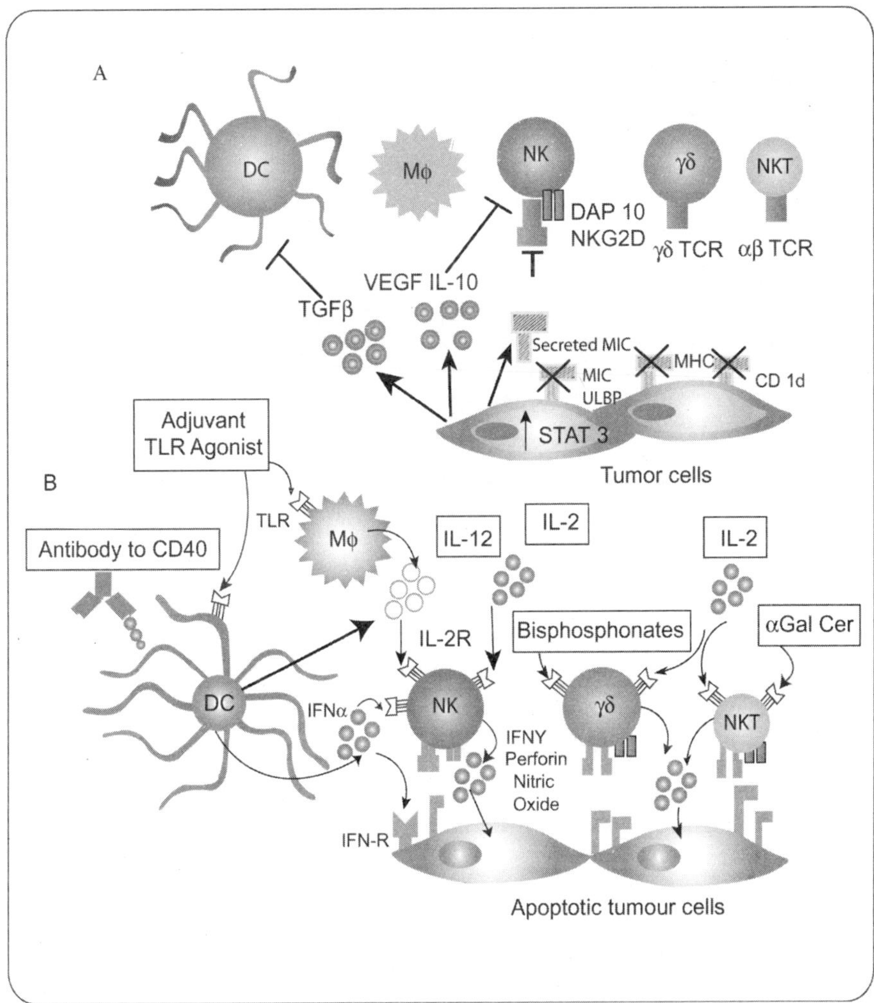

Fig. 7.4 MANIPULATING THE INNATE IMMUNE RESPONSE: A. Tumour cells can avoid activating innate responses by producing inhibitory cytokines and down-regulating or secreting ligands for activating receptors. Mϕ, macrophage; TCR, T cell receptor. B. Activation of innate responses can be enhanced by administering adjuvants, ligands for costimulatory proteins, cytokines, or drugs that directly trigger innate immune cells. αGalCer, α-galactosylceramide. (From Blattman and Greenberg, 2004, Fig. 1; reproduced with permission from AAAS).

Unlike innate immunity, in humoral immunotherapy (Fig. 7.5) B cell activation leads to the production of antibodies that can bind to immunogenic cell-surface proteins on tumour cells and initiate complement-mediated cell lysis, bridge NK cells or macrophages to the tumour for antibody-dependent cell-mediated cytotoxicity (ADCC), interfere with tumour cell growth by blocking survival or inducing apoptotic signals, or increase immunogenicity by facilitating the uptake and presentation of tumour antigens by APCs (Blattman and Greenberg, 2004). Enhancing B cell responses *in vivo* or providing large amounts of *in vitro*-generated antibodies can therefore potentially promote antitumour activity (Fig. 7.5).

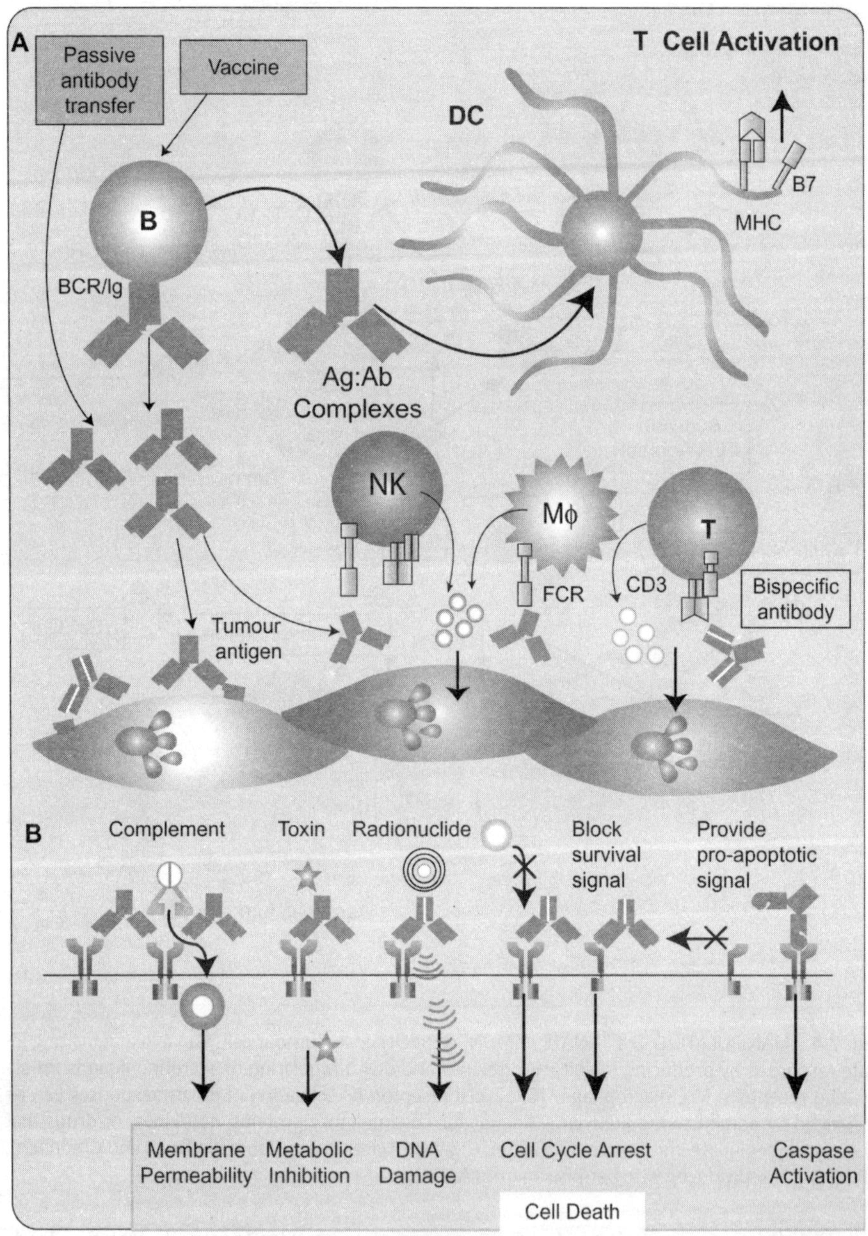

Fig. 7.5 MANIPULATING HUMORAL IMMUNITY: A. B cell responses can be augmented by vaccination with tumour antigens to induce antibodies that kill tumours or promote antigen presentation. Passively transferred mAbs or engineered bispecific antibodies can bind to tumours and activate effector cells. BCR/Ig, B cell receptor; AgAb, antigen:antibody; MAC, membrane attack complex. (B) Modified and unmodified mAbs can kill tumour cells by many mechanisms independent of recruitment of effector cells. (From Blattman and Greenberg, 2004, Fig. 2; reproduced with permission from AAAS).

Lymphocytes and Cancer

Lymphocytes have attracted much interest in cancer research, best exemplified by the B-cell tumour of humans known as Burkitt's lymphoma. Occasionally DNA strands break and are wrongly repaired. For instance, a piece of a chromosome may become attached to the broken end of another one and vice versa, during reciprocal translocation. Genes for making the heavy chains of antibodies (C_H) are located on chromosome 14, whereas those for the light chains are on chromosomes 2 and 22. These genes are expressed exclusively in B lymphocytes, because only these cells carry the required transcription factors to switch on their expression. In over 90 per cent of Burkitt's lymphoma cases, a reciprocal translocation moves the proto-oncogene *c-Myc* from its normal position on chromosome 8 to a location near the antibody heavy-chain genes on chromosome 14. In other cases, *c-Myc* is translocated close to the antibody genes on chromosome 2 or 22. In every case, *c-Myc* now finds itself in a region of active gene transcription and it may simply be the overproduction of the *c-Myc* product (a transcription factor essential for cell division) that pushes the lymphocyte towards cancer (Nossal, 2003). In the case of Burkitt's lymphoma, the tumour-promoting gene (oncogene) *myc* is translocated from its normal position on chromosome 8 right into the middle of the IgH chain locus on chromosome 14. In this highly active transcriptional environment, *myc* expression is switched on and eventually cancer develops.

DNA Vaccines

DNA studies have proved extremely valuable in vaccine research. Through gene cloning and expression, candidate antigens are identified and tested. Rapid nucleotide sequencing allows analysis of the genome of a pathogen and computer programs can search for sequences likely to encode outer membrane proteins, which are assessed as candidate vaccine molecules.

In fact, DNA itself can serve as a vaccine—the underlying principle is that the gene sequence for one or more candidate antigens should be introduced into an animal or person via some delivery vehicle (vector) along with a strong promoter that can switch on its expression in mammalian cells. Cells taking up the injected DNA transcribe and translate the gene and release the relevant antigen protein, against which the body can in turn make antibodies. This makes the body itself a vaccine factory (Donnelly et al., 1977). This approach has worked better in mice than in humans, but work is underway to make it work well for humans.

To enhance the immune response to a vaccine, it is often necessary to use an adjuvant substance—DNA proves useful here as well. Unmethylated CpG-rich DNA sequences represent a promising new category of adjuvant (Krieg, 2002).

Work in the past three decades led to clearing the puzzle of antibody diversity and mystery of T-cell recognition of antigenic peptides. The future of immunology will be all about how the system is regulated and how it makes decisions: whether to respond or not; whether to direct efforts towards antibody formation or cell-mediated immunity; and, if latter, whether more towards cytokine-secreting T cells or cytotoxic T cells (Nossal, 2003). It is expected that the complex signalling pathways, the feedback loops and the intricate rules governing cell division on the one hand or programmed cell death on the other, will be revealed soon, increasing the chances for finding new therapeutic targets and new 'miracle' drugs for various cancers. Potent cytokines and monoclonal antibodies directed against cell surface-associated structures are already conspicuous within a radically revised pharmaceutical agenda in areas such as cancer, autoimmunity, allergy and organ or tissue transplantation.

T Cells and Cancer

Many patients suffering from early-stage colorectal cancer do not receive chemotherapy. So, about 30 per cent have a relapse, which questions the validity of the general view that grape-sized tumours that have not spread need not cause much concern. There is some indication that in those 30 per cent of the patients who suffer a relapse, recurrence may have nothing to do with the tumour itself. Rather, poor prognosis probably comes from a weak immune reaction to cancer.

Traditionally, the treatment for most solid cancers, e.g., those in the breast, lung and colon, has focused on the tumour's size and whether or not it has spread. But there are significant differences in gene expression in tumour cells that have something to do with the prognosis to these patterns. Some immunologists in France, in the light of their earlier work suggesting a link between metastasis and a weak immune response, looked for T cells near colorectal tumours, depending on banked samples from 415 patients collected over the past 16 years, plus information about how those patients had fared. Search was focused on the T cells that attack bacteria, viruses and other pathogens and those that remember enemies they have encountered before (see Couzin, 2006). Their findings were surprising: the density of T cells near tumour cells was, in these patients, a better predictor of survival than traditional staging based on a cancer's size and spread.

The more T cells infiltrate the lesions, the better the survival. It is generally thought that a stronger, more robust immune system drives cancer rather than squelching it. For instance, conditions that induce chronic inflammation, such as colitis, seem to enhance cancer risk. However, some work also indicates that once a cancer forms, the immune system can also help combat it. Hopefully, if the above findings can be confirmed and found to be generally applicable and valid, T cell densities may be helpful in identifying apparently low-risk individuals who would benefit from aggressive treatment. Indeed, in principle, the finding could also lead to new treatments that stimulate these T cells to proliferate and contain a tumour.

Immunologists have believed that all T cells recognize peptide antigens bound to proteins of the major histocompatibility complex (MHC I and II) (see Adams et al., 2005; Mattner et al., 2005). It has recently emerged that T cells also respond to lipid antigens displayed by CD1 proteins (see Beckman et al., 1994; Borg et al., 2007). Borg et al. (2007) reported the crystal structure of an aβ-TCR bound to a glycolipid antigen that is in a complex with a CD1 protein. T-cell receptors (TCRs) are made of α- and β-chains that bind to a composite surface formed by an antigenic molecule complexed with antigen-presenting proteins from the MHC or CD1 families. In the classical mechanism of antigen recognition, both the α- and β-chains make contact with the antigen, so that their footprint covers the centre of the MHC platform. But as revealed by the crystal structure, a CD1-reactive TCR is rotated clockwise from the classical position and pushed laterally so that only its α-chain makes contact with the antigen.

The activation of T cells by CD1 and lipids has interested immunologists for two reasons. First, nearly all existing vaccines, adjuvants and immunodiagnostic tests based on

T cells are designed to stimulate MHC function and track responses to peptide antigens. But if human T cells commonly recognize CD1 and lipids in disease states, then current immunomodulation strategies could be missing many therapeutic targets (Moody, 2007).

The second reason is that T cells responsive to CD1 proteins operate in a borderline area between the two major modes of immune recognition: innate and acquired immunity. CD1-reactive T cells might harness the power of rearranged TCRs—containing many different types of TCR α- and β-chains sequences—to recognize virtually any lipid molecule bound to CD1 and so adapt the T-cell population after encountering lipid antigens. However, certain T cells, called invariant NK T cells, can be distinguished by their expression of nearly invariant TCR α-chains that recognize glycolipid antigens bound to CD1d (a member of the CD1 family). By sharing a limited receptor repertoire, many NK T cells can be activated in unison; they elicit very strong responses that change the outcomes of infectious, autoimmune, allergic, atherosclerotic and neoplastic diseases (Cui et al., 1997) in mouse models (see Moody, 2007).

T Cells for Therapy

Chester et al. (2002) described an ingenious but complex strategy to guide and deliver gene therapy to a tumour. Gene therapy for cancer was first attempted by the engineering of mouse fibroblasts (designated as 'producer or packaging cells') to produce retroviral vectors carrying an anti-cancer cDNA, such as the herpes simplex thymidine kinase (*tk*) cDNA (see Moolten, 1986). As these vectors are quite unstable, the producer cells within the tumour mass were first grafted in animal models and then in numerous clinical trials in humans. Following tissue availability for analysis from these trials, it was observed that the injected producer cells remained stuck very near the injecting needle and *tk* cDNA transfer by the retroviral vector was limited to a few cell layers away. Gene therapy's 'war' on cancer could not be won with such technology.

Later, more innovative strategies were developed for engineering cells other than mouse fibroblasts as vector-producing cells (Lynch et al., 1999). It was thought that cells of the immune system, stem cells, or even endothelial cells might provide a better delivery system for the retroviral vectors and so allow better targeting to tumours. An important advance was provided by engineering the T cells having a chimeric single-chain antigen receptor bearing a tumour-specific Fv and an appropriate signal domain; they facilitated specific T-cell binding to a desired tumour-cell antigen, leading to subsequent T-cell activation (Eshhar et al., 1993).

T cells are known to traffic into many different organs. Restricting the specificity of released retroviral vectors only to tumour cells may be biologically impossible. It is in this context that Chester et al. reported additional control mechanisms that could enhance tumour specificity *in vivo*. They engineered a T cell with a chimeric receptor that would recognize tumour cells expressing the tumour specific antigen, CEA (Fig. 7.6A). They believed that this binding would activate the IκBa/NF-κB signalling cascade (Fig. 7.6B). A retroviral vector genome in which multiple NF-κB promoter-binding sequences drive expression of the *tk* anti-cancer cDNA was then engineered within this T cell. Binding of translocated NF-κB enables transcription of the retroviral vector genome as well as production of retroviral vector particles (Fig. 7.6C). The retroviral vector is released very near the target tumour cell and, upon infection can integrate into the tumour cell's DNA

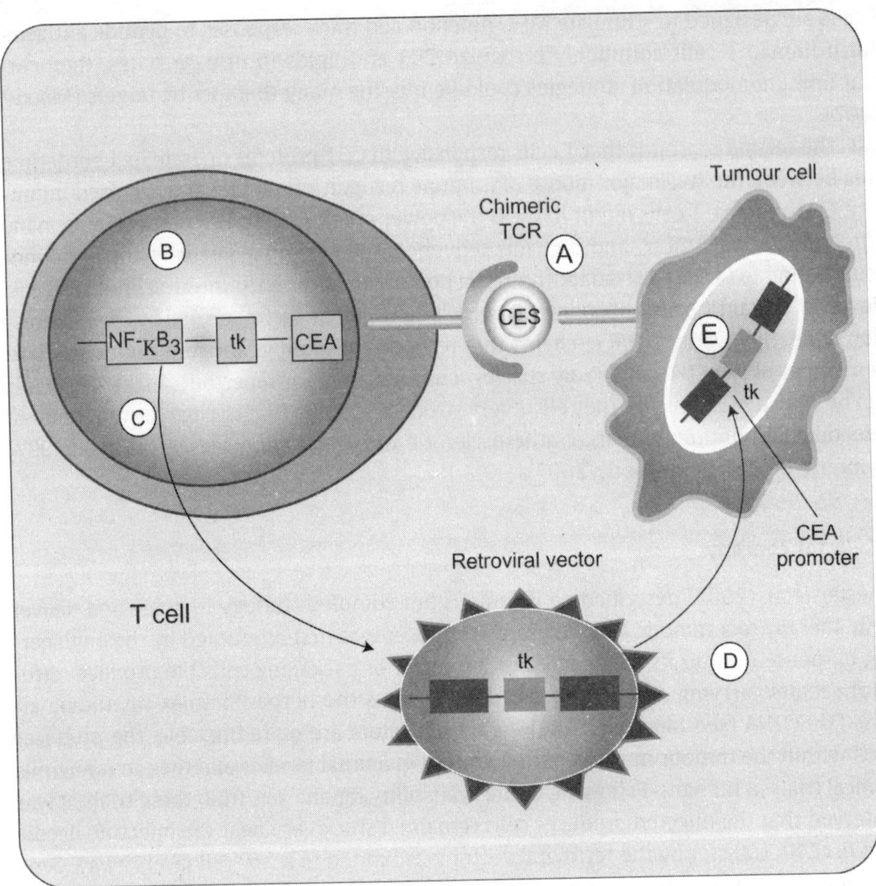

Fig. 7.6 USING T CELLS FOR THERAPY: Recognition of CEA antigen by chimeric TCR (A) leads to NF-κB activation and retroviral vector production by the 'producer' T cell (B and C). The vector is released in proximity to the target tumour cell and after infection (D), *tk* is integrated under the control of the CEA promoter (E) (after Chiocca, 2002).

(Fig. 7.6D). Engineering the last layer of selectivity involved placing the CEA promoter in the 3' region of the retroviral genome in the T cell. Upon infection and integration in tumour-cell DNA, this 3' sequence becomes duplicated in the 5' region (Fig. 7.6E). All these events equip the integrated tumour retrovirus with a *tk* cDNA under control of the CEA promoter. In fact, such a complex strategy covers three layers of selectivity: at the level of T-cell recognition of a tumour antigen; at the level of retroviral vector production because of this T-cell recognition; and at the level of anti-cancer cDNA transcription by a tumour-specific promoter (Chiocca, 2002).

Chester et al. performed both *in vitro* and *in vivo* experiments which show the feasibility of this strategy. *In vitro*, co-cultures of control T cells that recognize cancer embryonic antigen (CEA)-expressing tumour cells were seen to cause some tumour-cell death; however, co-cultures of vector-producing T cells with tumour cells caused a much greater decrease in tumour-cell survival, thereby pointing to the clear therapeutic value of this approach. Intravenous injection of these cells also greatly decreased liver metastases as compared with control injections. While activation of the chimeric T-cell receptor led to the death of the T cell, retroviral vector production was not prevented for about 20 hours.

One possible drawback of the above approach relates to the fact that the study was performed with human T cells attacking human tumour cells in an athymic mouse model. For clinical trial in humans, optimizing the ratio of injected T cells to estimated human tumour burden can be a challenging task. Other concerns relate to the biodistribution of the injected T cells, their trafficking into tumour tissue and the titers of vectors that they release in the few hours that they are alive *in vivo*. Addressing these issues critically may potentially help in designing a gene therapy approach that could provide selective targeting to multiple tumour foci with minimal side-effects (Chiocca, 2002).

Tumour Antigen Identification Through Reverse Proteomics

For developing anti-cancer therapeutic vaccines as well as for clinical diagnosis of cancer, tumour antigens need to be identified. SEREX (serological analysis of recombinant cDNA expression libraries) can be used to identify tumour antigens by screening sera of patients with cDNA expression libraries. SEREX-defined antigens serve as good markers for the diagnosis of cancers. These antigens are potentially valuable for diagnostics (Lee and Jeoung, 2007). In fact, SEREX can be a robust method for the development of anti-cancer therapeutics. The development of anti-cancer vaccines requires that tumour associated antigens (TAA) can elicit antigen-specific antibodies or T lymphocytes. Over 2000 antigens have been detected by SEREX. Peptides derived from some of these antigens have been clinically evaluated.

SEREX was designed by Sahin et al. (1995) for the identification of tumour antigens that are recognized by autologous serum IgG of cancer patients. It has facilitated identification of many provocative cancer antigens that have relevance to the etiology, diagnosis and therapy of cancer. The SEREX database (Cancer Immunome database: http://www2licr.org/ CancerImmunomeDB) contains over 2000 different antigens of more than 15 different tumour types. Immune recognition involves both cell-mediated and humoral immunity. It has become possible to dissect the humoral immune response to cancer and create a comprehensive picture of the immune repertoire against human cancer antigens. SEREX enables systematic and unbiased search for cancer-specific antigens and immunogenic proteins based on their reactivity with autologous patient serum (Lee and Jeoung, 2007).

SEREX analyses of renal, colon and breast cancers have led to the identification of 13, 32 and 40 different antigens, respectively, which react exclusively with sera from cancer patients, but not with those from healthy controls (see Scanlan et al., 1999, 2001, 2002).

Besides serological definition of human tumour antigens, dramatic advances have occurred in the structural identification of human tumour antigens that are recognized by the cellular immune systems as well. The work of van der Bruggen et al. (1991) enabled identification of peptide/protein antigens recognized by autologous cytotoxic T cells (CTL) and the list of new antigens identified in this way has grown rapidly, particularly in the case of malignant melanoma (Van den Eynde et al., 1995). However, this technique is applicable only to defining antigens on target cells that can be adapted to growth in culture, which express appropriate MHC molecules and are recognized by antigen-specific CTL lines.

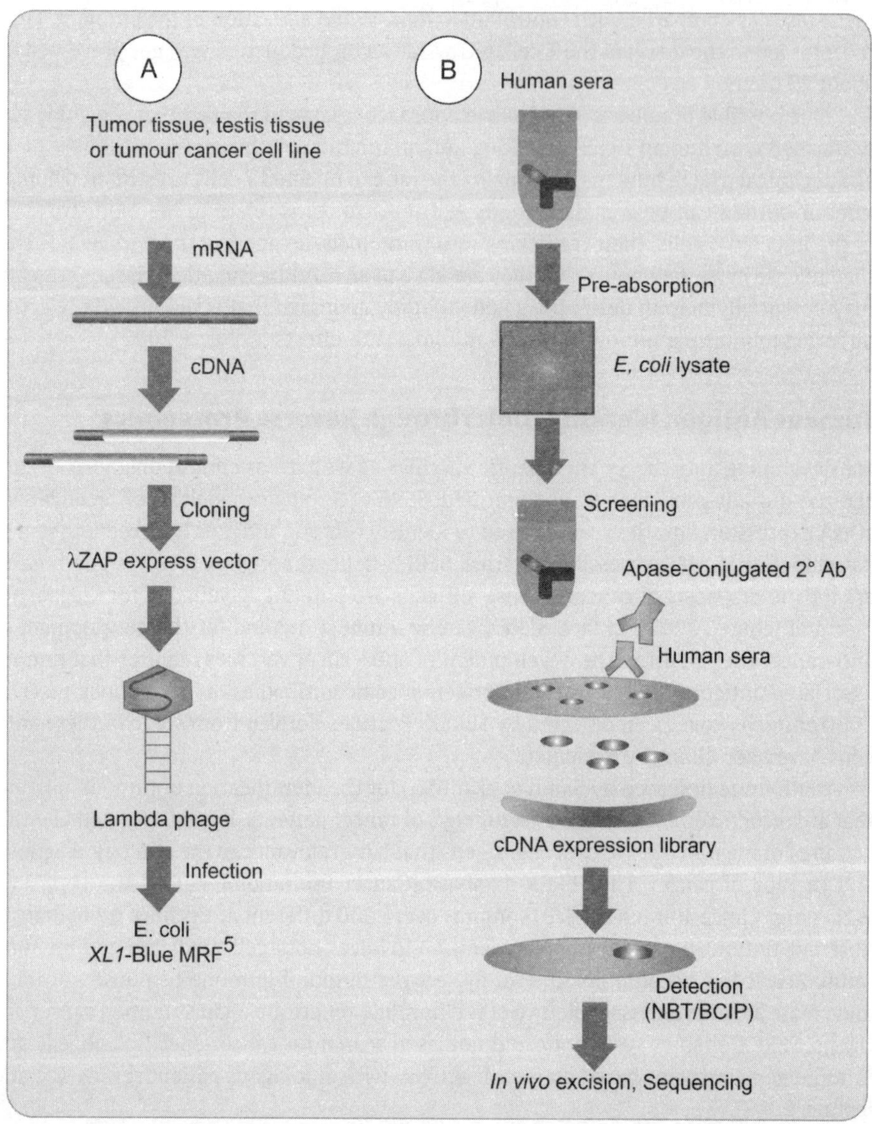

Fig. 7.7 IDENTIFICATION OF SEREX-DEFINED ANTIGENS AND ITS APPLICATION IN CLINICAL DIAGNOSIS: A. cDNA expression libraries are made from tumour tissues, tumour cell lines, or testis tissues. For this, 5 μg of poly $(A)^+$ RNA is converted into cDNA by reverse transcriptase. Thus obtained cDNA library is cloned into λ ZAP expression vector. Each library usually consists of 2×10^6 primary recombinants on average and 5×10^5 of them are used for immunoscreening. Each of these recombinant cDNA libraries is transformed into *E. coli*, to yield the recombinant cDNA expression library. B. Immunoscreening of the recombinant cDNA expression library. cDNA expression libraries are screened with pooled sera of patients with cancers. Immune-reactive clones are selected by reacting a nitrocellulose membrane containing recombinant clones with pooled sera of patients with cancers, followed by incubation with alkaline phosphatase-conjugated secondary antibody. Thus, selected clones are subjected to *in vivo* excision and sequencing to determine the identity of each immune-reactive clone. Sensitivity and specificity of each clone are determined by incubating each clone with the individual serum of cancer patients or healthy controls (after Lee and Jeoung, 2007; reproduced with permission from The Korean Society for Microbiology and Biotechnology).

Another very costly and technically-demanding method involves peptide elution from MHC molecules of tumour cells and the use of these purified fractions to stimulate CTL responses *in vitro*, to define antigenic structures recognized by T lymphocytes (Cox et al., 1994). Jager et al. (1998) and Sahin et al. (1995) showed that SEREX detects tumour antigens eliciting CTL immunity as well. As compared to other methods, SEREX is less technically demanding and can yield similar information regarding host immune responses to cancer (Lee and Jeoung, 2007).

SEREX

The SEREX approach (Fig. 7.7) offers the following valuable features: (i) use of fresh tumour specimens restrict analysis to genes expressed by the tumour cells *in vivo*; (ii) use of patients' sera allows for the identification of multiple antigens; and (iii) screening is restricted to antigens against which patients have raised higher-titer antibody responses (Lee and Jeoung, 2007).

Clinical Diagnosis Employing SEREX-defined Antigens

The identification of biomarkers for diagnosis, prognosis and therapy of human cancers has been a long-standing problem in cancer research. With regard to serum markers for cancer, a few clinically useful antigenic markers, such as carcinoembryonic antigen in gastrointestinal cancers, α-fetoprotein in hepatoma and germ-cell tumours, CA125 in ovarian cancer and prostate-specific antigen in prostate cancer (Theobald et al., 1995) have been defined. Much evidence indicates that the humoral immune system of cancer patients recognizes tumour-associated antigens (Sahin et al., 1995). Unlike detection of serum antigens, the detection of serum antibody responses to tumour antigens may turn out to be a new form of serum marker for cancer diagnosis (Scanlan et al., 1998). SEREX analysis has defined a subset of tumour antigens that react exclusively with serum antibodies derived from multiple cancer patients but do not react with sera from healthy persons.

SEREX analysis of renal cancer has resulted in the identification of 12 antigens as being associated with a cancer-related serological response in which 72 per cent of serum samples from the cancer patients had serum antibodies to at least one of these antigens, whereas sera from healthy individuals did not (Scanlan et al., 1999). Serum antibodies detecting this subset of tumour antigens therefore represent potentially valuable serum markers for cancer.

SEREX has been successfully applied to melanoma, renal cancer, Hodgkin disease and for the identification of the new tumour antigens in various tumours, including gastric cancer—one of the widely prevalent malignancies in the world. Gastric cancer exemplifies cancers that are resistant to both radiation and chemotherapy. This necessitates an alternative method of their treatment. SEREX may prove beneficial in this context (see Lee and Jeoung, 2007); it can facilitate identification of gastric cancer-associated antigens by using sera of patients with gastric cancers.

Recognition of SEREX-defined Antigens

The immune system appears to interact with tumour cells during the course of the disease (Fig. 7.8). Some general properties of cancer antigens (see Fig. 7.8) are the following:

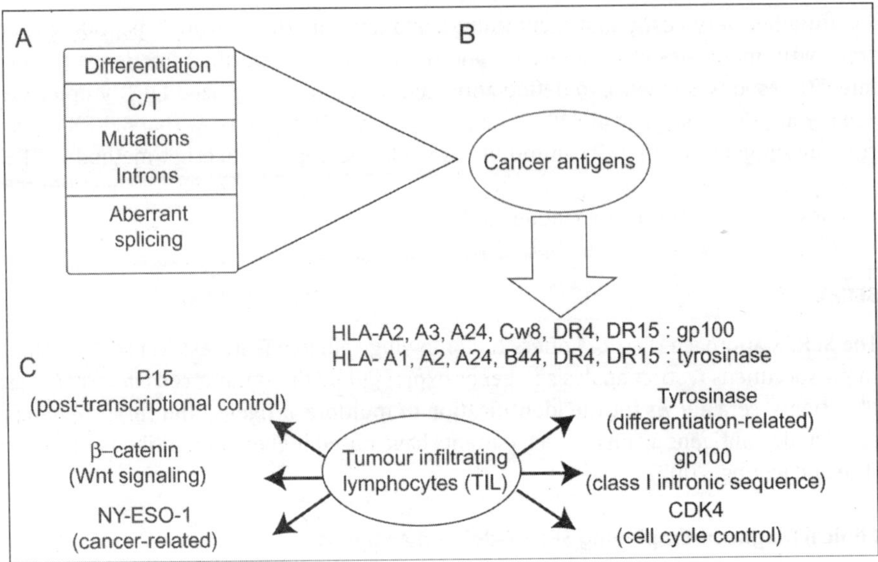

Fig. 7.8 PROPERTIES OF SEREX-DEFINED ANTIGENS (TAAS): A. Cancer antigens can arise from differentiation antigens, cancer/testis antigens, mutant antigens, intronic sequences and splicing variants. B. A single cancer antigen contains various epitopes that can be presented on many different alleles of HLA molecules. C. A single cancer patient usually develops immune response to multiple antigens (after Lee and Jeoung, 2007; reproduced with permission from The Korean Society for Microbiology and Biotechnology).

(i) cancer antigens contain epitopes binding to various HLA alleles; and (ii) tumour-infiltrating T lymphocytes (TILS) contain various cancer antigens. Several TILs from tumours greatly increased T-cell populations that could recognize cancer antigens. The presence of tumour-TILs is associated with better prognosis in individual patients, indicating that TILs recognize specific antigens expressed by the tumour (Fig. 7.8).

TILs when adoptively transferred along with IL-2 resulted in a significant tumour regression rate. Traditionally, before the identification of TAA by SEREX, immunotherapy used to focus chiefly on immunization with either autologous or allogeneic cancer cells or cancer cell extracts. This approach is not quite effective because of the very minute amounts of cancer antigens present in the intact cells. It also generates autoimmunity because many of the antigens overexpressed in tumours are also expressed in normal cells. Today, cancer antigens can be identified by SEREX and offer novel approaches to the development of anti-cancer therapeutic vaccines. Tumour cells express antigens that can be recognized by the host's immune system. These TAAs are then injected into cancer patients with a view to inducing a systemic immune response that can destroy the cancer growing in different body tissues (Lee and Jeoung, 2007).

Engineered Cells for Fighting Cancer

Immune cells from some patients are able to recognize spreading tumours and attack them. The genes governing the cancer-recognizing receptor in these immune cells have been cloned; these immune cells, called tumour-infiltrating lymphocytes, were taken from a patient who had successfully recovered from melanoma. This genetic information was introduced via retrovirus into regular T cells from 17 melanoma patients. After chemotherapy, the researchers infused the engineered lymphocytes back into their patients. It was found that such cells could persist, making up between 9 and 56 per cent of the T cell population one month after treatment in 15 of the 17 patients. Even better, the cancer disappeared in two patients, who continue to be disease-free 18 months after treatment and are showing high levels of the engineered immune cells in their blood (see *Science*, August 31, 2006 online).

Cancer Vaccines

Attempts are underway to develop vaccines that may help one's immune system to recognize cancer cells. Therapeutic vaccines are designed to treat existing cancers. Prophylactic vaccines prevent the development of cancer. Therapeutic vaccines are injected in a cancer patient. They may stop the growth of existing tumours, prevent cancer from recurring, or eliminate cancer cells which escaped killing by previous treatments. When administered early enough (when the tumour is small), cancer vaccines often eradicate the cancer.

Cancer cells may not be alien invaders but the immune system recognizes and attacks any molecules carried by cancer cells. Identifying these targets, or antigens, might help in devising cancer vaccines. It is possible to track down many of the antigens from abnormal cells that trigger an immune response at the Cancer Immunome Database at the international Ludwig Institute for Cancer Research. Visitors can peruse findings from a 2-decade project that has tested blood serum from cancer patients for antibodies against proteins from various types of tumours. One can search for data on more than 1000 genes or narrow the results by tissue or cancer type. Users can also add their results to the collection (see www2.licr.org/CancerimmunomeDB).

Prophylactic vaccines are given to healthy individuals before cancer develops. They stimulate the immune system to attack any carcinogenic viruses. By targeting these cancer-causing viruses, the development of certain cancers is prevented.

Nonspecific immunomodulating agents stimulate or indirectly augment the immune system. They target key immune system cells and cause secondary responses such as increased production of cytokines and immunoglobulins. Two common non-specific immunomodulating agents used in cancer treatment are bacillus Calmette-Guerin (BCG) and levamisole. A revolutionary cancer vaccine has been developed by Oxford BioMedica (UK). It can destroy and shrink deadly tumours, especially those of kidney and bowel by using the body's own immune system. The vaccine is likely to be licensed for use against kidney cancer within just three years.

The new vaccine is called TroVax and works in a totally different way to existing treatments. The patient is given a series of injections in the arm containing a harmless virus and a gene for a protein called 5T4. This protein is found on the surface of tumours but not on healthy cells. By injecting the gene into the body, it triggers an immune system response which kills the cancer cells but does no harm to healthy tissue. The vaccine may be given alone or in combination with other treatments such as interleukin-2. Phase-II trials have been highly successful in eliminating or shrinking tumours. Anti-tumour response was seen in over 90 per cent of the patients.

Synthesis of Glycoconjugate Antitumour Vaccines

One very promising approach to cancer immunotherapy is to use therapeutic vaccines derived from carbohydrate antigen-adjuvant combinations. The major limitation in this context is access to sufficient quantities of tumour-associated carbohydrate antigens and glycoconjugate adjuvants.

Currently, availability of the complex oligosaccharide constructs required for the systematic design and evaluation of novel vaccine formulations depends on *de novo* chemical synthesis. Happily, some emerging glycosylation technologies have led to significant advances in this field which allow the clinical exploration of carbohydrate-based antigens in the treatment of cancer (Galonic and Gin, 2007).

Some distinctive glycoprotein and glycolipid constructs are overexpressed on the cell surfaces of malignant cells (Livingston, 1995; Hakamori, 1996). Their identification has prompted the idea of exploiting these tumour-associated antigens for the development of anti-cancer vaccines (Slovin et al., 2005; Ouerfelli et al., 2005).

Tumour-associated carbohydrate antigens are attached to the cell surface either by a lipid tail or by a protein component (e.g., glycoproteins with an N-acetyl-galactosamine core (GalNAc) oligosaccharide, such as T_N, T and sialyl-T_N (ST_N). Glycoprotein and glycolipid carbohydrate epitopes have been tested as anti-cancer vaccines but they usually induce only weak T-cell independent B-cell (antibody) responses, in which only a small population of glycolipids seem to be presented to T cells.

It is possible to augment antibody response with three-component vaccine formulations. These constructs involve the covalent conjugation of various carbohydrate antigens to an immunocarrier protein such as keyhole limpet haemocyanin (KLH) (Helling et al., 1994) which, upon being processed and presented by antigen-presenting cells results in a strong T-cell immune response. This in turn leads to cytokine cascades which increase antibody response not only to KLH but also to the less immunogenic carbohydrate antigens to which it is bound.

Additional immune response potentiation of these antigen conjugates is achieved through co-administration with an immunological adjuvant such as QS-21 (Ragupathi, 1996). The early potential of carbohydrate vaccines in cancer immunotherapy has been discussed by Slovin et al. (1999). Many more 3-component anti-cancer vaccine formulations have since then undergone clinical trials (Ragupathi et al., 2005; Livingston and Ragupathi, 2006). Large randomized trials of polyvalent vaccines such as these can bring out the clinical impact of immunization against carbohydrate antigens (Galonic and Gin, 2007).

Several synthetic strategies have been developed for the preparation not only of complex oligosaccharide antigens but also of complex carbohydrate immunoadjuvants. Galonic and Gin have reviewed some glycosylation processes and strategies to the synthesis of tumour-associated carbohydrate antigens (TACA) and immunoadjuvants for use in anti-cancer therapeutic vaccines.

Glycosylation Strategies

Formation of the glycosidic bond is the primary means by which monosaccharide building blocks are assembled into more complex oligosaccharide structures (Davis, 2000; Nicolaou and Mitchell, 2001). An acetal exchange process (for details, see Galonic and

Gin, 2007) governs most existing chemical glycosylation processes. It effectively couples not only with simple nucleophiles but also with complex oligosaccharide, peptide and lipid glycosyl acceptors.

A more direct approach for glycosylation uses the class of Cl-hydroxy glycosyl donors in which an unprotected anomeric hydroxyl is exchanged under a controlled dehydration process. Cationic metal Lewis acids, sulphonium and phosphonium salts and activated sulphonyl halides are effective dehydrating reagents.

Glycal oxidation. The use of glycols as glycosyl donors has been studied in complex carbohydrate synthesis. Various methods enable the introduction of different functionalities in conjunction with anomeric bond formation (see Di Bussolo et al., 1998).

Acetal exchange couplings and glycal glycosylations have been widely used for the chemical synthesis of highly complex oligosaccharide conjugates. However, no single coupling method is effective for all glycosylations, especially for the extremely complex glycoconjugates identified for potential use in cancer immunotherapy, in which chemical glycosylation processes that are used to prepare these molecules show high substrate-specificity.

Synthesis of Tumour-associated Carbohydrate Antigens

Globo-H. Globo-H is a cell-surface glycosphingolipid expressed on several epithelial tumours, such as those of the breast, prostate and ovary (Hakamori and Zhang, 1997). It has a complex hexasaccharide which is a target of several total synthesis approaches (see Bilodeau et al., 1995; Park et al., 1996).

Sialylated gangliosides. Sialylated gangliosides are cell-surface glycolipids that are expressed in several neuroectodermal cancers, e.g., melanoma, neuroblastoma, sarcoma and small-cell lung cancer. Besides all the challenges facing the chemical synthesis of glycolipids, an added difficulty here is the incorporation of sialic acid residues such as neuraminic acid (NeuAc) into complex oligosaccharides (Boons and Demchenko, 2000). Glycosylations with sialic acid donors typically suffer from low yields.

Mucin-associated glycans. Mucin motifs represent another well-studied class of tumour-associated carbohydrate antigen (Hollingsworth and Swanson, 2004). Mucins are high-molecular-weight glycoproteins that are expressed on the surfaces of many epithelial cells characterized by the presence of GalNAc (N-acetyl-galactosamine core) moieties on the hydroxyl side chains of Ser and Thr residues (which are often clustered) in the protein. Further glycosyl transferase-controlled extension of the carbohydrate part feeds to the formation of oligosaccharides which, besides other functions, confer protection from proteolytic degradation and microbial infection. As a consequence of modified glycosyltransferase expression in tumour cells, premature termination of oligosaccharide biosynthesis is prematurely terminated and leads to the formation of shortened, often sialylated, saccharide antigens as well as the exposure of peptide epitopes (Müller and Hanisch, 2002). Some of these tumour-associated structural changes form a basis for the design of vaccines for selective eradication of tumours (Galonic and Gin, 2007).

Winterfeld et al. (2003) adopted a conceptually distinct approach to the production of mucin-type amino-acid-carbohydrate linkage which involves the formation of the critical sugar-amino-acid bond from the potassium tert-butoxide-promoted conjugate addition of protected Ser and Thr nucleophiles to a 2-nitrogalactal donor. Subsequent C2-nitro reductive acetylation and protective-group modification generates glycosylated building blocks, which can be further elaborated for glycopeptide synthesis (see Galonic and Gin, 2007). After their formation, the suitably protected glycosylated amino acids may be introduced into a growing peptide chain in a modular way. This allows the preparation of clustered carbohydrate antigen displays, a motif common to tumour cell surfaces. Various oligopeptide-tumour antigen conjugates have been made in this manner (see Seitz and Kunz, 1995; Liebe and Kunz, 1997; George et al., 2001).

Synthesis of Carbohydrate Immunoadjuvants

QS-21$_{Aapi}$ The third component that needs to be incorporated in clinically viable anti-cancer vaccines is a potent immunological adjuvant—something that is itself non-immunogenic but which enhances the immune response when administered together with the antigen-carrier conjugate. One very potent molecular immunological adjuvant commonly used in antitumour vaccines is QS-21A (Kensil et al., 1991). It is extracted as a complex saponin from the South American tree *Quillaja saponaria*. Microgram quantities of this amphiphilic saponin in combination with the antigen-carrier conjugate significantly and enhance both antibody and cell-mediated immune responses in many promising anti-cancer and antiviral vaccines (Kensil, 1996). The most serious problem with this saponin is the difficulty in extracting sufficient quantities in pure form—these natural products exist in a mixture of many distinct amphiphilic congeners that can only be partly purified by repeated high-performance liquid chromatography separation. Zhu et al. (2004) tackled this challenge by synthesizing oligosaccharide cores of the natural product through stereoselective glycosylation in the synthesis of fully protected versions of important moieties of QS-21$_{Aapi}$. Kim et al. (2006) have synthesized QS-21$_{Aapi}$.

In vivo immunological trials of synthetic QS-21A in vaccine formulations are currently progressing.

Advances in chemical glycosylation have greatly enhanced the role of organic synthesis as a provider of rare carbohydrate antigens identified as potential targets for cancer immunotherapy (Livingston and Ragupathi, 2006). In fact, chemical synthesis is now also facilitating the designing of novel versions of otherwise inaccessible antigen and adjuvant constructs, molecules that might be crucial to addressing major challenges in the induction of potent yet selective cellular and humoral responses (Galonic and Gin, 2007).

The recent synthesis of QS-21$_{Aapi}$ (Kim et al., 2006) is sure to boost the role of chemical synthesis to go beyond the arena of antigen construction to that of molecular adjuvant design in the preparation of new conjugate anti-cancer vaccines (Galonic and Gin, 2007).

DNA Tumour Viruses and Cancer

Cancer is a multistep process. Some oncogenic viruses have a key role in the development of human malignancies. The human population harbours a group of oncogenic DNA viruses whose members serve as infectious agents of cancer worldwide. This group includes the Epstein–Barr virus (EBV), Kaposi's sarcoma-associated herpesvirus (KSHV), human papillomaviruses (HPVs) and human polyomaviruses. Globally, about 20 per cent of all cancers are linked to infectious agents. Critical studies of DNA viruses have enhanced our understanding of the key molecular players in the transformation process, as also of the molecular mechanisms of tumourigenesis that are employed by these viruses

Table 7.3 Some human DNA tumour viruses and associated malignancies* (after Damania, 2006).

Virus	Disease	Presence in tumour tissue	Causal role	Cofactors
HPV	Cervical cancer	100%	Yes	Genetic
EBV	Lymphoproliferative	100%	Yes	Immunodeficiency
EBV	Hodgkin's lymphoma	40–50%	Nil	Not known
EBV	Nasopharyngeal cancer	100%	Yes	Genetic; environmental
KSHV	Kaposi's sarcoma; Primary effusion lymphoma	95–100%	Yes	Immunodeficiency
KSHV	Multicentric Castleman's disease	100% of AIDS and 50% of non-AIDS lymphomas	Yes	Immunodeficiency

*Abbreviations: EBV, Epstein–Barr virus; HPV, human papillomavirus; KSHV, Kaposi's sarcoma-associated herpesvirus.

(Goedert, 2000; Damania, 2006). Table 7.3 lists the various human DNA tumour viruses and associated malignancies.

Besides direct association of these viruses with cancer, some cofactors such as immune suppression and the environment are also implicated in the development of viral-associated malignancies. Infection with any or all of these viruses and with their cofactors can potentially lead to the development of cancer in the human population.

According to zur Hausen (1999), the following criteria can define a causal role for a cancerous infection: (i) epidemiological plausibility and evidence that a virus infection constitutes risk for the development of a specific tumour; (ii) the consistent presence and persistence of the genome of the microbe in cells of the tumour; (iii) the stimulation of cell proliferation following transfection of the genome (or portions of it) in corresponding tissue culture cells; (iv) the proof that the genome of the agent induces proliferation and the malignant phenotype of the tumour. For each infectious agent, the disease association, oncogenic properties and required cofactors need to be determined carefully.

Human Papillomavirus

Human papillomavirus (HPV) is associated with cervical, anal and skin cancer (Lowry and Howley, 2001). Certain strains of HPV are more oncogenic than others. The 'high-risk' strains include HPV-16 and HPV-18, being consistently associated with cervical and anal cancer. Although it is clear that HPV is the causative agent of cervical and most anal cancers, linking HPV to skin cancer is not definite because the virus can also be found in normal skin.

HPV, a member of the papovavirus family is a small double-stranded DNA virus, ~8 kb in size. Primary infection occurs in the basal stem cells of the epithelium, where after the virus migrates upwards and replicates in the terminally differentiated keratinocytes and is then shed from the stratum corneum (Howley and Lowry, 2001). The virus lacks a polymerase gene so the replication of its genome depends on the stimulation of cellular DNA synthesis in these cells. In most cervical carcinomas, HPV is integrated into the host genome, abolishes expression of the E2 viral gene (a transcriptional repressor of E6 and E7 gene expression) and causes enhanced expression of the E6 and E7 viral oncoproteins.

Sunlight and genetic backgrounds serve as cofactors in the development of skin carcinomas caused by some HPV strains.

Globally, cervical cancer is the second leading cause of cancer deaths in women and over 80 per cent of these occur in developing countries where access to screening programs is limited. Human papillomavirus (HPV) is a sexually transmitted virus that plays a crucial role in the pathogenesis of this cancer. Recently developed vaccines directed against the oncogenic virus strains have shown promising results in clinical trials aimed at assessing their ability to prevent high-grade precancerous lesions or cervical cancer in women who had not been exposed to HPV before vaccination (see *J. Am. Med. Assoc.* 298: 743, 2007).

Epstein–Barr Virus

Epstein–Barr (EBV) is associated with nanopharyngeal carcinoma (NPC), Burkitt's lymphoma (BL), subsets of Hodgkin's lymphomas and T-cell lymphomas, post-transplant lymphomas and gastric carcinomas (Rickinson and Kieff, 2001). NPC is an epithelial tumour commonly seen among many people in Southern China, Hong Kong, Singapore and Taiwan.

BL contains a chromosomal translocation that places the *c-Myc* oncogene under the control of the immunoglobulin heavy or light chain promoters; this results in the deregulation of *c-Myc* in these cells (Dalla-Favera et al., 1987). About 20 per cent of BL tumours are associated with EBV infection, but there are wide regional variations: whereas only 5 per cent of BLs in USA are associated with EBV, in eastern Brazil and Africa, nearly 90 per cent of pediatric BLs harbour EBV. Interestingly, the incidence of BL in African regions, which are also endemic for malaria, is quite high.

Hodgkin's lymphoma is a B lymphoproliferative disease in which 1 per cent of the tumour population is comprised of Hodgkin/Reed-Sternberg (HRS) cells, derived from germinal center B cells. The HRS cells are multinucleated giant cells with distinct nucleoli and marginated heterochromatin (Glaser et al., 1997).

EBV is a double-stranded DNA virus belonging to the γ subfamily of herpesviruses. Herpesviruses have a latent phase and a lytic phase in their lifecycle. Like other γ-herpesviruses, EBV generates a lifelong latent infection in its host's B lymphocytes. EBV codes for several viral proteins with transforming potential. Both EBV-associated BL and NPC show endemic patterns of incidence, strongly suggesting that both environmental and genetic factors contribute to the neoplastic process.

Kaposi's Sarcoma-associated Herpesvirus

KSHV/HHV-8 is linked to several malignancies including Kaposi's sarcoma (KS), primary effusion lymphomas (PELs) and multicentric Castleman's disease (MCD) in the human population. KS is a vascular tumour of mixed cellular composition and is commonly seen as a cutaneous lesion. KSHV is always found in the spindle cells of the lesion. KS is the most frequently detected tumour in AIDS patients.

PELs are malignant B-cell lymphomas representing a specific subset of body cavity based lymphomas (BCBLs) that appear as body cavity effusions (Nador et al., 1996). All PELs are KSHV positive, pointing to an intimate epidemiological link between the presence of KSHV and the induction of PEL. These lymphomas sometimes contain EBV also.

PELs are observed in both HIV-positive and HIV-negative individuals, with both types of PELs invariably containing KSHV viral DNA (Damania, 2006).

MCD refers to a B-cell lymphoproliferative disorder. It is characterized by vascular proliferation of the germinal centers of the lymph node. Nearly 100 per cent of AIDS-associated MCD is positive for KSHV, whereas ~50 per cent of non-AIDS-associated MCD contains KSHV viral DNA. AIDS-associated MCD is usually accompanied by the development of KS in the affected patients (Moore and Chang, 2003).

KSHV is strongly linked to KS, PELs and MCD and is essential for the development of these malignancies. Clearly, KSHV is a tumour virus with oncogenic properties (Damania, 2006). A member of the γ-herpesvirus family, it establishes lifelong latency in B cells. Its genome is ~160 kb in size, encodes >80 open reading frames (ORFs) and diverse genes involved in transformation, signalling, prevention of apoptosis and immune evasion.

In KSHV, K1 and viral G-protein-coupled receptor (vGPCR) genes carry oncogenic potential. The K1 protein can transform rodent fibroblasts *in vitro* and, upon being injected into nude mice, these cells induce multiple, disseminated tumours (see Tomlinson and Damania, 2004; Wang et al., 2004). As with other tumour viruses, HIV is a cofactor for the development of malignancy—the prevalence of KS in AIDS patients is abnormally high.

Human Polymaviruses

Human polymaviruses—JC virus (JCV) and BK virus (BKV)—are linked to a variety of different human cancers, e.g., JCV is associated with brain tumours in patients with or without progressive multifocal leukoencephalopathy (PML), glial tumours and pediatric medulloblastomas (Krynska et al., 1999). Its other associations include colon cancer and central nervous system (CNV) lymphoma (Laghi et al., 1999 Croul et al., 2003).

The genomes of these viruses do not encode their own replication machinery. To replicate, they express two proteins, large T antigen and small t antigen, which push the host cell into the cell cycle (Cole and Conzen, 2001). Large T antigen carries both Rb- and *p53*-binding domains which interact with these two tumour-suppressor proteins, inactivate them and release the E2F transcription factor from Rb suppression and activate cyclin promoters. The large T interaction with *p53* suppresses its apoptotic function and prevents the activation of inhibitors of the cellular cyclins (Pipas, 1992). Cells proliferate and precede oncogenic transformation. Small t antigen seems to co-operate with large T antigen in the transformation of differentiated cells.

BKV is highly oncogenic in rodents. Complete BKV genomic DNA or fragments that code for the large T and small t antigen can transform many cells including human embryonic fibroblasts; and cells cultured from the kidney or brain of rodents and hamsters. The transforming ability of JCV is seen mainly in cells of neural origin. JCV also shows high oncogenicity in primates.

Tumourigenesis is a multistep process and infection with the DNA tumour viruses can substitute for one or many of the mutational events that result in complete transformation, neoplasia and metastasis. Currently, most anti-tumour therapies against virus-induced cancers target cellular proteins having a role in these processes rather than viral proteins (Damania, 2006).

Future studies should be aimed at designing therapeutics that specifically target viral proteins—these therapies will be more specific and will reduce drug cytotoxicity. Vaccines need to be developed against these DNA tumour viruses. One vaccine against human papillomavirus is already available, but there is none against EBV, KSHV and the human polyomaviruses (Damania, 2006).

Virus-like Particles (VLP) for Vaccination, Gene Therapy and Drug Delivery

Pattenden et al. (2005) focused on virus-like particles (VLPs) which are being used in vaccination, gene therapy and drug delivery. Existing laboratory processes, when scaled, do not easily give a compositionally and architecturally consistent product. New process routes might ultimately be based on chemical processing by self-assembly, involving the precision manufacture of precursor capsomeres followed by *in vitro* VLP self-assembly and scale-up to required levels. A synergistic interaction of biomolecular design and bioprocess engineering (i.e., biomolecular engineering) is required if these alternative process routes and the full promise of new VLP products are to be realized.

Two major aims in biochemical engineering are: (i) to create a knowledge base that can economically and rapidly deliver new and increasingly complex biological products, e.g., VLPs to market in the shortest possible time; and (ii) to discourage the development of inefficient laboratory processes that are difficult or costly to scale and that cannot be improved because of costly regulatory constraints on late-stage bioprocess modifications. The second objective can be addressed by suitable scaled-down bioprocess technologies (Boychyn et al., 2000) which produce pre-clinical and clinical materials. Bioprocess manufacturing research can go on in parallel with early-stage product development research, so as to improve product processing characteristics. For example, protein processing can be improved by coupling biomolecular design with bioprocess engineering so that product molecules are selected with respect not only to functional, but also process criteria (Morreale et al., 2004).

VLPs differ from the more-complex pseudoviruses (PSVs). Recent innovations in VLP and PSV construction aim to develop novel VLPs and PSVs as contenders for use as vaccine and gene therapy products.

A VLP has been historically viewed purely as an assembly of structural proteins, organized into capsomeres that further organize into the capsid (Fig. 7.9). The VLP may be directly used as an 'empty' shell, or may be packaged *ex vivo* with a payload typically comprising DNA or some therapeutic small molecule or protein. Here, a VLP is a replication-incompetent macromolecular protein assembly which can be created from the minimal self-assembling structural proteins of bacteriophages and viruses (Brown et al., 2002).

VLPs can also be described as virus-inspired ensembles of proteins, lipids and nucleic acids that cannot technically be described as a virus. Although often used to describe replication-incompetent ensembles, the term is increasingly being applied to particles that undergo limited replication and *in vivo* packaging of viral genomes or host factors. Such particles are termed PSVs (Buck et al., 2004) and include attenuated or otherwise replication-limited emulations of viruses. The same principles for PSV bioprocessing apply as for VLPs.

Like viruses, the structural proteins that comprise a VLP or PSV can either self-assemble to form the 'shell', or assemble through intermediate steps involving a scaffold, a compartment, or a chaperone. The process is usually through multimeric biomolecular structures such as capsomeres that finally assemble to the higher order structures com-

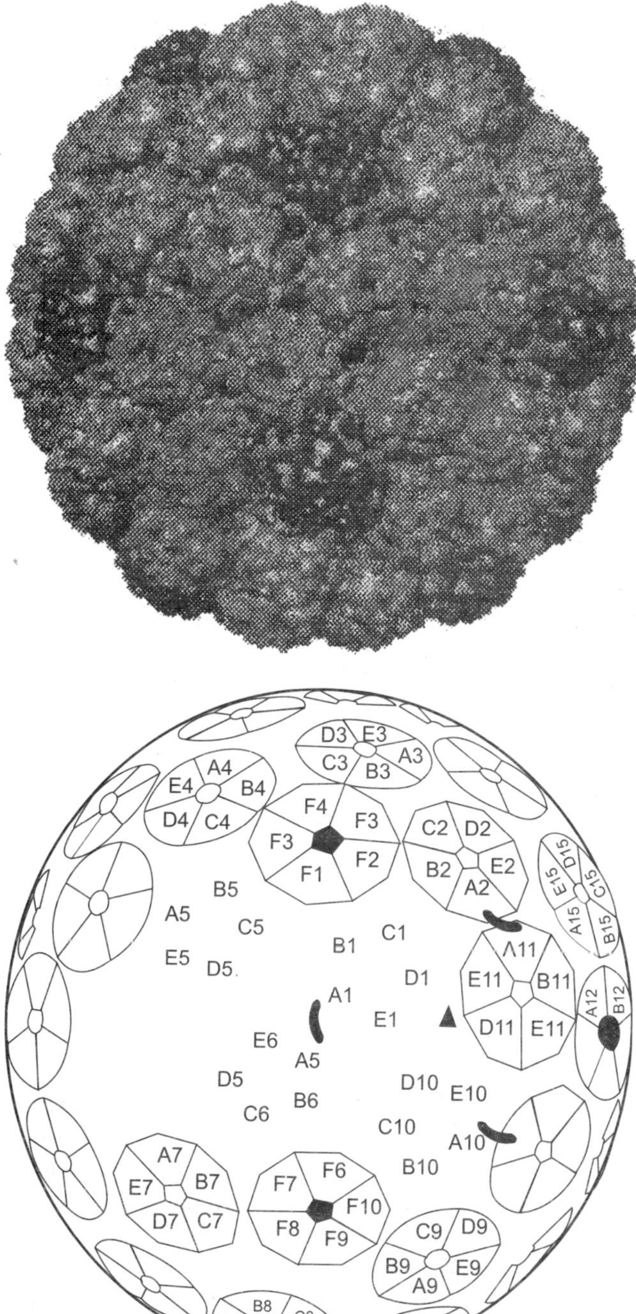

Fig. 7.9 Structure And Architecture of A Polyomavirus VLP. Each VLP (A, B) consists of 72 capsomeres. Macromolecular organization is a common feature of all VLPs, but the number of total monomeric building blocks and the overall geometric organization varies (After Pattenden et al., 2005).

prising the VLP. The capsomeres or particles can be expressed in a range of host cells (Table 7.4).

VLPs are primarily marketed as products for vaccination: Hepatitis B vaccines contain recombinant protein-based VLPs synthesized in controlled expression systems. Villa et al. (2005) showed that VLPs assembled from the major structural protein of human papillomavirus (HPV) reduce the incidence of HPV infection and cervical cancer. Some other diseases as targets for VLP vaccines include epidemic gastroenteritis, hepatitis C and malaria. However, the application of VLPs has so far been restricted to animal trials and proof-of-concept.

A new application not yet commercialized is to use VLPs as vectors in gene therapy. It is possible to use VLP or PSV specificity (tropism) to deliver a therapeutic agent either by systemic injection or oral administration (Takamura et al., 2004). In both cases, a foreign protein could be expressed within the targeted liver cells or intestinal mucosa *in vivo*. The control of tropism is a major focus of current research. PSVs may be constructed by exchanging the envelope protein from one virus with that of another—a process termed pseudotyping. For example, a combination of Ebola envelope protein and a lentiviral backbone created a PSV targeted against airway epithelia (the Ebola trait) and successfully infected non-dividing cells (the lentiviral trait) (Kobinger et al., 2001). It is also possible to exchange tropism by introducing a cell receptor recognition domain, (e.g., an antibody fragment) onto a VLP or PSV (Martin et al., 1999), which replaces the original tropism with the introduced binding preference. The removal of type-specific epitopes helps in gene therapy applications in cases where the epitope promotes the production of neutralizing antibodies, to derive VLPs and PSVs having improved bioavailability (Pattenden et al., 2005).

One effective method of creating novel PSV function involves generating a library of variants expressing the desired function; this is followed by selection for the desired feature by using *in vivo* screening, employing molecular evolution and using replication-competent viruses (Schneider et al., 2003). Viruses with a desired trait are only allowed to replicate under conditions of selection. Another option is to generate display libraries and select them independently from the virus (e.g., in phage display); these can then be incorporated into the VLP or PSV (Nicklin et al., 2004).

Bioprocess Engineering

We badly need to design and model novel bioprocesses that can rapidly manufacture VLP candidates at suitable scale and to make sure that the processes do indeed produce VLPs having the right characteristics for both function and regulatory registration (e.g., consistent architecture and composition). One good route for VLP bioprocessing depends on *in vivo* assembly and then separates the desired product from a large pool of morphologically related contaminants *ex vivo*.

Besides mammalian cell cultures which suffer from some problems and present many difficulties, other eukaryotic cells such as insect and yeast can be used for VLP production. This *in vivo* method involves the synthesis, ordered folding and quaternary association of capsid-forming proteins within the cell in a native-like environment where macromolecular assembly can occur either spontaneously in the cytoplasm by self-association, or at interfaces such as cell membranes, or upon key proteins where the interface might act as a scaffold.

Table 7.4 Hosts used to generate VLPs and PSVs (after Pattenden et al., 2005).

Host	VLPs and PSVs made in host	Comments
Bacteria	Polyomavirus, papillomavirus	Production system simple and efficient at producing bacterial phage proteins. Expression efficiency of viral protein components varies and the yield of soluble protein can be low. Does not normally assemble VLPs of mammalian viruses. Does not post-translationally modify proteins.
Yeast	Polyomavirus, papillomavirus, hepatitis virus	Efficient low-cost protein producers can assemble viral structural proteins into VLPs with low architectural consistency.
Insect cells	Polyomavirus, papillomavirus, rotavirus, calicivirus, norovirus	Fairly efficient protein producers able to express and assemble viral structural proteins into VLPs with higher architectural consistency than yeast, but at higher cost.
Mammalian cells	Retrovirus, adenovirus, adeno-associated viruses, Epstein–Barr virus	Used to produce PSVs for gene therapy tests. This method yields authentic virus at high cost. Unknown and variable contaminants can be incorporated into the PSV and variable post-translational modification can result.

Retaining the native expression system is crucial for more consistent VLP product formation or to retain important post-translational modifications (e.g., glycosylation and phosphorylation) required for function.

The *in vivo* approach has been usually based on virus and vaccine production/purification methods that economically separate individual capsid-forming elements because they require extensive removal of contaminants and biosafety monitoring (Rueda et al., 2000). VLPs assembled in eukaryotic systems contain fragments of contaminating cellular DNA (Gillock et al., 1997) which must be removed for pharmaceutical applications, necessitating *ex vivo* disassembly/reassembly processing (Volkin et al., 2001). This kind of post-expression processing is also essential for encapsidation of a specific molecule or the removal of cellular, morphological and structural contaminants. For gene/drug-delivery purposes, high reassembly yields are crucial for sufficient packaging and final product yield. Very often, very low DNA-packaging efficiencies within reassembled VLPs are quite low (Touze and Coursaget, 1998). This points to the inefficiency of the process and necessitates separation of the desired product from closely related contaminants.

A better approach is that of chemical self-assembly processing (Texter and Tirrell, 2001). An idealized *in vitro* process for the manufacture of VLPs may be that based on the precision manufacture of precursors (monomer proteins or capsomeres) with a high compositional consistency, followed by self, directed, or controlled supramolecular assembly to give consistent capsids and scaling up to desired levels. This process route also realizes a significant safety requirement not possible for PSVs produced with *in vivo* processes: the decoupling of the viral protein(s) and the viral genome eliminates the possibility of making replication-competent viruses by recombination, thereby overcoming a major risk factor in many gene therapy applications (Pattenden et al., 2005).

VLP self-assembly seems to involve hydrophobic, electrostatic and covalent (disulfide) interactions. Self-assembly is usually spontaneous under favourable environmental conditions but certain scaffold proteins are required as catalysts for some viral proteins to assemble in biological systems (Dokland, 1999). The process of VLP assembly comprises parallel and competing first- and second-order reactions of folding and aggregation, as well as a pathway of correct and ordered self-assembly, possibly requiring scaffolding catalysts. This makes self-assembly a multimolecular, dynamic association reaction in which unimolecular protein folding is involved, but is not the sole determinant. Addressing this problem of reaction engineering is a daunting task in chemical processing by self-assembly for the creation of VLPs.

The *in vitro* route to VLPs commonly generates large amounts of precursors which are then used in self-assembly processing. The major problem for VLP monomer production by a prokaryotic route is how to obtain soluble and full-length product free of toxin, heat shock proteins (HSPs) and chaperone proteins (Lai and Middelberg, 2002). In fact, the *in vitro* approach can be plagued by several process challenges, even though several of these problems have been solved in conventional biopharmaceutical processing or can be tackled by using standard biomolecular tools coupled with novel approaches to assembly.

Downstream simplification required to intensify the process for both the *in vivo* and *in vitro* routes can be achieved by cross-flow microfiltration or tangential-flow ultrafiltration to remove low-molecular-weight proteins, followed by affinity, ion-exchange, or size-exclusion chromatography to concentrate or isolate VLP products. Some new matrices can improve both yield and purity; those suitable for use in VLP bioprocesses include hydroxyapatite, Matrex Cellufine Sulfate (Millipore), Q-Sepharose RTM-XL (GE Healthcare) and Macroflow resins (BIA separations). In one such bioseparation CIM (Convective Interaction Media—BIA separation), a monolithic support is cast in a continuous, homogeneous phase for faster separation in shorter columns (Kramberger et al., 2004).

Biomolecular Engineering and Precision Precursor Manufacture

Precursor manufacture can be improved through the synergistic interaction of biomolecular design and bioprocess engineering (biomolecular engineering). Such engineering for chemical self-assembly processing entails biomolecular redesign by rational and/or evolutionary means, followed by the selection of appropriate product molecules with respect not only to functional but also process criteria.

Rational biomolecular design depends on extensive prior knowledge of a target protein including its high-resolution crystal structure. Computer-aided modelling facilitates analysis of enzyme active sites, docking surfaces with binding partners, or conformational changes.

Following the identification of suitable sites of biomolecular modification, site-directed mutagenesis (SDM) is used to introduce specific changes at chosen sites in the coding sequence. This enables the protein to be altered, for instance, by replacing non-polar residues with charged residues (or vice versa). This approach increases the solubility of human respiratory syncytial virus (RSV) major glycoprotein (from 27 per cent to 75 per cent, giving a dramatic improvement in process potential) (Murby et al., 1995). Other applications of SDM are optimization of codon usage, or the removal of specific protease cleavage sites to minimize proteolysis which increases the yield of full-length product (Rozkov and Enfors, 2004).

Another way to biomolecular redesign is to use different techniques to make large libraries of molecules. From these variants, those having desired properties can be selected. Peabody and Al-Bitar (2001) used error-prone PCR to generate a library of bacteriophage coat proteins containing random point mutations from which a variant with altered assembly properties could be selected. The trouble is that most mutations happen to be single base replacements so the result could be neutral because of codon redundancy.

Further, restrictions on library size could also limit this strategy. DNA shuffling is an alternative way of building a large library. It enables exchange of functional domains between two related proteins through recombination of homologous DNA sequences (Stemmer, 1994). Modern bioinformatics tools that can statistically generate locations of crossover in DNA shuffling experiments can prove helpful in this endeavour (Moore et al., 2001).

We urgently need new bioprocess technology to make VLPs clinically valuable products. Current manufacturing methods using eukaryotic cells generate VLPs with low compositional and architectural consistency, necessitating increased process complexity. The full use of the merits of VLPs requires the development of new large-scale bioprocesses having high yield, quick process time and reduced total cost. New process routes might ultimately be based on chemical processing by self-assembly, involving the precision manufacture of precursor capsomeres followed by *in vitro* VLP self-assembly and scale-up to required levels. Proficiency in biomolecular engineering is essential for activating these native process routes.

Use of the Defensive Sugars of HIV-1 for Drug and Vaccine Design

Our understanding of viral immunology has benefited greatly from the sustained effort in developing an antibody vaccine against HIV/AIDS. One strong barrier to antibody neutralization of HIV has been the dense carbohydrate (glycan) array that surrounds the exposed envelope antigens. These carbohydrates, which have evolved to protect HIV and promote its transmission, may also be effective therapeutic targets (Scanlan et al., 2007).

The HIV genome does not code for any gene products that synthesize carbohydrates—its surface antigens are glycosylated entirely by host cellular enzymes. This extensive glycosylation affects almost every aspect of virus biology. The folding of viral glycoproteins, the transmission of the virus and the nature of the immune response to infection are all greatly influenced by this glycosylation. The effect of coating of HIV with immunologically 'self' glycans (that is, those synthesized by the host cell) on viral immunogenicity is predictable: antibodies against most of the available antigenic surface of HIV do not normally occur. Scanlan et al. have reviewed the apparently contradictory roles of HIV glycans as powerful adaptations for viral survival as well as targets for therapeutic intervention. The fact that HIV relies so heavily on the human glycosylation pathway has revealed new vulnerabilities which can be targeted for both drug and vaccine design. Most of the viral envelope surface is covered by carbohydrates.

The antigenic surfaces of not only viruses but also prokaryotes and eukaryotes are covered by 'shields' of polysaccharides, glycolipids, or glycoproteins. Much, if not all, of this carbohydrate diversity is an outcome of antigenic selection or co-evolution (Blixt et al., 2004). The humoral immune system can effectively discriminate self from non-self carbohydrates (Seymour et al., 2004).

In viruses such as HIV, the relationship between host and pathogen is jeopardized by the fact that the carbohydrates on the pathogen are synthesized by the host. An exception could be the primary virions which cause the initial infection. These are glycosylated by the donor host and may bear non-self antigens; Lowe and Marth (2003) reported that HIV-1 from an AA or AO donor is susceptible to antibody-mediated, complement-dependent neutralization by BB, BO or OO host antibodies and vice versa. Possibly, transmission of viruses may be decreased between individuals (or species) with heterologous blood groups. A strategy that augments this natural phenomenon might contribute to herd immunity against HIV.

Glycosylation affects the binding of antibodies against gp120 (gp120 arises from the cleavage, mediated by furin proteases, of the envelope gene which is translated as gp160 and then cleaved into gp120 and gp41; see Cole et al., 2004). The acquisition (or loss) of a glycosylation site usually affects the immunogenicity of the surrounding protein surface.

Analysis of HIV envelope sequences has indicated that highly variable regions usually lie adjacent to N-linked glycosylation sites. Moreover, the positions of N-linked glycans usually shift during the course of infection. This has generated the concept of the 'evolving glycan shield' of gp120, in which modifications in N-linked glycosylation increase the rate of immune evasion (Wei et al., 2003).

Therapeutics Based on the HIV Glycan Shield

Several types of drugs inhibit key stages of mammalian glycan biosynthesis. Some imino sugars inhibit the trimming of $Glc_3Man_9GlcNAc_2$ to $Glc_1Man_9GlcNAc_2$ in the endoplasmic reticulum and prevent entry of its carrier glycoprotein into the calnexin/calreticulin folding cycle. Some create structural alterations in gp120 and viruses expressed in the presence of such drugs fail to undergo productive post-receptor-binding rearrangements or fusion with the target-cell membrane (Zitzmann et al., 1999).

The molecular mechanism of the enhanced sensitivity of viral, but not host, glycoproteins to glucosidase inhibitors is not clear. Helenius and Aebi (2004) suggested some link between lectin-mediated retention of glucosylated gp120 in the endoplasmic reticulum and complex disulphide bond network of gp120 needed for productive infection by T-cell thiol-reactive proteins. Another explanation may be that the sensitivity of gp120 to glucosidase inhibition simply illustrates the correlation between N-glycosylation density and calnexin/calreticulin dependence (see Kwong et al., 2000).

Lectin-mediated HIV Neutralization

The glycans of gp120 are suitable targets for exogenous lectins that prevent viral infection or transmission. These lectins competitively inhibit the association of gp120 with DC-SIGN (dendritic cell-specific intercellular adhesion molecule-3-grabbing non-integrin, see Nobile et al., 2005; Balzarini et al., 2007) or disrupt receptor-induced conformational changes and/or inhibit membrane fusion (Esser et al., 1999). Many plant, animal and microbial lectins have been assayed for efficacy against HIV. Some bind to the mannose residues of gp120; in others, monosaccharides (e.g., N-acetylglucosamine, galactose and fucose) are also candidates. Lectin specificity for HIV (not for host proteins), probably depends on the unusual density of the sugars found on gp120 and their specificity for terminal residues, such as mannose, that are not normally observed in mammalian proteins (Balzarini, 2006).

Besides the work to develop an effective vaccine for HIV/AIDS, other microbicidal lectins may potentially complement traditional barrier protection; Tsai et al. (2003) reported that cyanovirin is effective *in vivo*. This is a small bacterial lectin with specificity for α1-2-linked mannose residues. Systemic use of antiviral lectins has not been tested but their ability to prevent cell-cell virus transfer might make them a valuable therapeutic tool (Chiba et al., 2001). In fact, the more general specificity of lectins, as compared with that of traditional small-molecule inhibitors, makes them potentially strong antivirals.

Vaccines

Most antibodies against HIV-1 are either directed against non-neutralizing epitopes (e.g., those on monomeric gp120 but not on functional trimers) or exert some selection pressure which HIV can rapidly evade through changes in its envelope sequence (Pantophlet and Burton, 2006). Likewise, many immunogens based on the envelope proteins of HIV elicit a narrow antibody response that is specific only for non-neutralizing epitopes or those that are poorly conserved between strains (Gilbert et al., 2005). However, a few antibodies, isolated from infected individuals, do show a potent neutralizing activity against a wide variety of HIV isolates (Zolla-Pazner, 2004). Notably, in the face of the generally weak immunogenicity of several heterogeneous self glycans, one broadly neutralizing antibody, IgG1 2G12, binds directly and exclusively to the carbohydrates of gp120 (Calarese et al., 2003).

Synthetic mannose vaccines against HIV?

Chemical synthesis of molecular mimics of the 2G12 epitope has yielded antigens that interact with 2G12 (Geng et al., 2004). The merit of the synthetic approach lies in the potential variation in design for antigen optimization and presentation, but one potential problem associated with the chemical approaches for 2G12 is the degree of internal flexibility seen within the compounds (Scanlan et al., 2007).

Convergent Possibilities for Anti-cancer and HIV Vaccine Design

Increased or altered expression of self glycolipids, glycoproteins and sialyl-LewisA (SLeA), SLeX and SLeY epitopes is associated with many cancers (Freiere et al., 2006). The idea of normally clustering self antigens with a view to improving immunogenicity and the importance of carrier peptides such as keyhole limpet haemocyanin has been explored along with such strategies as immunization with peptide mimetics of glycan structures (Kagan et al., 2005; Reimer et al., 2006). Pashov et al. (2006) explored the same for HIV. These approaches have not so far been translated into clinical vaccines but it is clear that high-titre, class-switched antibodies against self carbohydrate epitopes can be elicited (Vliegenthart, 2006). This not only warrants research into carbohydrate vaccines against HIV-1 but also critical consideration of constructs, carriers and adjuvants that have proven successful for cancer antigens to be assessed for possible use in HIV vaccine development (Scanlan et al., 2007).

8 Diagnostics: Biomarkers and Omics

Introduction

Cancer is usually considered as a genetic disease. Despite the development of several drugs, the death rates for the most prevalent cancers have not declined significantly (Zhang et al., 2007). Mortality rates can be brought down if the disease is detected early enough. The majority of patients are diagnosed as having cancer at a fairly late stage. In fact, 72 per cent of lung cancer patients, 57 per cent of colorectal cancer and 34 per cent of breast cancer patients in the US are diagnosed at late stage. If these cancers could be diagnosed early, the survival rate may exceed 85 per cent (Gloeckler-Ries et al., 2003). For realizing the goal of early diagnosis, highly sensitive and specific assays for biomarkers are needed. The post-genome era has shifted research focus on biomarker discovery and the early diagnosis of cancer through the application of various omics technologies—transcriptomics, proteomics, metabonomics, peptidomics, glycomics, phosphoproteomics or lipidomics—on tissue samples and body fluids (Zhang et al., 2007). The biological samples being analysed include blood, urine, sputum, saliva, nipple-aspirate fluid, breath, tear-fluid, cerebrospinal fluid and tissue samples. These omics technologies have stimulated discovery of new biomarkers for the diagnosis, prognosis, therapeutic-response prediction and population screening of human cancers.

An exciting new field has emerged in biomedical science. Biological markers (biomarkers) have applications in the diagnosis, staging, prognosis and monitoring of disease progression, as well as in the monitoring of clinical responses to a therapeutic intervention and the development and delivery of personalized treatments to reduce attrition in clinical trials. The field is providing several examples of individual biomarkers which find application as indicators of disease pathophysiology, such as blood pressure, cholesterol levels and viral load in HIV. These biomarkers can also be used as a substitute for a clinical endpoint.

The complexity of the underlying pathophysiological pathways and interactions is widely known to biomedical researchers who are now greatly interested in the possibility of the identification of a pattern or profile of several biomarkers (representing, for instance, some combination of genes, proteins, organic molecules, or metabolites in a given condition)—an achievement that can potentially usher in a new era in disease diagnosis, classification, intervention and the assessment of therapeutic responses. Certain non-invasive biomarker strategies based on imaging technologies are exemplified by magnetic resonance imaging, single-photon emission computed tomography and positron emission tomography; these are already being employed in several therapeutic areas (Rudin and Weissleder, 2003; Ilyin et al., 2004).

Biomarkers can have a beneficial impact on health economics. The term 'biomarker' has been used widely across several therapeutic areas and many disciplines. In drug trials, biomarkers may find use in efficacy determination and patient population stratification, in deducing pharmacokinetic–pharmacodynamic relationships and in safety monitoring (see Frank and Hargreaves, 2003; Ilyin et al., 2004). Effective interfacing and integration of different technologies for data collection and analysis are crucial to biomarker identification, characterization, validation and application. 'Integrative functional informatics' is a novel direction in such technology integration (Ilyin et al., 2004).

Although biomarkers have attracted much interest, this has been accompanied by some confusion over definitions, types and approaches. Generally, a biomarker or biological marker is viewed as a factor that can be precisely measured and reliably points to a normal biological or pathophysiological process or a therapeutic response (Ilyin et al., 2004). BDWG (2001) developed suitable definitions as well as a conceptual framework and proposed the following standards:

- Biological marker (biomarker) is a characteristic that is objectively measured and evaluated as an indicator of normal biological processes, pathogenic processes or pharmacological responses to a therapeutic intervention;
- Clinical endpoint is a property or variable which reflects how a patient feels, functions or survives;
- Surrogate endpoint denotes a biomarker that may substitute for a clinical endpoint. A surrogate endpoint may predict clinical benefit (or harm, or lack of benefit or harm) on the basis of epidemiological, therapeutic, pathophysiological or other scientific evidence. Surrogate endpoints constitute a subset of biomarkers.

The steps involved in omics-based cancer diagnosis include Biological samples → Pretreatment → Omics experiments → Bioinformatics analysis → BIOMARKER DISCOVERY → Biomarker validation → Clinical Diagnostics (see Table 8.1).

Table 8.1 Comparison between various omics technologies for biomarker discovery (after Zhang et al., 2007).

Technique	Advantages	Disadvantages
Transcriptomics	Well-established technology; Fewer genes and/or transcripts (approx. 25,000 in humans) relative to proteins	Tissue materials required
Proteomics	Suitable for various biological samples	More proteins (>500,000 in humans) relative to transcripts or metabolites
Metabonomics	Suitable for biological samples; fewer metabolites (approx. 10,000 in humans) relative to transcripts or proteins	Technology not yet fully developed
Peptidomics	Low molecular weight	Proteolysis in *ex vivo* samples complicates results
Glycomics	Greater stability and solubility of glycoproteins relative to unmodified proteins	Glycosylation analysis is difficult (e.g., structure identification)
Phosphoproteomics	Sub-proteome: limits the amount of proteins that can be analysed	Identification of phosphorylated proteins is difficult
Lipidomics	Sub-metabonomics: limits the amount of metabolites that can be measured	Technology still being developed

Important Biomarker Techniques

Approaches to biomarkers based on genomics include different methods to measure the expression of genes and include micro-array - and polymerase chain reaction (PCR) analysis of gene expression analysis (Ilyin et al., 2003).

The integration of cDNA micro-array, high-density tissue micro-array and linked clinical and pathology data has become a robust approach for the molecular profiling of human cancers such as prostate cancer.

Pharmacogenetics deals with the role of genes in an individual patient's response to drugs. It covers research on basic drug discovery, the genetic basis of drug responses, pharmacodynamics, pharmacokinetics and metabolism and has substantial implications for new drug development, patient genetic testing and clinical patient management (Ilyin et al., 2004). Its aim is to predict a patient's response to a specific drug as a means of providing best 'personalized' medical treatment.

Proteomic technologies have been developed to provide information about protein abundance, location, modification and protein-protein interactions. Unlike the fixed genome of the cell, the proteome is very complex and remains in a constant state of flux. Protein analysis is able to consider post-translational modifications, which can markedly change the function and activity of a protein. Besides, the final amount of protein can differ greatly from the amount of mRNA transcribed from a gene of interest (Ilyin et al., 2004).

Metabonomics

The new discipline of metabonomics facilitates rapid *in vivo* screening of various factors, including those for drug efficacy and/or toxicity and underlying pathophysiological processes. The metabonomic approach complements proteomics and genomics and provides a chemical or biόchemical profile of a specific body fluid, organ or tissue during a continuous time-course analysis (Robosky et al., 2002). It aids in the tracking of metabolic profiles and the mapping of interactions between metabolic pathways across complete systems.

Till recently, bioinformatics was chiefly concerned with genome data storage, management and analysis, but it now has a much broader role in connecting and integrating more varied types of biological data as for instance, identification and validation of drug targets and for the development of biomarkers. Linking expressional data derived from genomic and proteomic approaches to biological pathways of interest greatly enhances our understanding of target biology. The major challenge here is that effective use of integrated techniques strongly depends on the ability to analyze the resulting complex datasets (Martinez-Cruz et al., 2003; Ilyin et al., 2004). Darrow et al., (2003) showed how industrialized robotic high-throughput screening enables quick and efficient screening of thousands of chemical compounds against a biological target of interest. For this purpose, miniaturization is very helpful but requires advanced liquid handling and automation, in addition to improvements in technologies for detection and data management.

Integration of Genomic and Proteomic Technologies

Proteomic knowledge is being rapidly built on the genomic outputs. Gene expression data determined by micro-arrays are being strongly linked with proteomic data so as to have valuable insights into critical disease events and to facilitate drug discovery (Ilyin et al., 2004). Combining both genomic and protein analyses to assess potential biomarkers yields much superior results than those obtained with only one technical approach (Hanash et al., 2002).

DNA Sequences to Protein Arrays

Another novel approach to biomarker discovery involving the integration of genomic and proteomic techniques exploits the production of protein chips. Here, cDNAs encoding tagged proteins are expressed and proteins are isolated and printed on a slide; slides are used to examine protein profiling, protein–protein interactions and antibody profiling (Schweitzer et al., 2003). These protein array techniques allow detection of potential novel biomarkers and also provide better understanding of the signalling pathways associated with the printed proteins.

But one possible drawback of protein chips is that the use of bacterial expression vectors for mammalian proteins can result in none of the post-translational modifications normally seen on the proteins expressed in the mammalian cell. Some of these concerns may, however, be addressed by using yeast expression systems, even though the post-translational modifications in yeast are not necessarily similar to those in mammals.

Integrative Functional Informatics and Bioinformatics

Regardless of which omics technology is used for biomarker development, bioinformatics tools are needed to extract the diagnostic or prognostic information from the complex data. Based on pattern recognition technologies, discriminatory patterns (a panel of gene, protein or peptide patterns) are identified for the diagnosis of individuals with and without a cancer. For transcriptomics investigations, there are several approaches to make diagnostic and prognostic predictions for cancer patients, based on gene expression profiles. Zhang et al. (2005) described the recently developed independent component analysis (ICA). For proteomics experiments, the computational issues involved in the processing and classification of protein mass spectra were reviewed by Hilario et al. (2006) and the relative performance of various methods was discussed by Shin and Markey (2006). For analysing metabonomic data, a principal component analysis (PCA) method has been used for the diagnosis of liver cancer (Yang et al., 2004).

'Integrative Functional Informatics', can potentially contribute substantially to the identification, characterization, validation and application of various cellular and molecular biomarkers. Table 8.1 lists some important biomarker techniques.

The ability to identify novel pathways, targets and potential biomarkers for drug discovery and clinical application has greatly increased. Micro-array analyses, for instance, are used to identify genes which are induced or suppressed in some disease states; these genes can be studied as potential biomarkers (Pinhasov et al., 2004). The rate-limiting step here is the functional validation of such newly discovered targets and biomarkers (Ilyin et al., 2004).

A novel experimental approach, termed 'integrative functional informatics' is based on the convergence and integration of proteomics, bioinformatics and high-throughput screening techniques (Bernal et al., 2003). It can speed up the discovery and validation of novel targets and biomarkers.

By using such integration and convergence, Xin et al. (2004) introduced highly selective changes into the cell proteome by using rationally developed libraries of small interfering RNA (siRNA) molecules and industrial high-throughput screening equipment. siRNAs inhibit the expression of target genes; the siRNA-mediated downregulation of the target genes can be monitored by micro-array, PCR and reverse transcription analysis. Transfection of the siRNA library results in modified cell populations which can be detected individually since they remain confined to separate wells (one population per well). If downregulation of a gene manifests in a phenotype of interest (as detected in a functional assay), then the event is recorded as a hit and can be followed up by a confirmation assay (Ilyin et al., 2004).

Integrative functional informatics has also proved to be a boon in the mass parallel processing of clinical samples (Pinhasov et al., 2004); potential biomarkers may be characterized and validated in preclinical and clinical models. In fact this approach may be an ideal tool for the validation of novel biomarkers.

One major problem is the over-fitting of data—when the parameters in a model are too many relative to the number of samples and the outcome is that the model fits the original data but often predicts poorly for independent data. Two methods frequently used to avoid data over-fitting are: cross-validation (applied to the entire data-analysis process) and validation of independent datasets (Zhang et al., 2007). Another problem is that different bioinformatic analyses tend to generate different predictive patterns, possibly because the number of samples is too small (Ein-Dor et al., 2006). Thousands of samples are needed for transcriptomic analysis to generate a robust gene list for predicting outcome in cancer. No such framework is available for estimating appropriate sample sizes in other omics research.

Two similarities among the various omics technologies are that they rely on analytical chemistry methods and generate complex datasets. MS technology is used commonly in all omics platforms except transcriptomics. Also, in omics research the development of robust data analysis approaches is crucial for generating discriminatory patterns (e.g., gene, protein or metabolite). Theoretically, at least, the bioinformatic tools developed for micro-array analysis should be transferable to such other omics as proteomics. Also, any lessons learnt from analysis of DNA micro-array data should prove helpful in designing new methods in proteomics (Kremer et al., 2005), but in reality they are limited owing to the unique attributes of proteomics data.

Cancer diagnostics will benefit greatly if we can advance from the use of a single omic platform to the integration of multiple omic platforms and finally to systems biology. However, a direct link between genes and/or proteins and metabolites cannot be easily established: multiple mRNAs could be formed from one gene; multiple proteins from one mRNA; multiple metabolites may be generated from one enzyme; and the same metabolite may participate in many different pathways. All these possibilities strongly complicate the interpretation and integration of the various omics data. To overcome this kind of constraint, Bernal et al. (2003) have developed integrative functional informatics, based on the convergence and integration of proteomics, bioinformatics and high-throughput screening techniques, to accelerate the discovery and validation of novel biomarkers. This novel approach makes possible high-throughput testing of potential biomarkers without compromising high-specificity and sensitivity; this makes it a valuable tool for the validation of novel biomarkers (Llyin et al., 2004). Li et al. (2006) have made use of an integrative omics approach (genomics, transcriptomics and proteomics) to directly identify two genes as potential biomarkers for the diagnosis and therapy of lung cancer.

While omics technologies do offer several opportunities in biomarker discovery and cancer diagnostics, the data generated by these technologies is not reproducible or robust enough to be used clinically. Validation of omics findings in prospective, well-controlled clinical studies of diverse patients across multiple institutions is very difficult in view of the large number of patients required. Another challenge is the integration of biochemical, genetic, clinical and various omics data to better understand organisms and disease states. The greatest challenge is how to introduce and use these data in clinical practice. To achieve these goals, it is hoped that simple, fast, robust, portable and cost-effective clinical diagnosis devices can be moved from the bench to the bedside in near future (Zhang et al., 2007).

Cancer Biomarkers

Emerging genomic technologies can generate novel biomarkers that predict how individual cancer patients will respond to various treatments. Reliable identification and validation of cancer biomarkers still face certain technological, political and cultural hurdles that, if not addressed, could derail many of the anticipated benefits of biomarker research.

Survival rates for patients with the most common cancers, especially those detected at an advanced stage, are typically quite low—less than 10 per cent of patients with metastatic colon cancer and about 5 per cent of patients with pancreatic cancer survive 5 years or more (see Dalton and Friend, 2006).

Cancer therapies are still virtually 'one size fits all'; all patients within a given diagnostic category—usually based on tumour type and stage of disease—receive the same treatment despite the high biological heterogeneity from patient to patient. In their quest for better ways to match the right treatment with the right patient, many investigators are now turning to the promise of cancer biomarkers.

Biomarkers are quantifiable measurements of biologic homeostasis (i.e., what is 'normal'), so providing a reference frame for predicting or detecting what is 'abnormal'. Cancer biomarkers occur in several different forms, for instance, physiologic (patient performance status), images (mammograms), specific molecules (prostate-specific antigen, PSA), genetic alterations (*BRCA* mutations), gene or protein expression profiles (serum protein electrophoresis for detection of monoclonal gammopathies) and cell-based markers (circulating tumour cells). The range of cancer biomarkers has increased greatly to cover identification of single-nucleotide polymorphisms (SNPs), genomic profiling, transcriptome analysis and proteomic analysis (Simon and Wang, 2006). The new molecular technologies enable researchers to advance from a linear, single event-based concept of cancer pathogenesis to a better understanding of how changes in entire biosystems contribute to disease.

Three benefits that accrue from the implementation of molecularly based cancer biomarkers into patient care are: (a) their great potential to predict who will develop cancer and/or to detect the disease at an early stage (Hernandez, 2005); (b) biomarkers can guide treatment decisions; thus, cancer patients with biomarkers that predict a poor outcome may be selected for more rigorous treatments to increase their chance of survival, whereas those with biomarkers predicting a good outcome could be spared unnecessary or debilitating treatments; (c) biomarkers can help identification of new targets for drug development (see Dalton and Friend, 2006).

A wider use of cancer biomarkers can potentially usher in an era in which doctors need not make treatment choices based on population-based statistics but rather on the specific characteristics of individual patients and their tumour.

Personalized cancer care should be viewed as a continuous cycle which starts with the discovery of specific molecular alterations in tumours that are then linked to specific patient outcomes in clinical trials. Obtaining molecular profiles and clinical information at the level of individual patients allows translation of the information into more personalized cancer care. The underlying relational databases and health information systems in turn ensure more informed delivery of cancer therapies to future patients and can also guide the discovery of new therapies (Dalton and Friend, 2006).

Molecular Imaging

Medical imaging technologies now play a central role in clinical oncology. But the truly transformative power of imaging in the clinical management of cancer patients will take place in the coming few years. Molecularly targeted imaging agents could broadly expand the capabilities of conventional anatomical imaging methods. Molecular imaging will allow clinicians to not only see where a tumour is located in the body, but also to visualize the expression and activity of specific molecules (e.g., proteases and protein kinases) and biological processes (e.g., apoptosis, angiogenesis and metastasis) that influence tumour behaviour and/or response to therapy (Weissleder, 2006). This information may have a strong impact on cancer detection, individualized treatment and drug development. It will enhance our understanding of how cancer arises.

Biomarkers: Strengths and Weaknesses

Drug and diagnostic companies are keenly interested in the ability to predict the future. Instead of having to wait for several years and studying many patients, they would like to be able to identify those who have a disease, who can benefit from what drug and whether a drug will have unintended side effects. To meet these requirements, predictive tests are now entering the market. The first DNA micro-array test, called the AmpliChip Cytochrome P450 Genotyping Test has been developed by Roche Molecular Systems of Pleasanton, California. It measures how quickly an individual will metabolize a range of drugs; this helps physicians to select the optimal drug and dosage. Paik et al. (2004) discussed the Oncotype Dx test, which can assess tumour expression of 21 genes and predict how likely certain breast cancers are to recur and respond to chemotherapy. Assays that show whether tumours over-express marker proteins (e.g., HER2 and EGFR) help in assigning cancer treatments.

Table 8.2 shows some markers for various predictive tests that could prove useful for everything from target identification to patient care. Biomarkers are not only crucial for more efficient drug development but also in deciding patient-specific treatments.

While higher throughput technologies facilitate data collection, the irritating bottleneck is the long time required to understand and characterize new biomarkers. Also, while the 'omics' revolution offers several decision making tools, what is much more important is to know how to use them. One serious problem is finding biomarkers that

Table 8.2 Types of biomarkers (after Baker, 2005).

Role of biomarkers	Description	Examples
Disease diagnosis	Indicate the presence or likelihood of a particular disease in patients or in animal models.	High blood levels of proteins (troponin, C-reactive protein) associated with risk of stroke or heart disease, genotypes and gene expression profiles linked with cancer.
Surrogate endpoints	Serves as a substitute for desired clinical outcome and often can be measured long before meaningful clinical endpoints like mortality or morbidity.	Blood pressure, tumour shrinkage, psychometric testing, pain scales, CD4 blood count for HIV AIDS.
Efficacy or outcome	Correlate with the desired effect of a treatment, but the validation is not as high as surrogate endpoints.	Pain scales, lung function tests, electrocardiogram readings, bone density, blood or urine levels of proteins and other analytes associated with disease.
Mechanism	Suggest a drug affects the desired pathway.	Reveal downstream effects of the drug, such as activation or deactivation of enzymes and receptors.
Pharmaco-dynamic	Used in early clinical trials to determine the dose that has the highest response. This dose is often below the maximum tolerated dose.	Blood or urine levels of proteins and other analytes associated with disease.
Target	Show that a drug interacts with a particular target in *in vitro* studies, preclinical studies and, increasingly, in *in vivo* imaging studies.	PET imaging studies to show residence time on a receptor.
Toxicity	Indicate potentially harmful effects of a drug in cell-based, preclinical or clinical studies.	Q-T prolongation; induction of cytochrome P-450.
Bridging or translational	Used in both preclinical and clinical studies, may also be disease, efficacy or toxicity biomarkers.	Any of the above examples that can be assessed in both humans and animal models of disease.

can be extrapolated from animal models to humans. Inhibiting an enzyme in a mouse may have a strong effect whereas inhibiting the corresponding enzyme in humans may not have any clinical impact whatsoever (see Baker, 2005).

In some cases, use of biomarkers to predict clinical outcome can mislead (Frank and Hargreaves, 2003). A treatment can sometimes affect a biomarker but is irrelevant to a disease. One example: drugs that lower blood levels of prostate specific antigen (PSA) may or may not slow prostate cancer. Or the biomarker may not reflect clinically important effects of treatment, particularly if a drug works through several mechanisms (Baker, 2005).

The quintessence of finding biomarkers is to look for differences between groups that respond to a treatment and those that do not. Multivariate analysis or machine learning can spot differences or clusters of differences that distinguish members of one group from those of the other, at least for that particular sample set. However, the issue is so highly complex with many variations that some can discriminate the treatment group from control groups by chance and give misleadingly high statistical significance (Baker, 2005). Statistics and genomics are useful in finding biomarkers that identify patients most likely to benefit from treatment; and single nucleotide polymorphisms (SNPs) and statistics can usually separate nonresponders from responders, but the crucial point about biomarkers that predict drugs' efficacy is not a requirement for a more sophisticated statistical methodology but rather an understanding of how well the biomarker reflects the mechanism of disease. We want a drug to treat a disease, not a biomarker!

Unless a biomarker is identified, we usually cannot know whether it points to a specific disease or simply poor health. Biomarkers need to be confirmed in independent studies before being used to make decisions; the level of certainty required varies with the biomarker's purpose. For example, an immunohistochemical study might reveal whether a drug candidate blocks a particular kinase and hence warrant the decision to move the candidate into preclinical studies. Such a target biomarker would in fact be insufficient by itself to move a compound into clinical trials. The decision would rather depend on mechanism biomarkers that can detect downstream effects of the target and on even more rigorously validated outcome biomarkers which measure clinical aspects of the disease (Table 8.2).

One possible way to improve biomarker-enabled efficacy of drug development may involve replacing the idea of biomarker validation with one of qualification. The latter covers both the data backing a biomarker as well as its intended use, whereas the former implies an either/or kind of statistical correlation. There is need to create a framework that outlines increasing levels of confidence in a biomarker's predictions based on several lines of evidence and one that will allow different biomarkers to be considered together. A very specific biomarker could, for example, be combined with a very sensitive one.

Biostatisticians know that clusters of variables can be used to differentiate responders from nonresponders or people at high risk of disease from those at low risk. This is why panels of biomarkers have often been singly considered as more accurate than individual biomarkers. But the number needs to be critically considered. If the number of analytes to be measured is very large and very expensive, it may not provide useful additional information. According to some experts, predictive benefit falls completely between five and eight markers, with five generally being the most cost-effective (see Baker, 2005).

Multiple biomarkers can help in anticipating questions relating to drug behaviour or patient response. Combinatorial biomarkers will provide us the predictability needed in the clinic. Indeed, eventually even surrogate endpoints might be a composite of biomarkers. Since no clinical biomarker can capture all of the clinical benefits, companies should seriously think about multiple biomarkers with complementary predictive properties.

Biomarkers can potentially reshape the drug market, as has already happened in some cancer drugs: Herceptin (trastuzumab, a monoclonal antibody against HER-2 developed by Genentech in South San Francisco, California and Roche) got regulatory approval using Carpenteria; California-based DakoCytomation's test to select patients most likely to respond to the drug based on the levels of HER-2 expressed by the tumour. Novartis's Gleevec (imatinib) got quickly approved by focusing initially on a small patient population of nearly certain responders who had the Philadelphia chromosome, a translocation causing a kinase to become active.

Sooner or later, it appears certain that biomarker assays for noncancer therapies will move out of clinical trials and into the market where they will be used to classify disease and match patients with the most appropriate drug. The ultimate success of biomarkers will only be possible by changing the focus from finding them to understanding their physiological relevance.

Surrogate Endpoints

Some good examples of the most trusted and highly studied biomarkers are: blood pressure, LDL cholesterol levels and HIV load (see Fleming and DeMets, 1996; Woodcook, 2004). And yet, enthusiasm for using surrogate endpoints is waning with the realization that the expectations of clinicians about drugs' effects could be wrong. Two obvious problems of using a surrogate are that it may not predict the clinical outcome as expected; and that the surrogate measures only one of the many effects that a drug might have.

In vivo Diagnostics in Clinical Practice

The recent availability of promising new *in vivo* diagnostic agents has generated enthusiasm in the utility of *in vivo* diagnostics in clinical practice (Frangioni, 2006). There is a strong excitement over molecular imaging agents. *In vivo* diagnostic agents are exogenous compounds that are introduced into the body in order to detect and/or quantify a molecular or cellular target (Table 8.3).

Unfortunately, many promising *in vivo* diagnostics fail to reach the patients. Ideally, molecular imaging should permit detection and quantification of single cells, but it does not—the sensitivity is too low. Improved sensitivity is a must before imaging at the single-cell level in patients becomes a reality.

Only four clinical imaging modalities are capable of imaging all parts of the human body: computed tomography (CT), magnetic resonance imaging (MRI), single-photon emission CT (SPECT) and positron emission tomography (PET).

Ultrasonography and optical imaging are suitable only for certain organs and in restricted clinical situations. For various technical reasons, none of the four whole-body modalities is able to 'see' less than approximately 10^9 cells after the introduction of an exogenous targeted agent; to sense even that high number, all the cells must be present as a single, solid mass.

Molecular imaging has not yet advanced to a level where it can solve many important clinical problems, e.g., quantification of pancreatic β-cells during the progression of diabetes, detection of cancer before the incidence of angiogenesis or as small metastases and tracking of stem cells distributed diffusely throughout the body.

Fortunately, however, with further improvements in detector technology and innovative techniques for improving agent sensitivity, *in vivo* cell detection could improve

Table 8.3 *In vivo* diagnostic contrast agents approved by the FDA over the past few years (see www.fda.gov).

Year	Generic name	Targeted	Indication
2001	Perflutren lipid microspheres	No	Intravascular contrast for echocardiography (ultrasound)
2002	Perflexane lipid microspheres	No	Intravascular contrast for echocardiography (ultrasound)
2004	Gadobenate dimeglumine	No	Gadolinium-based intra- vascular contrast for MRI
	^{131}I-tositumomab	Yes(CD20)	SPECT agent for dosing of therapeutic monoclonal antibody

significantly in the near future. In the meanwhile, agents that have already passed preclinical scrutiny need to be translated to the clinic. Clinical translation faces several roadblocks. All diagnostic agents must undergo extensive preclinical and clinical testing before regulatory approval is granted. The failure to produce more than a few *in vivo* imaging agents to date can be attributed to at least five factors: inadequate preclinical critique and acceptance of small effect sizes; financial and time costs of navigating the regulatory system; intellectual property (IP) and patenting related issues; fear of litigation; and unpredictable industry timetables (Frangioni, 2006).

The most successful *in vivo* diagnostic agents so far have been nonspecific and general purpose but in the future we may see many novel agents specific for particular cells and their products, permitting agents to be chosen based on the needs of individual patients. For cancer, big profits or markets do not exist and although the orphan drug model provides benefit to a small number of patients, it does so at a huge cost to society.

Barriers to Innovative Diagnostics

Technology adoption and adequate remuneration seem to act as barriers to innovative diagnostics (Billings, 2006). The results of diagnostic tests are important for answering key questions like who should be hospitalized. Does a patient have a significant illness? Or, what specific treatments are indicated? The answers to these queries are not only crucial to patients but also quite costly. Yet the quantum of investment in diagnostics is meagre as compared to the huge investments in pharmaceuticals and in-patient care.

Some have pointed to an era when it would be possible to prevent or delay illness and to personalize medical care. In our march to that era, healthcare systems everywhere will need to cross at least three major hurdles: first, the difficulty in convincing that new tests should be adopted; second, the difficulty in obtaining appropriate payment for an innovative diagnostic that is equitable to the investment in research and development; and finally, convincing people that the benefits of diagnostic-driven health are not outweighed by privacy and discrimination fears (Billings, 2006).

Disease Proteomics

A sequence-based framework is now available for mining proteomes; this has aroused keen interest in applying proteomics to foster a better understanding of disease processes, develop new biomarkers for diagnosis and early detection of disease and speed up drug development (Petricoin et al., 2002; Hanash, 2003).

Some promising areas of research in disease proteomics include: delineation of altered protein expression at the whole-cell or tissue levels, in subcellular structures, in protein complexes and in biological fluids; the development of novel biomarkers for diagnosis and early detection of disease; the identification of new targets for therapeutics and the potential for accelerating drug development through improved strategies for evaluating therapeutic effect and toxicity. Current proteome profiling technologies emphasize the need for sensitivity and throughput. But no singular technology can meet the needs of all types of proteomics-based investigations, from expression proteomics to functional proteomics, particularly as they relate to disease.

Several studies have identified disease-related changes in protein expression, primarily using 2D PAGE and mass spectrometry (see Van Eyk, 2001; Hanash, 2003). Online

2D gel-derived databases of protein expression in the myocardium for human and other species have been created (Evans et al., 1997). These databases allow investigators to compare data and establish reference standards. Although only a small fraction of the proteome has been analysed, marked changes in the composition of the cardiac proteome have been detected—changes that affect proteins with diverse functions. Altered overall levels of specific proteins or of post-translational modifications of proteins such as myosin light chain 2 have been reported in the failing heart (van der Velden et al., 2001). Protein-expression studies have also revealed proteins that showed new disease-related post-translational modifications with predicted functional relevance (Evans et al., 1997).

In the advanced version of 2D PAGE, immobilized pH gradients (IPGs) in which the pH gradient is fixed within the acrylamide matrix can be formed. IPGs allow making of gels that cover a defined pH range, from wide to narrow, or the use of 'zoom gels' in which the protein contents of an individual sample are first fractionated into narrow pH ranges under low resolution, where after each fraction can be efficiently separated by 2D PAGE (Zuo and Speicher, 2002). The pre-fractionation of serum using this new approach has allowed detection of low-abundance and potentially new circulating disease-marker proteins. Another innovation is differential in-gel electrophoresis (DIGE): two pools of proteins are labelled with different fluorescent dyes (Patton, 2002) and the labelled proteins can be mixed and separated in the same 2D gel. Zhou et al. (2001) used 2D DIGE to quantify the differences in protein expression between oesophageal carcinoma cells and normal epithelial cells. Several different proteins are either upregulated or downregulated in cancer cells (Hanash, 2003).

Unfortunately, the usefulness of even improved 2D gels is limited by their requirement for a fairly large amount of sample. In this respect, various non-gel-based approaches that rely on liquid-based separations of proteins or peptides, with or without tagging, may have greater utility for disease proteomics, particularly due to their high potential for automation.

Advances in microfluidic technology can enhance automated separation of proteins in complex lysates using much reduced sample amounts. Other notable recent developments are exemplified by non-separation-based strategies, including direct profiling using mass spectrometry or the use of protein micro-arrays. Mass spectrometry can be applied to the *in situ* proteomic analysis of tissues—this allows imaging of protein expression in normal and diseased tissues. Tumour analyses using this approach have revealed differences in protein expression between normal and tumour tissues that may have specificity for different tumour types (Stoeckli et al., 2001).

DNA and Protein Micro-arrays

Profiling of gene expression by using DNA arrays has exerted a tremendous impact on biomedical research. Unsuspected associations between genes and specific clinical features of disease have been uncovered and are helping devise new molecular-based classifications of disease. DNA micro-arrays have helped in examining pathologically homogeneous sets of tumours so as to identify clinically relevant subtypes, pathologically distinct subtypes of tumours of the same lineage to identify molecular correlates, or tumours of different lineages to identify molecular signatures for each lineage (see Brenton et al., 2001; van de Vijver et al., 2002).

DNA micro-array studies have great utility for revealing clinically informative patterns of gene expression. However, the use of DNA micro-arrays does not eliminate the need for other types of profiling technologies that go beyond measuring RNA levels, particularly for disease-related investigations and also that DNA micro-arrays have limited utility for the analysis of biological fluids. Many changes can occur in proteins that are not reflected in changes at the RNA level; this warrants direct analysis of gene expression at the protein level. Attempts are underway to develop micro-arrays or biochips that allow the systematic analysis of thousands of proteins.

Unlike DNA micro-arrays, which provide a measure of gene expression (i.e., RNA levels), protein micro-array strategies that address several different features of proteins altered in disease are badly needed. These include, on the one hand, determination of their levels in biological samples and, on the other, understanding their interactions with other proteins, antibodies, drugs or various small ligands. The pressing need for protein chips has spurred new strategies for producing biochips having utility for biomedical investigations. New classes of capture agents have been designed. For assays of protein interaction, biochips containing either peptides or proteins are being produced (Pellois et al., 2002).

Profiling studies of disease tissue that have used protein micro-arrays are now emerging. Paweletz et al. (2001) developed a reverse-phase protein array approach for immobilizing a tissue's proteins. Application of protein micro-arrays can help in the identification of proteins that induce an antibody response in autoimmune disorders (Robinson et al., 2002) such as systemic lupus erythematosus and rheumatoid arthritis, as well as cancer.

One major problem in making biochips for global analysis of protein expression is the lack of comprehensive sets of antibodies. Another complication stems from the fact that proteins undergo post-translational modifications which can affect their functions (see, however, Madoz-Gurpide et al., 2001).

Disease Biomarkers

Proteomics are used for the identification of disease markers. Comparative analysis of protein expression in normal and diseased tissues is used to identify abnormally expressed proteins that may represent new markers, analysis of secreted proteins in cell lines and primary cultures and direct serum protein profiling (Hanash, 2003). Mass spectrometry facilitates serum analysis (Petricoin et al., 2002) to have profiles of peptides and proteins in biological fluids without protein separations. Such an approach is well suited for marker identification as its sample requirements are low and throughput high. The surface-enhanced laser desorption/ionization technology may have potential application.

Also, cancer markers have been identified through the analysis of serum for autoantibodies against tumour proteins. An immune response to cancer in humans has been demonstrated by the identification of autoantibodies against certain intracellular and surface antigens detectable in sera from patients with different cancer types (Hanash, 2003a). The identification of tumour antigens that elicit an antibody response may be useful in cancer screening, diagnosis or in establishing prognosis and in immunotherapy against the disease.

Indeed, there are several approaches for the detection of tumour antigens that induce an immune response. Antigens have been detected by screening expression libraries with patient sera or, by using a random peptide-library approach (see Yamamoto et al., 1996; Soussi, 1996; Old and Chen, 1998). For most antigenic proteins, it appears that post-translational modifications contribute to the immune response (Le Naour, 2001). Micro-arrays containing proteins derived from tumour cells carry the potential of significantly increasing the rate of discovery of tumour antigens and yielding a molecular signature for immune responses directed against protein targets in different types of cancer (Madoz-Gurpide et al., 2001).

Disease-related Functional Proteomics

Some technologies for direct functional analysis of altered levels or post-translational modification states of proteins in disease, are exemplified by the need to analyse protein complexes and their disruption in disease, to a high-throughput assay of the activity of various classes of proteins and to manipulate the levels and activities of individual proteins in a cellular context, so as to find their role in biological processes and disease states (Hanash, 2003).

Although several strategies are in use for studies of protein complexes and protein-protein interactions, there has been only limited application of activity-based proteomics to disease investigations, in its early stages (Vondriska and Ping, 2002). Activity-based assays of normal and diseased tissue will probably be limited to the analysis of one class of proteins at a time.

Certain approaches are being designed to make directed protein manipulations other than by decreasing or increasing their overall amounts, as can be done by gene manipulations. These approaches can inactivate a specific site in a protein in a time-dependent and localization-restricted manner, as with chromophore-assisted laser inactivation (CALI) that allows assessment of the disease relevance of the site and enables one to revert a cellular phenotype to a more normal state. Inactivation of protein targets involved in different signal-transduction pathways in cancer using CALI has also been reported (Rubenwolf et al., 2002).

Proteomics for Drug Development

The pharmaceutical industry has a keen interest in proteomics—most drugs target proteins and so proteomics could have great utility for drug development. Under favourable conditions, the use of proteomics may advance many aspects of drug development by identifying new targets and facilitating assessment of drug action and toxicity.

Lewis et al. (2000) combined functional proteomics with selective activation and inhibition of certain kinases with a view to identifying cellular targets; they discovered some new targets, pointing to new roles for a signalling cascade in cellular processes of nuclear transport, nucleotide excision repair, nucleosome assembly, membrane transport and cytoskeletal regulation. Likewise, McKerrow et al. (2000) have identified some proteases most suitable for drug targeting.

Activity-based screening offers a basis for selecting targets in the development of inhibitors to specific proteases. Protein biochips may well provide a high-throughput platform for target identification. Biochips developed for interaction studies may be important in lead-compound optimization and so could speed up drug development by facilitating evaluation of lead compounds for specificity and selectivity in binding to drug targets. According to Hanash, proteome alterations in disease possibly occur in different ways that cannot be predicted from genomic analysis. A better understanding of these alterations should have a substantial impact in medicine. Although a fairly useful basket of proteomics technologies is available for disease-related applications, there is need for continuing technological innovations to increase sensitivity, reduce sample requirement, increase throughput and more effectively detect protein alterations such as post-translational modifications. The use of these technologies will go a long way in meeting the need for better diagnostics and to shorten the path for developing effective therapy.

Protein Chips to Map Yeast Kinase Network

Recent research into the molecular communications between proteins that govern the lives of yeast cells has scored another victory for high-throughput biology. A Yale University team, led by Michael Snyder used glass chips arrayed with thousands of yeast proteins to track down the molecular targets of the organism's protein kinase. These enzymes modify the function of other proteins by tagging them with a phosphate group. About 160 interactions between specific yeast kinases and their targets had already been identified earlier. The chip study added more than 4000 and allowed the Yale researchers to map out a complex signalling network within yeast cells. Drug makers are enthusiastic in reviewing this new bounty of results to find similar kinase interactions in human cells that they can affect (Service, 2005).

Snyder et al. at first developed protein chips displaying the majority of yeast proteins. Invitrogen in Carlsbad (California), which makes these chips commercially, provided ones that harbour 4088 of yeast's 6000 or so proteins for Snyder's new research. Snyder could express and purify 87 of yeast's 122 protein kinases. Each kinase was washed over a different chip along with radiolabelled ATP which provides the phosphate group that kinases attach to a targeted protein. An autoradiography instrument then imaged sites on the chips where a radiolabelled phosphate group had modified a protein.

The results showed 4192 interactions between the yeast kinases and some 1300 different protein targets. Snyder was surprised at the targets of a widely studied family of three protein kinases. It was previously concluded that these three were redundant, i.e., if one or two were absent, the third took their place and allowed the yeast cells to survive. That suggested that they phosphorylate the same proteins. But Snyder found that each kinase had a very different profile of targets.

Besides teasing out individual kinase-protein interactions, the research team integrated their results with other yeast protein data sets, including that for the transcription factors that turn genes on and off. This enabled them to build a complex map of protein encounters that regulate life in yeast cells. Snyder reported that eight particular patterns of protein interactions showed up repeatedly. For instance, so-called adaptor proteins interact with both a kinase and a protein they modify. These adaptor proteins probably help to control the rate at which other proteins are activated.

Pharmaceutical companies are most interested in the implication of this work. Protein kinases are very important drug targets, with kinase inhibitors such as the cancer drugs Herceptin and Gleevec accounting for billions of dollars an year in sales. Even though the Yale group's yeast research does not reveal the critical kinases at work in humans, it does give drug companies a clue to identifying equivalent kinase interactions in humans and possibly clues about how to block them (Service, 2005).

Carbohydrate-based Diagnostics

Our understanding of the different glycoconjugates bound to cells, proteins and organisms has lagged far behind advances in genomics and proteomics. Carbohydrate sequencing and the synthesis of defined oligosaccharides have catalyzed considerable progress in glycomics research. Synthetic tools and high-throughput experiments such as carbohydrate arrays are now beginning to impact biological research—these techniques can now be applied to the development of carbohydrate-based diagnostics, vaccines and therapeutics (Seeberger and Werz, 2007).

Glycomics deals with the study of the structural and functional aspects of the various glycoconjugates present on proteins, cells and, in some cases, even whole organisms. Its more developed counterparts are genomics and proteomics which deal with nucleic acids and proteins, respectively. The term glycoconjugate covers diverse kinds of biooligomers and biopolymers.

Such different natural products as glycoproteins, glycolipids, glycosaminoglycans and glycosylphosphatidylinositol anchors are summarily known as sugars (Varki et al., 1999). Even oligosaccharide chains, being branched, are highly complex as compared to the typically linear peptides and oligonucleotides. Further, since they are not under direct genetic control, glycoconjugates are usually more heterogeneous.

Amplification methods analogous to the polymerase chain reaction (PCR) for nucleic acids or bacterial expression systems for protein production are not available for glycoconjugates; this is why until recently, isolation of carbohydrates used to be the only way to procure these natural products.

Indeed, overall progress in glycobiology has suffered greatly from a lack of tools such as those for studying nucleic acids and proteins, including automated sequencing, automated synthesis, high-throughput micro-array screening and detailed structure elucidation, including X-ray analyses (Hunkapiller et al., 1991; Grant et al., 1997; Caruthers, 1985; Merrifield, 1997). Also, carbohydrate synthesis methods are tedious and time-consuming (Ernst et al., 2000). Laroy et al. (2006) have discussed glycome mapping by using DNA sequencing equipment.

Biomarkers and Trade-off Optimization

Biomarkers can be measured in a patient's blood, tissue, urine and cerebrospinal fluid for use in various clinical settings. Besides the several successful biomarkers already developed, advances in genetics and proteomics have the potential to develop novel and informative biomarkers that could transform the application of molecular biology to human disease. In this effort, the application of biomarkers to cancer is in the forefront because of the unique association of genomic changes in cancer cells with the disease process (Hartwell et al., 2006).

DNA-based biomarkers have been incorporated into routine patient management and enhance the utility of appropriate diagnostic tests. Cancer being a highly complex disease, the application of suitable biomarkers to different patients as well as different states of the disease enables physicians to distinguish among the different possibilities as well as the multistep nature of cancer treatment.

Biomarker-based diagnostics for cancer can be used for: (a) risk assessment, (b) noninvasive screening for early-stage disease, (c) detection and localization, (d) disease stratification and prognosis, (e) response to therapy and (f) screening for disease recurrence. In this series, cost and potential morbidity increase progressively from (a) to (f).

The objectives in applying diagnostic tests include: (i) identification of individuals harbouring potentially life-threatening cancers at the earliest stage possible, (ii) avoiding false-positive tests and diagnosing of cancers that would otherwise not threaten a person's well-being or expose him to psychological stress and unnecessary treatments and (iii) minimizing the overall cost of the program. However, no single test may fully satisfy all these objectives. This means that sensitivity, specificity and cost tend to become trade-offs in the application of diagnostics to disease management.

For cancer screening, besides sensitivity and specificity, overdiagnosis also has to be considered—there may be no need to detect cancer that would never manifest into observable symptoms during a person's lifetime. An example (see Thompson et al., 2005) is that of prostate-specific antigen, a biomarker with fairly low sensitivity; it becomes more problematic by its weak ability to distinguish latent cancers that would never cause symptoms from cancers that are aggressive or lethal. Overdiagnosis not only increases healthcare costs but also provides no positive health benefits and can cause a net loss of health owing to the side effects of unnecessary treatment. Specificity refers to the ability of a test to rule out cancer in individuals who do not have cancer. Specificity is important because false-positive screening tests can lead to costly additional testing that may even carry a morbidity risk.

One method for optimizing trade-offs of sensitivity, specificity and cost is to use multiple biomarkers: a biomarker with high sensitivity and low specificity (which would detect potentially lethal cancers but would result in many false positives) may be combined with a second biomarker that shows less sensitivity but higher specificity (Hartwell et al., 2006).

As discussed by Hulka (1988), several different criteria determine whether some particular diagnostic screening test will succeed or fail. Some of these criteria are listed below. It is very important that all these criteria are carefully considered for critically evaluating biomarkers for cancer screening.

1. The disease should represent a substantial burden at the public health level and should have a prevalent, asymptomatic, non-metastatic phase.
2. It should be possible to recognize the asymptomatic, non-metastatic phase.
3. The screening test should show reasonable sensitivity, specificity and predictive value. It should be of low risk and low cost. It should be acceptable to both the screeners and the person screened.
4. The curative potential of early stage cancer should be much better than that of advanced stages of disease.
5. Treatment of patients whose disease is detected by screening should decrease cause-specific mortality (see Hulka, 1988; Hartwell et al., 2006).

Stratification of risk proves helpful for selecting abnormal findings for biopsy. Biomarkers are very important in stratification of screening results to reduce invasive follow-up procedures, as for instance, initial cervical cancer screening with pap smears; this screening is quite cheap, but dysplastic results require follow-up by colposcopy with cervical biopsies. Human papillomavirus typing of pap smears read as 'atypical cells of uncertain significance' facilitates identification of low-risk lesions and decreases the number of colposcopies in those women who are least likely to have significant pathology (Kim et al., 2002). Newer imaging methods involving biomarkers (see Mankoff and Krohn, 2006) can characterize cancer and direct its treatment. However, the ability of imaging to identify *in vivo* tumour characteristics likely to lead to aggressive behaviour and therapy resistance, such as hypoxia or drug efflux transporter expression, can move patients toward therapies that circumvent resistance (Rajendran and Krohn, 2002; Sasongko et al., 2005).

Imaging complements tissue-based biomarkers for stratification and prognosis. Biomarkers based on assay of biopsy samples can be useful even for very small deposits of cancer—such deposits are often below the detection threshold for cancer imaging. The identification of tumour-derived DNA in local body fluids carries considerable diagnostic promise for several solid tumours.

Markers for Therapeutic Response

Improved diagnostics can accelerate novel drug development by shortening clinical trials, identifying responsive patients and revealing toxic side- effects. Biomarkers in malignant tissues are also often used to predict therapeutic response. One example: the presence of epidermal growth factor receptor (EGFR) mutations is associated with the response to EGFR inhibitors in lung cancer (Lynch et al., 2004).

Functional imaging enables detection of early response by measuring molecular changes, rather than waiting for a change in tumour size. Therapeutic approaches can be tested quickly; if they do not work, they can be abandoned (Weber, 2005).

Surveillance for Disease Recurrence

The risk of cancer recurrence is quite high in patients who have previously had cancer, even for patients who were in remission for over five years. Cancer survivors fall in a high risk group that could benefit from surveillance for early detection of disease recurrence. False-positive surveillance tests should be avoided. In this context biomarkers could prove useful. The characteristics of the initial tumour being already known, biomarkers could in some cases be designed to detect the patient's tumour cells, thereby maximizing specificity (Hartwell et al., 2006).

Indeed, biomarkers that can detect recurrent cancer early could also provide effective treatment for a selected subset of solid-tumour patients with metastatic disease (see Robbins, 2006). Biomarkers capable of detecting micrometastatic disease recurrence may enable definitive clinical trials to test the curative potential of systemic therapies.

Systems Approach to Biomarker Assessment

Ideally, any new biomarker employed for management of a particular cancer should be assessed directly by measuring its impact on survival and costs in a prospective, randomized, controlled experiment. But the high costs, together with regulatory and healthcare market constraints and pressures usually preclude such assessments. As an alternative, simulation modelling is being increasingly used to predict effects of new biomarker technologies on overall outcomes (Quaranta et al., 2005). A simulation approach optimizes the sensitivity, specificity and cost trade-offs at each step and identifies critical points where more definitive biomarkers should be used.

Companion Diagnostics for Mutation-targeted Therapies

Although cancer cells can differ from normal cells in many respects, it is only the genetic differences that unequivocally distinguish the former from the latter. Not surprisingly, therefore, many recent therapeutic advances are based on agents that specifically target the products of the genes that are mutated in cancer cells. These advances are facilitating identification of the patients most likely to benefit from such therapies. Development and use of companion diagnostic tests can simplify the drug discovery process (see Torrance et al., 2001; Komarova and Wodarz, 2005), make clinical trials more efficient and informative and be used to personalize therapy of individual cancer patients.

Cancer cells can outgrow neighbouring cells, change the structure of the tissue in which they appear and survive adverse environments that are hypoxic, hypoglycemic or lack growth factors. Mutations in three types of genes are involved in the ability of cancer cells to survive in their hostile environment: oncogenes, tumour-suppressor genes and stability genes. Mutations in oncogenes and tumour-suppressor genes can directly promote net cell growth by stimulating cell birth or inhibiting cell death. Mutations in stability genes indirectly promote tumourigenesis by allowing the accumulation of mutations at higher than normal rates, thereby facilitating more rapid acclimatization of cancer cells to new microenvironments (Papadopoulos et al., 2006).

The products of mutated oncogenes are either constitutively active or active under conditions in which the normal gene product is inactive. Activating mutations include translocations, amplifications and point mutations that can affect the regulation or activity of the gene product. Usually, a mutation in one paternal or maternal allele can suffice for activation. On the other hand, as tumour-suppressor genes are inactivated by mutations or epigenetic mechanisms, both the maternal and paternal alleles need to be inactivated to remove the inhibitory potential of tumour-suppressor gene products. Most recent therapeutic efforts have targeted the products of oncogenes that are activated in various cancers.

All currently used chemotherapeutic drugs are 'targeted' in the sense that they interact with specific intracellular components. Some examples are: docetaxel (Taxotere) that binds to tubulin; methotrexate inhibits dihydrofolate reductase; and cisplatin binds to DNA. In contrast, mutation-targeted therapies interact with proteins that are different in the cancer cell than in any normal cell—as a result of somatic mutation, the amino acid sequence or the concentration of the mutant gene product differs from that in normal cells. Moreover, the aberrant proteins activate downstream pathways under conditions in which the pathways would be inactive in normal cells. This explains why mutation-targeted therapies selectively inhibit cancer cell growth. As a corollary, mutation-targeted therapeutic agents may not be active against those cancers which lack mutations of their target. This contrasts sharply with conventional chemotherapeutic agents, in which it is impossible to predict which cancers will respond before clinical trials. The optimal use of these agents requires early development of companion diagnostic methods to determine which tumours contain genetic alterations of the target.

At least three requirements for an effective companion diagnostic test are: first, availability of material suitable for testing; second, mutations that are predictive of a therapeutic response; and third, a reliable and cost-effective method for identifying mutations. Some currently used methods in companion diagnostics are described in Table 8.4. Choice of the warranted assay for the detection of genetic alterations depends on the

Table 8.4 Relative strengths and weaknesses of currently adopted cancer diagnostic methods (after Papadopoulos et al., 2006).

Advantages	Disadvantages
Immunohistochemistry	
Detect fewer mutant-containing cells amongst many normal cells; routinely performed in hospital labs; fast and cost effective.	Not quantitative. The fraction of cells expressing the antibody-reacted protein can be determined, but the level of protein within individual cells can only be crudely estimated; does not distinguish between expression due to gene amplification versus other, nongenetic causes.
Cytogenetics	
Quantitative. Provides clear evidence of genetic alterations.	Only a few cells can be analysed as large numbers of mitotic cells are difficult to obtain. Process is tedious and time consuming.
FISH	
Quantitative. Provides clear evidence of genetic alterations. Large number of cells can be analysed.	Time consuming. Requires special equipment. More expensive than other tests.
qPCR	
Very sensitive with large dynamic range.	Careful controls are essential for reliable interpretation of data. Results depend on sample quality. Does not distinguish between a lot of cells with a little transcript or a few cells with a lot of transcript.
DNA sequencing	
Provides clear evidence of somatic mutations.	Does not detect some important mutations such as deletions of an entire exon or amplification. Insensitive, as detection requires the mutation to be present in at least 20 per cent of the DNA templates in the sample.
Indirect mutation analysis	
Cost effective and usually more sensitive than sequencing when neoplastic cells represent a minor fraction of the total cells in the clinical sample.	Some mutations cannot be detected, even when present in a large fraction of the cells; extensive optimization required to detect mutations in individual genes or PCR fragments; in general, the presumptive mutation needs to be detected and defined by sequencing.
Mutation specific assays	
Cost effective and usually more sensitive than sequencing when neoplastic cells represent a minor fraction of the total cells in the clinical sample.	Can only identify a few predefined mutations rather than any mutation that happens to be present in the cancer. Requires considerable optimization.
Micro-arrays	
Massive, parallel, high-throughput interrogation of many genes; patterns of gene expression are useful for prognostication.	Companion diagnostic tests generally need to interrogate only one or a few genes per sample and micro-arrays are not suitable for this purpose. Requires careful controls to ensure reproducibility.

Box 8.1: Currently used methods for cancer diagnostics (after Papadopoulos et al., 2006).

1. **Immunohistochemistry** Using antibodies against target proteins to determine whether proteins are present in cells within the specimen.
2. **Cytogenetics** Mitotic cells are analysed to find any gross chromosomal abnormalities such as translocations and amplifications.
3. **FISH** Use of fluorescent or colorimetric probes to detect specific changes such as translocations and amplifications (see also Hicks and Tubbs, 2005).
4. **qPCR** This amplifies a specific gene or transcript and quantifies the amplified template molecules. It can be used to determine amplification of a gene or the presence of a translocated gene.
5. **DNA sequencing** The gene(s) are first amplified by PCR, whereafter certain direct methods are employed to determine the sequence of the entire PCR product.
6. **Indirect mutation analysis** The target sequence is at first amplified by PCR. Physical or enzymatic methods are then used to distinguish mutant from wild-type PCR fragments.
7. **Mutation-specific assays** These involve the use of probes which bind to mutant, but not wild-type sequences, single base extension, oligonucleotide ligation and various hybridization-based methods.
8. **Micro-arrays** Labelled DNA or RNA from clinical specimen is hybridized to ordered arrays of nucleic acids (usually oligonucleotides) representing thousands of genes. Micro-arrays point to amplification when used with DNA and overexpression when used with RNA (Papadopoulos et al., 2006).

Notes: FISH, fluorescent *in situ* hybridization; PCR, polymerase chain reaction.

type of mutation to be detected: when the targeted gene can be mutated in multiple different ways, direct or indirect sequencing methods are appropriate. But if the goal is to identify one or a small array of predefined mutations, then a mutation-specific method should be employed. If an increased copy number of the target gene, rather than a subtle change in amino acid sequence is being sought, then fluorescent *in situ* hybridization (FISH) or (q)PCR will be suitable (see Box 8.1).

There are robust connections between various new cancer therapies and diagnostic tests for the genetic alterations that the drugs target (see also Komarova and Wodarz, 2005). Companion diagnostic tests are indispensable for directing the conduct of clinical trials and eventual treatment of cancer patients with such drugs. Papadopoulos et al. have illustrated the use of companion diagnostics in the provision of five drugs approved by the US FDA that target the products of genes that are mutated in cancers. Table 8.5 shows the drugs, their targets and the companion tests.

The drug Gefitinib at first quite effectively treats certain types of lung cancer, but most cancers soon develop resistance to it. It appears that Gefitinib inhibits the enzyme EGFR kinase and around half of the resistance cases are due to mutations in this target. Among the rest, Jänne et al. (2007) found that some resistant cells show increased expression of a tyrosine-kinase receptor named MET. This activates the same signalling pathway that EGFR kinase triggers—a pathway that mediates cell survival. According to these researchers, the MET gene had multiplied rather than mutated and that inhibiting MET restored the cells' sensitivity to Gefitinib.

As rightly pointed out by Papadopoulos; the five drugs represent only the first step toward the development of mutation-specific therapeutics. These drugs inhibit the mutant form of the target and also interact with or inhibit the wild-type form. The model employed to explain the response to these agents (see Papadopoulos et al., 2006, for details) involves 'addiction' (Weinstein, 2002)—the idea that cancer cells evolve specific

Table 8.5 Five anti-cancer drugs that target mutant genes (after Papadopoulos et al., 2006)*.

Brand name; manufacturer	Mechanism of action	Known target protein	Targeted mutation	Diagnostic test	Disease	Purpose
Imatinib mesylate (Gleevec; Novartis)	Tyrosine kinase inhibitor	BCR-ABL	Translocation	Cytogenetics, FISH, PCR*	CML	Suitability for therapy
		BCR-ABL	Missense mutations/ presence of RNA	Sequencing/ PCR	CML	Monitor response to therapy and drug resistance
Trastuzumab (Herceptin; Genentech)	Antibody	ERBB2	Amplification	Immunohisto-chemistry, FISH	Breast cancer	Suitability for therapy
Cetuximab (Erbitux; ImClone Systems)	Antibody	EGFR	Amplification	Immunohisto-chemistry, FISH	Colo-rectal cancer**	Suitability for therapy
Gefitinib (Iressa; Astra-Zeneca)	Tyrosine kinase inhibitor	EGFR	Activating mutations in the kinase domain	Sequencing	NSCLC	Suitability for therapy
Erlotinib (Tarceva; OSI Pharma-ceutical/ Genentech)	Tyrosine kinase inhibitor	EGFR	Activating mutations in the kinase domain	Sequencing	NSCLC	Suitability for therapy#

* BCR-ABL, Breakpoint cluster region—Abelson; ERBB2, v-erb-b2 erythroblastic leukaemia viral oncogene homolog 2; EGFR, epidermal growth factor receptor; CML, chronic myelogenous leukaemia; NSCLC, non-small cell lung cancer; FISH, fluorescent *in situ* hybridization; qRT-PCR, quantitative reverse transcription polymerase chain reaction.

** see Barber et al. (2004);

see Tsao et al. (2005)

genetic alterations because these mutations confer some selective growth advantage which allows them to survive under unfavourable conditions. The cancer cells depend on these mutated gene products for their survival; any interference with signalling from these genes prohibits growth. Normal cells, in contrast, are not so dependent on such signalling (Papadopoulos et al., 2006).

The BRCA1 tumour-suppressor is associated with hereditary breast and ovarian cancer and helps in maintaining genomic stability (Venkitaraman, 2002). It contains an N-terminal RING domain, a Ser-Gln (SQ) cluster domain and two BRCT (BRCA1 C-terminal) repeats; all these make up a phosphopeptide recognition domain that binds peptides containing a phospho-SXXF motif (S is Ser, F is Phe and X varies) (Yu et al. 2003). The domain is needed for tumour suppression. By dimerizing with BARD1 (BRCA1-associated RING domain protein) through the RING domain, BRCA1 forms an E3 ubiquitin ligase (Ruffner et al., 2001). With a view to identifying those proteins which bind BRCA1 BRCT domains, Wang et al. (2007) combined peptide affinity purification, stable isotope labelling with amino acids in cell culture and mass spectrometry; the aim was to quantify phosphopeptides that directly bind to BRCA1 BRCT domains.

Phosphopeptide affinity proteomic analysis identified a protein, Abraxas, that directly binds the BRCA1 (BRCA1-associated C-terminal helicase) and CtIP (CtBP-interacting protein), forming a third type of BRCA1 complex. Abraxas recruits the ubiquitin-interacting motif (UIM)-containing protein RAP80 to BRCA1.

Both Abraxas and RAP80 were required for DNA damage resistance, G_2/M checkpoint control and DNA repair. RAP80 was required for optimal accumulation of BRCA1 on damaged DNA (foci) in response to ionizing radiation and the UIM domains alone were capable of foci formation. The RAP80-Abraxas complex may help recruit BRCA1 to DNA damage sites partly through recognition of ubiquitinated proteins (Ruffner et al., 2001).

It is well-known that DNA repair involves several molecular recognition steps that enable DNA damage response proteins to localize at and near DNA lesions. Failure of these responses causes genomic instability and predisposition to malignancy (Wang et al., 2005). Binding of the mediator of DNA damage checkpoint 1 (MDC1) protein to the phosphorylated tail of histone H2AX (γH2AX) facilitates the formation of BRCA1 nuclear foci at DSBs (double strand breaks) (Stewart et al., 2003).

Mutations affecting the BRCT domains of tumour-suppressor BRCA1 disrupt the recruitment of this protein to DNA DSBs. The molecular structures at DSBs recognized by BRCA1 are not known.

Sobhian et al. have studied the interaction of the BRCA1 BRCT domain with RAP80, a ubiquitin-binding protein. RAP80 targets a complex containing the BRCA1-BARD1 (BRCA1-associated ring domain protein 1) E3 ligase and the deubiquitinating enzyme (DUB) BRCC36 to MDC1-γH2AX-dependent lysine^{6}- and lysine^{63}-linked ubiquitin polymers at DSBs. These events are required for cell cycle checkpoint and repair responses to ionizing radiation, implicating ubiquitin chain recognition and turnover in the BRCA1-mediated repair of DSBs.

Kim et al. (2007) have identified receptor-associated protein 80 (RAP80) as BRCA1-interacting protein in humans. RAP80 contains a tandem ubiquitin-interacting motif domain, which is required for its binding with ubiquitin *in vitro* and its damage-induced foci formation *in vivo*. Moreover, RAP80 specifically recruits BRCA1 to DNA damage sites and functions with BRCA1 in G_2/M checkpoint control. Together, these results suggest the existence of an ubiquitination-dependent signalling pathway involved in the DNA damage response (Kim et al., 2007; see also Sobhian et al., 2007; Wang et al., 2007).

Indeed, it appears that many cell cycle checkpoint proteins, including ATM, Chk2, BRCA1 and *p53* perform crucial roles in maintaining genomic stability. Their mutation can result in increased tumour incidence and highlights the importance of the integrity of DNA damage pathways in tumour suppression. As a BRCA1-associated protein involved in DNA damage checkpoint control, RAP80 may also function as a tumour-suppressor and it may be dysregulated or mutated in human patients.

Probes to Detect Gene Expression

Such imaging tools as X-rays, positron emission tomography (PET) and magnetic resonance imaging (MRI) enable physicians to examine the inner workings of the body and they show fundamentally the same organs and tissue masses. This ability has now been extended to medical imaging that looks beyond general anatomy into the molecular workings of tissues. Probes that give off a detectable signal upon encountering a specific molecule, such as the product of a particular gene have been developed (see Bogdanov and Weissleder,

1998). Researchers hope to pinpoint a tissue's exact metabolic state. This strategy has been used to track the transfer of genes in gene therapy experiments and map the distribution of an animal's own proteins. Work is underway to develop the ability to image the effectiveness of cancer therapy to map when different genes get turned on during development - all without any surgical operation or testing in the lab (Service, 1998).

Novel molecular probes are being developed to track gene therapy and cancer treatment. Genes involved in cancer and other diseases are being unmasked as also the exact shape of the proteins for which they code. That knowledge, in turn, enables researchers to design specific new molecular imaging probes that can illuminate one gene or protein while all else remains dark. To turn on this light, use is made of true imaging techniques such as PET, which tracks gamma rays from tiny amounts of radioactive elements injected into the body. In an improved version of PET, neuroscientists can add the radiolabels to organic compounds that bind selectively to particular types of receptors that decorate the outside of nerve cells in the brain. This approach has enabled mapping the distribution of nerve cells that use dopamine and serotonin. It is hoped to reproduce this level of selectivity throughout the body.

PET has already been used to image the expression of a transplanted gene in live animals (this is not possible with autoradiography). Researchers have also developed a technique in which a transplanted gene induces cells to express molecules on their surface that bind to a radioactive probe—the goal is to use these tracer genes to mark the expression of a therapeutic gene; the tracer gene is spliced into a stretch of DNA alongside the therapeutic gene and a promoter that causes both to be expressed at the same time. Where the tracer gene shows up, we know the therapeutic gene is being expressed as well. As a PET-based technique has far broader applications such as imaging the expression of native genes, one aim is to develop radioactive tags that would home in on and bind to specific messenger RNA molecules which turn on cellular synthesis of a protein. This technique could greatly impact diagnostic imaging, enabling doctors to know if patients are expressing particular genes. By looking for declines in the activity of genes involved in cancer cell proliferation, doctors could measure the effectiveness of therapy.

Several biotech companies develop antisense RNA that would bind to mRNAs from such genes, blocking the production of the proteins they encode. Some imaging researchers have piggybacked on this technology, by attaching radioactive labels to the antisense molecules. Some have already radiolabelled antisense molecules and tracked them through the body (Service, 1998).

Another approach has used light instead of radiation or magnetic resonance to detect the signature of specific enzymes associated with tumours—a novel set of probes that fluoresce only when they react with the target enzymes.

Rational Therapies

Biotechnology has been applied with great success in designing drugs that are used as adjuncts to conventional cancer therapies. This is best exemplified by the two blockbusters, erythropoietin-α and granulocyte-macrophage colony stimulating factor which ameliorate the adverse effects of cytotoxic chemotherapy regimes. Until a few years ago, interferon-α was the preferred agent used with traditional chemotherapy in certain leukaemias and multiple myeloma. It has now been overtaken by 'molecularly targeted' biotech drugs—monoclonal antibodies and small molecules that inhibit protein kinases activated by mutations and chromosomal rearrangements occurring in tumours. Enthusiasm about these newer therapies has been strongly boosted by the approvals of monoclonal antibodies Herceptin (trastuzumab) and Erbitux (cetuxiamb) and of the small molecule Tarceva (erlotinib); all three targeting mutated receptor tyrosine kinases.

An increasing number of different kinases are being targeted by drug developers. More than 30 kinase inhibitors are in clinical development and more than 500 protein kinases have been identified in the human genome—much to the liking of drug companies. Indeed, kinase inhibitors may even be the main reason for the biotech industry's continuing success.

However, not all kinases may be equally promising—some kinase inhibitors have not turned out to be clinically very effective. AstraZeneca's Iressa (gefitinib) has also elicited certain adverse responses in non-small cell lung cancer patients.

Some kinase inhibitors that are initially effective lose their effect with the emergence of resistance in patients to monotherapy, most often as a result of mutations in the ATP-binding pocket of the kinase. It may be better to use combinations of inhibitors that either target inactive and active conformations of the same kinase or that compete for binding with both ATP and the kinase's protein substrate.

When combined with conventional cytotoxic agents, some kinase inhibitors have in certain cancers not conferred much therapeutic benefit. Today, drugs are being developed against a background where the underlying cancer biology (and the role of kinases in that biology) is poorly understood. Even when preclinical work establishes a mechanism of action, new targets sometimes emerge. It is extremely important to understand fully the molecular basis and targets of promising compounds that interact with kinases before they can distinguish themselves as rational therapies. This is because the clinic is a crowded area where molecularly defined therapies compete for attention with cytotoxic therapies, life-cycle-managed variants of those therapies, cellular and genetic approaches, 'alternative medicine' prescriptions and several pretender nostrums whose place on the roster is based as much on clinical despair and hope as on any form of underpinning scientific rationale.

Cell Cycle Checkpoints

In eukaryotic cells, genotoxic stresses that either damage the DNA or inhibit its synthesis activate cell cycle checkpoints, leading to diverse cellular responses including cell cycle arrest, DNA repair and cell death. These responses help to prevent genomic instability, a chief cause of cancer. The cell cycle checkpoints activated by damaged or unreplicated DNA in turn activate signalling pathways that ultimately block the cyclin-dependent kinases (CDKs). CDKs together with their cyclin partners are key regulators of cell cycle progression (Sagata, 2002). When their activity is inhibited, the cell becomes arrested or delayed at specific phases of the cell cycle, enabling the DNA to replicate or be repaired (Zhou and Elledge, 2000).

'Omics' Diagnostics

The burgeoning information treasure from studies of the human genome and proteome has led to the emergence of molecular ('omics') diagnostics. Although so far, much of the growth has been in infectious disease, cancer is emerging as the next big growth area (Baker, 2006).

Table 8.6 Some private and public companies developing 'omics' diagnostics for cancer (after Baker, 2006).

Company (year founded, location)	Description (Use)	Marketed tests or tests being developed
Private Companies		
Agendia (2003), Amsterdam	Gene expression profiling and computer algorithms to predict risk of cancer spread, cancer recurrence, response to certain drugs or primary site of a tumour	MammaPrint (breast cancer recurrence), CupPrint (primary tumour identification)
Aureon Laboratories (2001), Yonkers, NY, USA	*In situ* RNA and protein imaging plus other clinical factors to predict recurrence and stage cancer	Prostate Dx (prostate cancer recurrence)
Corelogic Systems (2000), Bethesda, MD, USA	Develops tests through a patented pattern recognition approach by using pattern discovery and recognition software, mass spectrometry and proprietary lab procedures. Validating tests in breast, colon, ovarian and prostate cancers	OvaCheck (early detection of ovarian cancer)
Orion Genomics (2002), St. Louis, USA	Methylation micro-arrays to detect, type and stage cancers	None yet
Public Companies		
Ciphergen (1993), Fremont, CA, USA	Protein markers for diagnosing ovarian cancer and other diseases	ProteinChip System (SELDI biomarker discovery tool)
Chondrogene (1998), Toronto, Canada	Detects changes in gene expression in the blood to diagnose bladder cancer, colon cancer and other diseases	ChondroChip profiling services
Genomic Health (2000), Redwood City, CA	Identifies gene expression patterns in tumour samples to predict response to treatment and risk of recurrence	OncotypeDX
Genzyme Genetics (1986), Westborough, MA	Markers and tests to type cancer and other conditions	Sells tests assessing EGFR expression, Gleevec resistance, irinotecan toxicity, etc
Monogram Biosciences (1995, formerly Virologic), South San Francisco	Identifies activated protein signalling pathways in cancer cells	-
OncoMethylome (2003), Liege, Belgium	Gene methylation patterns to detect cancer, predict response to therapy and predict recurrence	Developing tissue- and urine-based assays for early diagnosis of multiple cancers

The 'omics' diagnostics are expensive but can get the right drugs to the right patient. Meanwhile, some other resources that are becoming more available include clinical samples backed by years of patient information, tools to probe gene and protein expression in these samples and the computing power to identify meaningful patterns in them.

The DNA micro-array technology is one of the best representatives of 'omic' science. It admirably serves as the platform for massively parallel gene- expression profiling. The US Food and Drug Administration (FDA) has approved the 'AmpliChip' to help physicians tailor patient dosages of drugs that are metabolized differentially by cytochrome P450 enzyme variants.

However, there are some doubts about the reproducibility of micro-array experiments at different sites, the comparability of results on different platforms and even the variability of micro-array results in the same laboratory. Lack of resolution of these issues is hampering translation of micro-array technology into the regulatory and clinical settings.

The Micro-array Quality Control (MAQC) Consortium is a unique community-wide effort, directed by FDA scientists. It seeks to experimentally address the various issues surrounding the reliability of DNA micro-array data. In one major project, ~60 hybridizations were carried out on each of the seven micro-array platforms: >1300 micro-arrays were used during this project. MAQC concluded that, with careful experimental design and appropriate data transformation and analysis, micro-array data can indeed be reproduced and are comparable among different formats and laboratories, irrespective of sample labelling format.

The variations observed between micro-array runs by MAQC were quite low and could be attributed to cross-platform differences in probe binding to alternatively spliced transcripts or to transcripts showing much cross-hybridization to probes other than their own. In fact, experimental variability appears manageable.

Another finding is that statistical analysis in regulatory submissions and clinical diagnostics may differ from that used in basic research (for instance, the simple two-sample *t* test). There is no one-size-fits-all statistical solution.

The MAQC study represents a milestone in DNA micro-array research because it provides the researchers with a well characterized reference data set against which new refinements in platforms and probe sets may be compared. From a clinical perspective, it validates the DNA micro-array as a tool that is sufficiently robust and reliable to be accepted for use on hard-to-obtain human tissue samples (see *Nature Biotechnol.* 24(9): 1039 (2006). Some companies that originated in the era of genomics and proteomics plan to create a technology for discovering and validating markers, develop it as a test and commercialize it.

Genomic Health (Redwood City, CA, USA) represents one of the most advanced in the growing cadre of companies that are designing tests to guide therapy decisions. Its test to predict whether some breast cancers will recur costs more than $3,000—much more than the $48 (plus processing fees) that US Medicare pays for a HER2/neu test used to predict whether cancer will respond to Herceptin (trastuzumab; Genentech, South San Francisco, CA, USA).

As diagnostics become more and more firmly tied to therapy decisions, their prices can determine the cost of the therapies. In the coming years, the role for diagnostics will increase and so diagnostics will need to demonstrate their value on the strength of generating more data.

Entry to the market can be fairly quick because most innovative tests do not require FDA approval. Like other diagnostic companies, Aureon Laboratories (Yonkers, NY) offers its Prostate Dx test for sale even when its clinical validity has not yet been clearly proved. This test is based on a collection of disparate markers, ranging from the location of particular proteins within cells to a patient's clinical information and converts them into a single score to indicate the risk that prostate cancer will recur. To predict prostate cancer recurrence, Aureon's algorithms use multiple inputs, including image analysis of prostate tissue, to quantify the locations of proteins such as within a cell androgen receptor, CK18 (cytoplasmic marker), nuclei and α-methylacyl-coenzyme A racemase (AMACR); which are overexpressed in prostate cancer cells.

Validation of Cancer Drug Targets

The only reliable way to validate a cancer drug target is the demonstration that a given therapeutic agent is clinically effective and acts through the target against which it was designed.

But in some cases an early-stage drug target may be declared 'validated' before making heavy investment in a drug discovery program dedicated to it. Cancer research programs can benefit greatly from the outcome of validation studies. But universal validation criteria have not been established so far (Benson et al., 2006).

Targeted therapy refers to the development of drugs that influence the action or activity of a specific signalling pathway or its constituent. The three interrelated elements essential for implementing such targeted drug discovery projects are: (a) a reasoned belief that a given target (a specific gene or protein against which a drug will be developed) is causally related to cancer—that is, a hypothesis must be formulated with respect to the target; (b) reliable data relevant to this hypothesis is collected and evaluated; this includes evaluating the effects of modulating the activity of a given target in available experimental models and (c) clinical determination of the impact of intervention via the target. The process involved in evaluating potential cancer targets in this way is termed 'validation' and the targets that emerge can be declared in general terms, as 'validated'.

Conceptual Framework for Therapy

The ultimate aim of cancer drug discovery is to design effective, non-toxic therapies. Metabolic enzymes, the focus of drug discovery efforts half a century ago, led to the development of folate and methotrexate as 'targeted' therapies at that time. Later, improved understanding of DNA structure and the molecular basis of DNA replication prompted the development of therapies directed against DNA polymerases and topoisomerases. Understanding of hormone signalling catalyzed the design of cancer therapies targeting nuclear hormone receptors in breast and prostate cancer.

Determination of the roles of many kinase signalling pathways in cancer, including growth factor receptors and their effectors, plus the identification of kinases as a druggable target class, has been the focus of productive target-based oncology drug discovery in the past few years.

Identifying specific changes in cancer cells has inspired elegant hypotheses about the differences between them and their normal counterparts and the relevance of such differences to the aetiology of the cancerous phenotype. Modern cancer research involves the quest to identify such distinguishing characteristics emerging from gene rearrangements, mutations, stable epigenetic changes, lineage legacies and identities, or other accrued genetic (or metabolic) liabilities.

Research is focused on genes for which activity, expression or dependence might have increased. On the basis of the major principles of cancer dependencies, Benson et al. defined four different subtypes of cancer target, viz., genetics, synergy, lineage and host (Fig. 8.1 and Table 8.7).

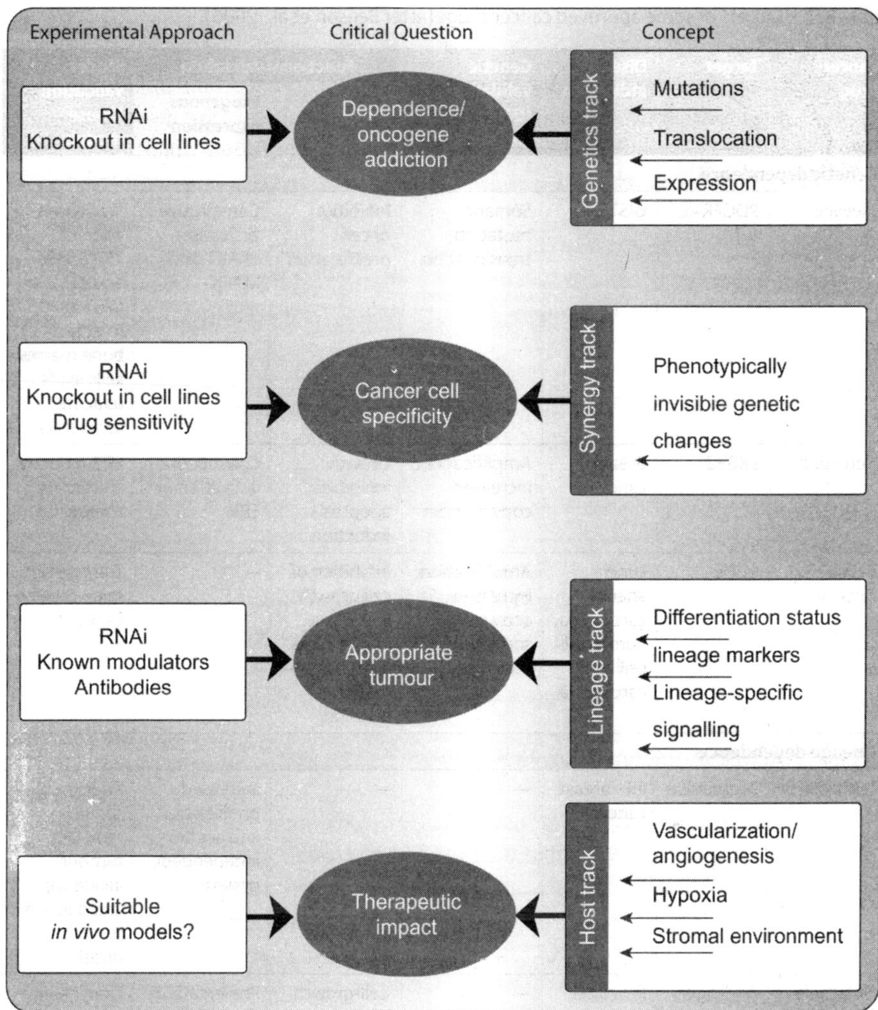

Fig. 8.1 General outline of the four cancer drug discovery tracks defined by Benson et al. (2006). The crucial issue that needs to be addressed for target-validation purposes varies by track and determines the appropriate experimental approaches for the evaluation and validation. RNAi: RNA-mediated interference (after Benson et al., 2006).

Genetics Track

Analysis of the sequence, copy number and expression levels of individual genes within cancer cells and simultaneous interrogation of many genes in multiple independent tumours versus normal tissues suggests that such data may facilitate the reliable identification of therapeutically exploitable differences between cancerous and normal cells.

The association of gross chromosomal rearrangements with leukaemias proved that genetic lesions could cause cancer. Besides genetic alterations that change the encoded proteins in cancer cells, stable changes in gene expression, usually through the amplification of specific genes, have not only guided therapeutic development but also helped

Table 8.7 Targets of some approved cancer drugs (after Benson et al., 2006).

Cancer drug	Target	Disease indication	Genetic validation (DNA changes)	Functional validation		Model validation Mouse models
				SiRNA/ shRNA	Exogenous expression	
Genetic dependence						
Gleevec	PDGFR-α, KIT	GIST	Somatic mutation, translocation	Inhibition of cell proliferation	Constitutive activation of AKT and MAPK	Transplantation of KIT(G559)- and KIT (V814)-infected bone marrow cells leads to acute leukaemia
Herceptin	ERBB2	Breast cancer	Amplification, increased copy number	Growth inhibition, apoptosis induction	Constitutive activation of ERK	ERB-induced mammary tumours
Iressa, Tarceva	EGFR	Lung adenocarcinoma, non-small-cell lung carcinoma	Amplification, increased copy number, somatic mutation	Inhibition of cell growth, induction of cell-cycle arrest, suppression of invasion	—	Transgenic mice develop cancer
Lineage dependence						
Letrazole	Aromatase	ER+ breast cancer	—	—	Increased proliferation and anchor-independent growth	Knockouts show reduced tumour incidence and delayed tumour onset
Flutamide, Biclutamide	Androgen receptor	Prostate cancer	—	Cell-growth inhibition	Prevents TGF-β1-induced growth inhibition and apoptosis	Transgenic mice develop prostate cancer
Host dependence						
Avastin	VEGF receptor	Colon cancer, pancreatic cancer	—	Inhibition of proliferation, induction of apoptosis	—	—

Notes: (a) AKT, protein kinase; B, ALL, acute lymphoblastic leukaemia; APML, acute promyelocytic leukaemia; EGFR, epidermal growth factor receptor; ERK, extracellular signal-regulated kinase; ER, oestrogen receptor; GIST, gastrointestinal stromal tumours; KIT, stem cell-factor receptor; MAPK, mitogen-activated protein kinase; PDGFR-α, platelet-derived growth factor receptor-α; shRNA, short-hairpin RNA; siRNA, short-interfering RNA; TGF-β1, transforming growth factor-β1; TNF-α, tumour necrosis factor-α; VEGF, vascular endothelial growth factor.

(b) Protein expression is overexpressed in all listed cases.

to identify patients who might benefit from such treatments—the fact that the epidermal growth factor receptor-2 (*ERBB2*) gene is amplified and that its encoded receptor protein is aberrantly expressed in some breast cancers, triggered the development of trastuzumab (Herceptin), an effective antibody therapy (Emens, 2005).

Synergy Track

Synthetic lethal genetic interactions are often viewed as significantly deleterious or lethal phenotypes resulting from the combination of mutations that do not produce such phenotypes individually. Certain gain-of-fitness changes in cancer cells can allow their survival or confer some growth advantage; the same changes might also inadvertently sensitize the cells to other stresses that would not affect normal cells but prove lethal in combination with the tumourigenic changes. Cells bearing such unique combinations have special liabilities that might be exploited therapeutically (Kaelin et al., 2005).

Chemical inhibition of the function of a gene product is analogous to a genetic loss-of-function mutation. As such, the identification of specific drug targets in cancer cells that are synthetic lethal in combination with mutant genes could possibly destroy cancer cells while leaving normal cells intact.

Farmer et al. (2005) observed that inhibiting poly(ADP-ribose) polymerase (PARP) together with mutations that inactivate the breast cancer (*BRCA*) gene, results in tumour cell death in experimental settings.

Since the PARP and BRCA proteins have important roles in different DNA damage-repair processes, loss of both these functions could spell disaster for the cell. Thus, cancer cells that have undergone homozygous somatic loss of BRCA function differ from other cells and might be typically susceptible to PARP inhibition.

Rapamycin sensitivity of cells in which loss of PTEN (phosphatase and tensin homologue) or gain of phosphatidylinositol-3-OH kinase (PI(3)K) function has occurred also exemplifies a synthetic lethal phenotype that is applicable to cancer therapy (Mills et al., 2001).

Many cancer cell lines have lost essential protective cellular mechanisms while becoming tumourigenic. An example: loss of apoptotic signals (those mediated by B-cell leukaemia/lymphoma 2 (BCL2) family members) is necessary for survival of pre-malignant or tumour cells. In cases where cancer cells defy apoptotic signals, restoring the function of apoptotic signalling pathways might conceivably result in selective death of such cells (O'Neill et al., 2004).

Lineage Track

Comparative analysis of gene expression has suggested that patterns of gene expression from tumours of the same cell type not only resemble each other but also their normal counterparts more closely than either cancer cells or normal cells derived from different tissue types. Cancer cells tend to maintain many traits of the cells from which they are derived. The implication here is that it might be possible to exploit such residual or legacy features in targeted cancer therapy, i.e., a kind of lineage addiction. One notable example of the fairly nontoxic targeted therapy is the therapeutic efficacy of oestrogen receptor antagonists, such as tamoxifen and letrozole (Femara), in the treatment of breast cancer (Jensen and Jordan, 2003). Other good examples are the dependence of many prostate tumour cells on androgen receptor (AR) signalling, which is required for the survival of normal prostate secretory epithelial cells and the therapeutic efficacy of AR antagonists (Jenster, 1999).

Host Track

Other strategies for targeted therapy do not address tumour cells as such, but focus on the tumour environment or context. Many tumours seem to sponsor *de novo* blood vessel development. This points to angiogenesis mediators as potential therapeutic targets. Bevacizumab (Avastin)—a monoclonal antibody that inhibits vascular endothelial growth factor (VEGF) receptor exemplifies an effective angiogenesis-directed therapy for the treatment of colorectal cancers. Clinical efficacy against renal cell carcinoma and gastrointestinal stromal tumours has also been reported for small-molecule inhibitors such as sorafenib (Nexavar) and sunitinib (Sutent), which target the tyrosine kinase activity of VEGF receptor (Marx, 2005).

Conceivably, by evolving within a particular physiological niche, tumours might become dependent upon certain growth factors or other environmental elements (e.g., stromal cells) for their growth or survival. These concepts need to be experimentally tested.

Validation Strategies

The modern definition of target validation is the experimental evaluation of the role of a given gene or protein in cancer as the basis for determining whether it is a promising target validation or simply a process of hypothesis generation and testing. Criteria for evaluating the validity of a target can range from observing altered mutation or expression status in tumours, to proof that activity of a given target promotes cancer cell growth in experimental systems. Three major strategies for validation are genetic approach, functional cell-based assays and validation in animal model systems (Table 8.7). These strategies can be used to assess the four types of targets shown in Figure 8.2.

Genetic Validation

Patterns of somatic mutations in a specific gene in a given tumour type provide strong evidence that the mutant form of the gene (and perhaps even its wild-type counterpart) has an aetiological role in that tumour type. When such mutations take place in genes associated with signalling cascades, both the mutant gene product itself and downstream effectors of that pathway can be potential therapeutic targets (Benson et al., 2006). Some specific examples have been discussed by Walker and Olson (2005) and Janne (2005).

Epidermal growth factor receptor (EGFR) is a good example of a genetically validated target; it is a causal factor in non-small-cell lung cancer (NSCLC), leading to the development of two EGFR tyrosine kinase inhibitors: gefitinib (Iressa) and erlotinib (Tarceva). Unfortunately, in spite of the presence of EGFR aberrations in many NSCLC tumours, therapeutic inhibition of EGFR has given significant tumour regression in no more than 20 per cent of patients (see Janne et al., 2005).

It is very difficult to predict response to therapy only by studying expression levels and/or the genetic status of a particular gene. Nevertheless, knowledge that a gene is genetically changed and selected for in cancer cells might warrant initiating a drug discovery project. Complementary validation (or at least a parallel path) by using other suitable experimental models can enhance our understanding of the function and role of genetically identified targets in cancer.

Target Validation in Cell-based Systems

Introducing and expressing exogenous genes in non-transformed cells led to the discovery of the first transforming mutation in human cancer (Shih and Weinberg, 1982). The ability to express and knock out genes in mice provided model systems that have advanced knowledge of the biology of cancer in a physiological setting.

The more recent application of RNA-interference (RNAi) technologies allows the 'knockdown' of expression of specific genes transiently by short-interfering RNA (siRNA), stably by short-hairpin RNA (shRNA) or in an inducible fashion via regulatable shRNA (Silva et al., 2004).

In principle, gene-specific loss of function in suitable experimental systems should predict the outcome of using a specific inhibitory compound in tumour cells and might be extended to testing several genes or compounds in cell lines with various defined genetic backgrounds. These approaches should preferably be used before starting a small-molecule therapeutic discovery program; they may even help in the exploration of synthetic-lethality concepts.

A common practice in early stage evaluation of potential cancer targets is to use cancer cell lines in tissue culture. These lines can be used to test growth rate, immortalization, loss of contact inhibition, two-dimensional colony formation, colony formation in soft agar and reliance upon growth factors.

However, the inability to maintain or grow many tumour-derived cells in tissue culture limits the utility of these techniques. Yet, despite limitations, these systems have been valuable tools for the discovery and evaluation of some potential cancer targets (Benson et al., 2006).

Animal Models

Transgenic mouse models have proven useful in understanding cancers of the lymphoid and hematopoietic systems—the highly complex and diverse lineages of cells and cancers in these systems cannot be replicated in the laboratory. In fact, such mouse models have greatly facilitated important researches implicating stem cells in cancer (Mazurier et al., 2003).

However, one drawback of conventional transgenic models (knockout or knock-in systems) is that the deletion of many cancer-relevant target genes kills the embryo. Also, while constitutive ectopic oncogene expression might lead to tumours in mice, these models do not necessarily represent initiation and progression of tumours in humans. To address these problems, inducible mouse models have been developed in which the expression of certain genes can be changed at specific times (Benson et al., 2006).

Many functions associated with the proliferation or survival of cancer cells are known to be conserved in diverse organisms (Brumby and Richardson, 2005). One notable example of the impact of a model organism on cancer research is programmed cell death (apoptosis) (Hengartner and Horvitz, 1994). The recognition of apoptosis as a valid biological phenomenon was first achieved in nematodes, in which maps of cellular destiny documented the loss of specific cells at specific stages of development. Discovery of the molecular players that regulate apoptosis (including BCL2) and the observation that such players are involved in the survival of cancer cells, has strongly changed concepts of how these cells die.

Discovery of inhibitors of BCL2, as well as modulation of other apoptotic signalling and execution pathways is now an active area in the discovery of novel cancer therapeutics (Benson et al., 2006).

9 Prevention and Support

Introduction

The word cancer still terrifies people despite the fact that modern medicine has made substantial progress in its diagnosis and treatment. Cancer is still the second leading cause of death in the United States. More than 100 people die of cancer per 100,000 population. Thanks to impressive strides in cancer diagnosis and treatment, the five-year-survival rate for breast cancer rose from 72 percent in 1940 to 96 percent in 2000 (see *Cancer*. WebMD, 2001).

Cancer refers to more than 100 diseases that attack virtually every area of the body. Normally, in a healthy individual, cells divide and grow in an orderly manner but if and when the genes controlling this cellular division falter, cells multiply uncontrollably. A group of such uncontrolled cells is termed a tumour. Tumours may be harmless (benign) or malignant (cancerous). The former sooner or later stop growing. In contrast, malignant tumours outcompete and crowd out healthy cells, adversely affect bodily functions, consume and deplete the body's stores of nutrients and often spread throughout the body (i.e., metastasize).

Carcinogenesis involves the accumulation of genetic mutations that make cells defy homeostatic regulation and grow in an unregulated manner. The loss of functional tumour-suppressor genes is especially important in this context (Macleod, 2000; Boland and Goel, 2005); it prevents the development of abnormal growth by, for example, inducing repair, senescence or cell death in damaged or mutated cells (Wodarz and Komarova, 2007). Cells which have lost these safeguards tend to acquire mutations that make a tumour malignant.

Cancer cells can inactivate tumour-suppressor genes and progressively become unable to respond to DNA damage or mutation (Kinzler and Vogelstein, 1998).

Many researchers have studied the effect of cell death on cancer progression. It is generally thought that the loss of programmed cell death is required for carcinogenesis. Wodarz and Komarova (2007) have, however, argued that the situation is more complex and that the loss of apoptosis can have the converse effect, preventing cancer progression. If the death rate of cancer cells is low, fewer cell divisions are needed for the tumour to reach a certain size, resulting in the presence of fewer mutant cells. This means that the chances of overcoming potential selective barriers are reduced, rendering the failure of pathogenic progression probable. However, if there is a higher cell death rate, more cell divisions are required for the tumour to reach a certain size, resulting in the presence of more mutant cells and in an increased probability of overcoming selective barriers and cancer progression.

While a few (5–10%) cancers are thought to be hereditary, the commonest causes (or contributors) of cancer are smoking, excessive exposure to sunlight and improper diet. Fortunately, the commonest contributing factors can be controlled fairly easily. Also, if one already has cancer, changing these factors can improve one's chances of full recovery. Approximately three-fourth of the world's population depends on herbal botanicals for health care.

Herbs have specific tonic activities, cleansing actions and other striking healing properties that support the immune system, stimulate self-healing and strengthen the body's ability to eliminate and rid itself of cancer cells and tumours.

Our body is bombarded every day with a large number of harmful substances. As they enter the bloodstream, toxins build up in our body and contribute to a sluggish and unhealthy liver. They also affect our ability to properly metabolize and use the nutrients. Cancer can develop as the result of a depressed immune system, deficiencies in vital nutrients and imbalances in the organs. Cancer may therefore be prevented by cleansing the blood, liver and immune system so as to strengthen them once again.

Dietary fat is strongly believed to be linked to various cancers, particularly of the breast, colon and prostate gland. According to McKelvey et al. (2000), trans-fatty acids from partially hydrogenated vegetable oil may increase the risk of colon cancer.

Diets that are high in saturated fat, total fat and sodium and low in fibre are associated with increased risk for cardiovascular disease (including hypertension) as well as some types of cancer. A diet low in fruits and vegetables is associated with cancer risk because of various mechanisms, such as absence of protective nutrients, phytochemicals and other unknown compounds in fruits and vegetables, as well as the fact that a diet low in fruits and vegetables is generally low in fibre and often high in fat (WCRF, 1997).

The USDA (2000) recommended that intake of saturated and total fat for adolescents should be less than 10 per cent of total energy from saturated fat and no more than 30 per cent of energy from total fat. In many developed and industrially advanced countries, however, these recommended intakes are being exceeded, especially among adolescents (youth).

Fibre intake is also linked to some types of cancer. The recommended intake for fibre is age of child plus 5 g per day for youth aged 2 to 18 years (Williams, 1995).

Low levels of fibre and high levels of saturated fat, total fat and sodium are often related to the low intake of fruits and vegetables by adolescents. Fruits and vegetables are important sources of fibre and are low in fat, saturated fat and sodium; their intake by adolescents is usually not adequate.

Cancer cells produce unusually high levels of reactive oxygen species which somehow sustain cancerous growth. But these ROS can be turned against cancer cells (see *Cancer Cell* 10: 241–252, 2006). Very high levels of ROS are unusually toxic to cells, so cancer cells need antioxidant systems to counteract these effects. Huang et al. (2006) found that β-phenylethylisothiocyanate, a molecule found in some vegetables can kill cancer cells *in vitro* by disabling the cells' antioxidant systems. Normal cells are not killed, probably because they contain a low baseline level of ROS. Mice with cancers and treated with β-phenylethylisothiocyanate survive nearly twice as long as untreated mice.

Critical analysis of several long term studies involving 320,000 women by Smith-Warner et al. (1998) showed that women who drank two to five alcoholic drinks a day had a 41 per cent higher risk of developing breast cancer as compared to nondrinkers. Even one drink a day increased breast cancer risk by nine per cent.

Exercise

A moderate amount of exercise or other physical activity goes a long way in preventing cancer. Thune et al. (1997) conducted a study involving 25,624 women and found the lowest risk of breast cancer among lean women who exercised at least four hours per week. The greatest benefit was noted for pre-menopausal women rather than post-menopausal women.

While the above comment about exercise is applicable and valid for most countries of the world, it may be totally superfluous and unnecessary for many people living in India where in many states the condition of the roads (whether rural or urban—more especially urban!) is so bad that anybody who commutes from his/her home to/from workplace over a distance of at least 2–3 km everyday, by any means of transport such as car, bus, auto-rickshaw, manual rickshaw, bicycle, or even on foot, is guaranteed to get jolts, jerks and shocks of such high intensity that make any traditional exercise look like peanuts. Further, to exercise different parts of the body, one usually needs different kinds of exercises. If you live in Uttar Pradesh and Bihar, you need not do even a single exercise: mere commuting on the disgusting roads will exercise all parts of your body including the deepest bones and nerves. But, of course, in India also not everybody commutes to/from work everyday. For them, regular exercise of the conventional type is essential.

One general effect of physical inactivity is obesity. This increases the risk for some cancers.

Combating Cancer Through Diet

A substantial fraction of cancer patients die of malnutrition. People with cancer face three threats: sluggish appetite; their body uses up more nutrients than ever; and a sharp rise in their nutritional requirements.

The American Cancer Society has proposed the following guidelines on diet and lifestyle (see www.impakt.com). These recommendations can protect people against cancer and hasten recovery if one already has cancer:

- Eat five or more servings of fruits and vegetables every day.
- Eat other foods from plant sources, such as grain products or beans, several times every day.
- Avoid foods rich in saturated fat or trans-fatty acids (e.g., snack foods, baked goods).
- Reduce intake of high-fat meats.
- Be moderately active for 30 minutes or more at least four days a week (This does not apply to those living in cities/towns where the roads are full of pits, curves, pit-wells, depressions/elevations, contours and curves).
- Maintain a normal healthy weight range.
- Avoid drinking alcohol.

Cancer-combating Nutrients

Some notable cancer-combating nutrients are outlined below.

Folic acid Sellers et al. (2001) suggested that folic acid (a B vitamin) may reduce breast cancer risk in women who drink moderately. But those who drink too much do not derive any benefit from folic acid. The recommended dose is 400 mcg daily.

Coenzyme Q10 CoQ10 is found in almost every living cell, especially in the mitochondria. Dietary CoQ10 seems to protect against breast cancer.

Vitamin C This has been generally accepted as protecting against the side effects of some anti-cancer drugs. The daily requirement of healthy people is 250 mg but higher amounts may be indicated for those who suffer from cancer.

Omega-3 oils These represent an essential fatty acid and seem to protect against skin tumours (see Liu et al., 1998). For good health, omega-3 oils should make up 1 to 2.5 per cent of totally daily calories.

Carotenoids All green vegetables and fruits contain these nutrients which are converted to vitamin A in the body. Important carotenoids include lutein, zeaxanthin, beta-cryptoxanthin, lycopene, alpha-carotene and beta-carotene. Deficiency of carotenoids appears to increase breast cancer risk. No recommended dose for carotenoids has been established.

Vitamin E (alpha-tocopherol) may be beneficial in treating skin cancer (see Burke et al., 2000). The natural form of alpha-tocopherol is more bioavailable than is the synthetic compound (Acuff, 1998).

Other Potentially Useful Nutrients Including Micronutrients

Some other potentially useful nutrients including micronutrients which are needed only in small amounts include selenium, N-acetyl-cysteine, niacin, L-carnitine, MGN3, IP6 and quercetin. All these may be helpful not only for cancer treatment but also cancer prevention.

Beta Carotene and Antioxidants

The risk of developing cancer can be greatly reduced by consuming foods rich in beta carotene, a strong antioxidant. It is only the natural carotene found in foods that lowers the incidence of cancer; any synthetic carotene is not effective.

Peto et al. (1981) showed that people who maintain adequate levels of β-carotene tend to have quite low incidence of various types of cancer, especially oral. More than 500 different forms of carotene (carotenoids) have been detected in plants belonging to different plant families or groups and people should consume as many different varieties of carotenoids as possible. This is best done by eating a diversity of fruits and vegetables of as many different colours as possible (Kumar, 2004).

In many parts of India, people habitually chew betel (*paan*) which contains arecanut, cardamom, fennel, lime (calcium hydroxide), mint and some other ingredients. Some *paans* also contain tobacco which can induce oral cancer. Beta carotene from fruits and vegetables, especially carrots, prevents such cancer (Liede et al., 1998). A combination of raw (untreated) turmeric (*Curcuma longa*), carrots, other seasonal vegetables and fruits can be a treatment of choice for early stages of oral and other cancers. The turmeric harvested from the field should only be peeled and washed before eating. About 1 gram of peeled and washed fresh turmeric can be chewed daily for 2–3 months in a year to obtain good preventive effects against cancer. Some important natural sources of β-carotene are spinach, other dark green leafy vegetables, drumstick fruit (*Moringa oleifera*), broccoli, carrots, strawberry, papaya and various other yellow, orange and pink fruits and vegetables (Kumar, 2004). In fact, besides avoiding smoking, consuming a healthy diet is the single most important factor in preventing cancer. Beta carotene and vitamins C, D and E are particularly important in this context (Graewal, 1995).

Wonder Vitamin

Vitamin D is a wonder vitamin (see Bikle, 2007; Lips, 2007; Bonjour et al., 2007; Grant et al., 2007). A daily dose of vitamin D seems to substantially reduce the risk of breast and colon cancer (Jimenez-Lara, 2007; Knight et al., 2007; Lin et al., 2007). It has been shown to play a vital role in heart disease, cancer, diabetes, high blood pressure, schizophrenia and multiple sclerosis. It is also essential for bone health (see Fraser, 2007). Vitamin D appears to have a highly preventive and protective role in some internal cancers, especially those of colon, breast, prostate and ovaries. Garland et al. (2006) concluded that 20 out of 30 studies on colon cancer, 9 out of 13 on breast cancer, 13 out of 26 on prostate cancer and 5 out of 7 on ovarian cancer reported a significant benefit of vitamin D, its serum metabolites, sunlight exposure or some other marker of vitamin D status on cancer risk or mortality. Van der Rhee et al. (2006) found a significant inverse correlation between sunlight exposures and the incidence or mortality of prostate, ovary and colon cancers, but the data on non-Hodgkin lymphoma gave conflicting results. Vitamin D might confer protection by controlling cell proliferation, inducing terminal differentiation of tumour cells and inhibiting angiogenesis.

For internal cancers, a protective role for vitamin D status has been postulated for some autoimmune diseases such as multiple sclerosis (MS), diabetes mellitus type 1, rheumatoid arthritis (RA) and inflammatory bowel diseases (IBDs) (see Norval et al., 2007).

As reviewed by Ponsonby et al. (2005), poor vitamin D status can be prospectively associated with the onset of MS diabetes (I) and RA in humans. However, it is possible that some factor other than vitamin D, which is also linked with sun exposure, may be involved in modulating immune responses. Suggested factors include the UV-induced release of the neuropeptides, α-melanocytic-stimulating hormone and calcitonin-gene related peptide, or the light-induced suppression of melatonin levels (Ponsonby et al., 2005).

Many people in the northern hemisphere suffer from deficiency of vitamin D which probably accounts for several thousand premature deaths from cancers alone. A twenty minute daily exposure of the hands, arms and face to the sun provides an adequate dose. In winter, in the temperate countries the only way of maintaining levels is by taking cod liver oil or supplements (see Mullin et al., 2007; Schwartz and Skinner, 2007). Evidence for the benefits of vitamin D has been accumulating recently. The Association of Cancer Councils of Australia admitted two years ago that some exposure to the sun is essential to achieve adequate vitamin D levels.

It takes 20 minutes in full sunlight for a person with white skin to synthesize the maximum amount of vitamin D that can be formed in one day; but there is need to exercise caution and begin with just a few minutes' exposure (see Bouillon et al., 2006).

If one feels any unpleasant burning or baking sensations, one should cover up, apply high-factor sunscreen or move to shade.

Some experts suggest allowing children to play in weak sunlight, but to avoid exposure around midday. Others believe that children should be exposed in a swimsuit to full midsummer sunlight for 15 to 30 minutes a day, provided they do not feel a burning sensation (see John et al., 2007; Lappe et al., 2007).

Some other potentially useful nutrients including micronutrients which are needed only in small amounts include selenium, N-acetyl-cysteine, niacin, L-carnitine, MGN3, IP6 and quercetin. All these may be helpful not only for cancer treatment but also cancer prevention.

Herbs

Cellular detoxification can be achieved by eliminating cellular toxins that we have absorbed, ingested or inhaled during our lifetime. The commonest substances include prescription drugs, over-the-counter medications, recreational drugs, alcohol, tobacco, heavy metals, man-made chemicals (found in personal care products), food additives, herbicides, pesticides, petroleum products, solvents and commercial cleansing products, formaldehyde, household chemicals, fluoride and chlorine, as well as other chemicals in the air and tap water (Keith, 2006).

Various herbs form an integral part of a healthy lifestyle. They cleanse and detoxify right down to the cellular level. They efficiently influence the entire body, gathering and flushing out accumulated toxins, thus allowing for cellular renewal and cleansing and detoxifying our blood, liver and lymphatic system. They stimulate the immune system, enhancing the body's ability to defend itself. They provide excellent nutrition in the form of vitamins, minerals and enzymes.

Notable Herbs

Some notable herbs are listed below.

Blessed thistle (*Cnicus benedictus*) It is a strong blood purifier and promotes healthy cellular function by improving nutritional status. It not only purifies the blood but also supports the immune system. It enhances liver and bile functions and acts as an antioxidant.

Kelp It is a large brown seaweed. It contains all the minerals and vitamins considered vital to health. Researches in Japan revealed a direct relationship between the ingestion of algin found in kelp and the prevention of breast cancer. By affecting the T-cells, alginates enhance the immune system function.

Red clover (*Trifolium pretense*) It is an excellent blood purifier, provides many vital minerals and vitamins for all forms of degenerative disease, including cancer.

Sheep sorrel (*Rumex acetosella*) It is a traditional folk remedy for cancer. Rich in vitamins and trace minerals, it nourishes the glandular system and promotes digestion. It is a detoxifier and helps in destroying tumours.

Turkish rhubarb root (*Rheum palmatum*) It has a long history of use in China. It shows impressive detoxifying properties, especially in the liver and antibiotic and antimicrobial properties. The root purges the body of wastes and toxic matter and has antitumour properties (Keith, 2006).

Watercress (*Nasturtium officinale*) It is chiefly used as a tonic. It is a treasure of natural vitamins, minerals and trace elements, a powerful intestinal cleanser and purifier and builder of blood. Rich in vitamin C, it is strongly alkaline due to its high potassium content. It is used for treating acidity and purifying the blood (Keith, 2006).

Cancer-combating Medicines Derived or Extracted from Plants

Some cancer-combating medicines derived or extracted from plants are:

Garlic (*Allium sativum*) It shows anti-cancer properties, probably due to its allyl sulphur components. It decreases nitrosamine formation, which is implicated in cancer (Milner, 2001).

Green tea (*Camellia sinensis*) It protects against recurrence of breast cancer in its early stage (Inoue et al., 2001). It also seems to protect against skin cancer.

Astragalus (*Astragalus radix*) This plant boosts the immune system and exerts an anticancer effect on mice with cancer (Kurashige et al., 1999).

Echinacea (*Echinacea purpurea*) It appears to suppress spontaneously occurring leukaemia, probably by enhancing nonspecific immune or cellular immune systems, or both.

Mistletoe (*Viscum album*) It seems to prolong the lives of individuals with cancer (Grossarth-Maticek et al., 2001).

Reishi, shiitake and maitake mushrooms According to Kidd (2000), polysaccharide-K (PSK), which is a specific glucan from these mushrooms, extends survival by five years or longer for patients of cancers of the stomach, colon-rectum, oesophagus, nasopharynx, lung and breast. Another compound, polysaccharide-P (PSP) improves quality of life, provides substantial relief and enhances immune status in 70–90 per cent of patients with cancers of the stomach, oesophagus, lung, ovary and cervix. The merits of these mushrooms are their high tolerability, proven benefits to survival and quality of life and compatibility with chemotherapy and radiation therapy.

Immune System-supporting Herbs

Some other immune system-supporting herbs are turmeric and ginseng (*Panax ginseng*). These may be useful for both treatment and prevention of cancer. A complex illness such as cancer requires an equally complex mix of treatments. Whereas conventional therapies target the cancer itself, nutritional, herbal and other complementary treatments nourish and strengthen the body to enable it to cope with both the illness and the difficult treatments.

A judicious combination of conventional and alternative therapies can produce highly beneficial results while minimizing toxicity. Listed below are some tips which can boost our body's immune system naturally (see also Keith, 2006).

1. The immune system needs about 9 hours of sleep to recharge completely.
2. Learn to deal with stress and emotions by communicating and controlling our feelings. Excessive anger, frustrations and fears undermines our immune function.
3. The body should be detoxified periodically with a cleansing diet, detoxifying herbs or some form of juice fasting.
4. Our diet should be supplemented with phytonutrients and nutritional supplements to supply antioxidants such as selenium and vitamins A, C and E that help the body detoxify and reduce cancer risks.
5. Chemical exposure from food, work environment and around our home should be avoided as much as possible.
6. We should eat a healthy diet that is high in fibre, low in fat and rich in fruits and vegetables. Five to 10 servings of fruits and vegetables every day lowers the risk of cancer by half.
7. Minimize exposure to electromagnetic radiation; computers, TV sets, cellular phones and microwaves. Also, avoid inhaling noxious gases emitted by diesel-operated generators.
8. We should habitually consume herbs that have powerful immune-boosting and cancer-prevention properties such as garlic, cumin, turmeric, green tea and diverse mushrooms.
9. Some moderate exercise (about 30–45 minutes per day), three to five times per week enhances the overall function of the immune system. In areas where the urban and rural roads are full of potholes, there is no need for special exercise because daily commuting to /from workplace provides the needed exercise *gratis*.

Lactic Acid Bacteria for Cancer Prevention

Many human cancers arise through infection, inflammation, smoking and improper diet. Adoption of effective preventive strategies can reduce cancers (Lee and Lee, 2006). A proper diet based on fruits and vegetables can greatly reduce the risk of cancer (Surh, 2003).

Lactic acid bacteria (LAB) act as an effective chemopreventive against several cancers. LAB are Gram-positive, non-spore forming, nonrespiring bacteria that produce lactic acid as the major end product during the fermentation of carbohydrates. Some more common LAB genera in food fermentations are *Carnobacterium*, *Enterococcus*, *Lactobacillus* (*Lcb*), *Lactococcus* (*Lcc*), *Leuconostoc* (*Leu*), *Pediococcus*, *Streptococcus* (*S*), *Tetragenococcus* and *Weissella*.

The genus *Bifidobacterium* (*Bif*), not strictly a LAB, uses a unique metabolic pathway for sugar metabolism and its species are often considered to be LAB in view of their probiotic action while living in the gastrointestinal tract of humans and animals (Stiles and Holzapfel, 1997).

Lactic acid bacteria not only enhance the nutritional value of food and control serum cholesterol levels but also prevent against certain cancers. Several *in vitro*, *in vivo* human and epidemiological studies have demonstrated chemopreventive effective of LAB on colon, bladder, liver, breast and gastric cancers (see Kim et al., 2007). These effects manifest through diverse mechanisms such as changes in the gastrointestinal microflora, enhancement of the host's immune response as well as antioxidative and antiproliferative activities.

Colorectal Cancer

The major research focus on the relationship between LAB and cancer has been on colorectal cancer. *Bifidobacterium* species decrease the growth rate and increase differentiation by increasing the activity of differentiation-related enzymes such as dipeptidyl peptidase IV and alkaline phosphatase in the HT-29 human colon adenocarcinoma cell line (Baricault et al., 1995). *Lcb. plantarum* treatments have significantly reduced DNA damage in this cell line (Burns and Rowland, 2004). Kim et al. (2003) reported that the cytoplasmic fraction of *L. lactis* spp. *lactis* inhibits the proliferation of the SNUC2A human colon cancer cell line by arresting the cell-cycle S-phase. As early as 1990, Kubota had shown that in clinical tests, the number of *Bifidobacterium* species was significantly reduced in the fecal intestinal flora of patients with colon adenoma. *Lcb. casei* prevents the development of colorectal cancer—a daily intake of live *Lcb. casei* suppressed atypia of colorectal tumours in 398 men and women who were free from tumours and who had got at least two colorectal tumours removed (Ishikawa et al., 2005).

Bladder Cancer

Smoking, employment in rubber, chemical and leather industries and chronic bladder infection are the major causes of bladder cancer. While this cancer is somewhat easy to treat, it tends to recur and regrow more malignantly (Tolley et al., 1996). According to Ohashi et al. (2002), habitual intake of *Lcb. casei* strain *Shirota* reduces the risk of bladder cancer. LAB also effectively decrease the rate of recurrence.

Liver Cancer

Liver cancer is fairly uncommon in North America and Western Europe but in Korea it is the third leading site of diagnosed cancers (after gastric and lung cancers) (Bae et al., 2002). Hepatic metastases are quite common from cancers of the gastrointestinal tract, lung and breast due to the large blood flow through the liver. As hepatic disease usually arises from hepatitis, which is caused by liver damage due to viruses, alcohol and chemical compounds (e.g., aflatoxins, nitrosamines and azo compounds), the hepatitis can lead to cirrhosis and finally to cancer. Therefore, liver cancer may be prevented by avoiding liver damage. LAB can reduce liver damage. Alteration of the gastrointestinal microflora caused by LAB and the LAB's antioxidant effects reduce this damage. According to Han et al. (2005), *Lcb. acidophilus* gives greater protection than a commercial hepatoprotective agent, dimethyl diphenyl bicarboxylate, against liver damage. A mixture of *Lcb. rhamnosus* LC705 and *Propionibacterium freudenreichii* protected the liver from aflatoxin: its exposure was reduced by 55 per cent in 45 healthy young men taking a dietary supplement containing LAB as compared to another 45 men on a placebo (El Nezami et al., 2006). This implies that preventing liver damage by LAB lowers the incidence of liver cancer.

Breast Cancer

In the Netherlands, Van't Veer et al. (1989) reported that the consumption of fermented milk products was significantly less among 133 breast cancer women than among 289 healthy females, suggesting that LAB prevents breast cancer.

Gastric Cancer

Helicobacter pylori is a Gram-negative, spiral-shaped, microaerophilic bacterium that colonizes the human gastric mucosa by producing urease. Urease hydrolyzes urea to ammonium which alters gastric pH, causing inflammatory diseases such as chronic gastritis. Gastric cancer is strongly related to a transition from normal mucosa to gastritis and can eventually lead to adenocarcinoma (Peek and Blaser, 2002). This is why *H. pylori* is regarded a class I carcinogen. LAB prevent or retard the growth and colonization of *H. pylori* (Gotteland and Cruchet, 2003). Most studies of gastric cancer related to LAB have involved their inhibitory effects against *H. pylori* (Felley and Michetti, 2003). Kim et al. (2004, 2007) reported that cytoplasmic fraction of *L. lactis* spp. *lactis* induces apopto-

Table 9.1 Anti-cancer effects of LAB (after Kim et al., 2007; reproduced with permission from The Korean Society for Microbiology and Biotechnology).

Target organ	Strain/species	Effect
Colon	*Bifidobacterium*	Reduce cell growth Increase differentiation
	Lactobacillus plantarum	Reduce DNA damage
	Lactococcus lactis spp. *lactis*	S-phase cell cycle arrest
	Bifidobacterium longum	Reduce aberrant crypts Reduce β-glucuronidase Reduce ammonia concentration Reduce Ras mutation
	Bifidobacterium longum	Reduce tumour incidence
	Lactobacillus acidophilus	Reduce tumour incidence
	Lactobacillus casei	Reduce atypia
	Lactobacillus rhamnosus GG	Change faecal microflora
	Bifidobacterium lactis Bb12	Reduce proliferation
Bladder	*Lactobacillus rhamnosus* GG	Reduce cell growth
	Lactobacillus casei strain *Shirota* *Lactobacillus rhamnosus* GG	Increase in spleen CD3, CD4 and CD8a, T lymphocytes and NK cells
	Lactobacillus casei strain *Shirota*	Reduce bladder cancer
Liver	*Lactobacillus rhamnosus* GG	Reduce endotoxemia Reduce liver injury
	Lactobacillus acidophilus	Reduce liver damage Reduce β-glucuronidase
Breast	*Lactobacillus rhamnosus* LC705	Reduce aflatoxin exposure
	Bifidobacterium infantis	Reduce cell growth
	Bifidobacterium bifidum	
	Bifidobacterium animalis	
	Lactobacillus acidophilus	
	Lactobacillus pracasei	
	Lactobacillus helveticus R389	Reduce tumour growth Increase cytokines
Stomach	*Lactobacillus plantarum* MLBPL1	Reduce growth of *Helicobacter pylori*
	Lactobacillus casei strain *Shirota*	Reduce colonization of *H. pylori*

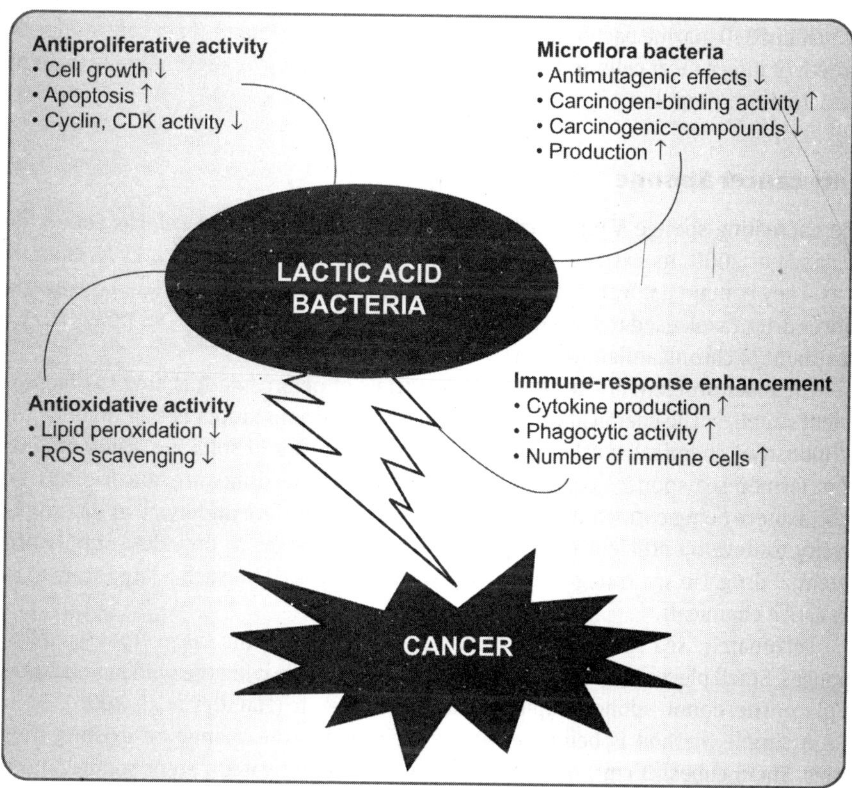

Fig. 9.1 Possible mechanisms underlying chemo-preventive effects of LAB against cancers (after Kim et al., 2007; reproduced with permission from The Korean Society for Microbiology and Biotechnology).

sis in the SNU-1 human adenocarcinoma cell line; arginine deiminase being the active compound that induces the apoptosis. Table 9.1 summarizes the chemoprotective effects of LAB on various types of cancer. Although the precise mechanisms of the anti-cancer effects of LAB are not well understood, possibilities may include changes in the gastrointestinal microflora, enhancement of the host's immune response and antioxidative and antiproliferative effects (Fig. 9.1).

Marine Bacteria

Extremely adaptable marine bacteria could be our next rich source of new anti-cancer drugs. Marine bacteria are found throughout the oceans, from the seafloor to the insides of fish stomachs. They live in many distinct habitats, such as deep-sea sediments, underwater mountains and even the outside of an algal cell. These microbes have developed unique mechanisms to survive adverse conditions, including very salty to merely brackish water and temperatures ranging from 35°C in tropical waters to –5°C in the polar and deep-sea waters. These unique survival mechanisms make marine bacteria highly promising as a source of new biological active substances for industrial processing, medicines and foods. Novel antibiotics and anti-cancer drugs have been identified from marine bacteria.

Out of 330 marine bacteria recently screened in New Zealand, 7 per cent stopped the growth of lung cancer cells and did not affect healthy cells. Work is underway to identify the actual compounds.

Anti-cancer Sponge

The encrusting sponge *Mycale hentscheli* was first collected from Pelorus Sound (New Zealand) in 2000. Its extracts showed activity against some cancer cells in laboratory tests. They contain a novel chemical—peloruside A—that operates in a similar way to the cancer drug Taxol, used to treat ovarian and breast cancer. Taxol also has potential in the treatment of chronic inflammation.

The chief problem affecting the clinical trials of peloruside A is how to obtain sufficient supplies. The chemical can either be extracted from sea sponges, or manufactured by industrial chemical synthesis. The marketing benefits of sourcing a potential drug from farmed sea sponges could match those from the leading anti-cancer drugs Taxol and Taxotere being extracted from the yew tree. Attempts are underway at Victoria University to develop efficient farming of enough sea sponges to provide a supply of the potential drug. No sea sponge has previously been cultured on such a large scale to supply active chemicals.

Fortunately, sea sponges can grow from living fragments taken from established sponges. Small pieces of sponge can be taken for culture, leaving the wild parent sponges in place. The 'donor' sponges rapidly heal and regenerate (Handley et al., 2006).

A simple method is being developed for growing the sponge on existing mussel farms. Small cubes (3 cm^3) of sponge are cut from a cultivated parent sponge and tied onto fishing mesh and then suspended at optimum depths under water. *Mycale* is an ideal candidate for aquaculture, growing almost 15-fold in size during winter and spring.

Only a small proportion of the cultured sponge is harvested to supply the raw material for peloruside A extraction for the pre-clinical trials. Enough raw sponge material is retained to re-seed the farm the following year.

Sponge aquaculture also faces problems. When its density increases, weeds and fouling organisms such as the colonial sea squirt *Aplydium*, appear. To control some of the ascidians, divers 'weed' out the farmed sponges. This is time consuming. For success in commercial aquaculture of *Mycale*, methods need to be developed that minimize fouling competition and speed up bulk production of the sponge. Labour costs can be reduced, for example, by mechanizing the seeding of sponges on to ropes (Handley et al., 2006).

After extraction and purification, the final yield from 200 kg of raw sponge may be no more than 2 g of pure peloruside A. Industrial-scale processing technology will be needed for extracting clinical-scale quantities of peloruside A. Alongside this extraction effort, some pharmaceutical companies are interested in developing industrial synthesis technology.

The likely benefits of the development of a pharmaceutical drug from a cultured sponge could be tremendous. But it is possible that industrial synthesis of the drug may overtake an aquaculture supply. Thus, a two-pronged push ahead may be useful for providing sufficient peloruside A for clinical trials: aquaculture plus extraction, as well as industrial synthesis ('Peloruside A' on the Marine Biotech website: www.marinebiotech.org/ pelorusidea.html).

Ayurvedic Biology

The traditional, ancient healing science of Indian Ayurveda needs to be critically scrutinized from the perspective of modern science, from molecular biology to nanotechnology, especially in the context of practices ranging from correlates of *tridoshas* to the possible connection between the preparation of *bhasmas* and their efficacy.

Both Ayurveda and Ayurvedic Biology are now witnessing a global resurgence of interest as exemplified by a vigorous churning in the areas of mind-body interaction, of alternative medicine, of philosophies and sciences of healing. Ayurvedic biology provides many effective ingredients especially in herbal medicine and Ayurveda is a valuable storehouse of possible new drugs or chemical formulations. While this activity is inevitable and necessary, some overarching scientific questions can help advance both scientific understanding and human welfare in major ways.

Epidemiological transition in advanced and developed countries has led to the realization that the elimination of infectious diseases by antibiotics has been hindered by the development of bacterial resistance and, more importantly, non-communicable diseases such as atherosclerosis, cancer and mental disorders are multifactorial in origin and not amenable to 'one antibiotic—one microbe' approach. This has shifted interest in traditional medicine in the hope that 'holistic treatment' may be more appropriate and effective in managing various complex diseases especially in old people. The thalidomide tragedy and the increasing aversion towards chemically synthesized drugs, especially in Europe, reversed medical interest towards traditional systems. Such reversal was also aided by the fact that the pharmaceutical industry is stressed from the twin burdens of huge cost of developing a marketable drug and the risk of crippling litigation in the post-market phase. Not surprisingly, MNCs shifted their focus to natural products, adopting a less expensive, less risk-prone route to drug development. The unfortunate aspect of this strategy is that scientific studies in Ayurveda have been few and far between. The need of the hour is to redress this lacuna and expose Ayurveda to critical scientific scrutiny.

Health is the most important determinant of development and nutrition is an important determinant of health. Environment and, to a lesser extent, genetics also play a role. Developing countries like India face the double burden of pre-transition diseases such as malnutrition and infections and post-transition diseases like obesity, hypertension, diabetes and cardiovascular problems. Recent studies have shown a link between the two. Individuals who have suffered intrauterine malnutrition and are born with low birth weight are more prone to the post-transition lifestyle-related diseases. The need for nutritional well being of women and children cannot be overstressed.

Serious gaps exist in our understanding of the mode of action of several nutrients, the link between biochemical and pathological manifestations of deficiencies and determining nutrient requirements. A multidisciplinary approach using knowledge and skills of modern biology can bridge the gaps. India has a wealth of traditional knowledge and should gainfully exploit the health-promoting phytochemicals (nutraceuticals) found in plant foods.

Indian diets are deficient in pulses, vegetables, fruits and animal foods. Nutrient-dense millets have been replaced by paddy. Dietary diversification to include these foods, paralleled by a corresponding diversification in agriculture, is the need of the hour. A model for diversification from water guzzling crops like paddy and sugarcane to mixed gardens of fruit trees and vegetables and application of organic methods has been developed in villages of Medak district to enhance nutritional and environmental security. Models have also been developed to improve healthcare outreach by training rural women as health entrepreneurs and community mobilizers. A model for wastewater disposal using double soakage pit has helped to reduce water stagnation. These models also provide scope for skill-based employment of women.

Life Style and Cancer

There is a great deal of evidence that a healthy lifestyle can reduce the risk of cancer in general. A cancer preventive diet is one that is high in fibre, low in fat and includes various fresh fruits, vegetables, wholegrain cereals and beans. Excessive alcohol consumption increases the risk of liver cancer. Moderate exercise has a positive impact on health.

Bhasmas

Bhasmas are an important and potent group of formulations. They are used more extensively in the *Siddha* system than in Ayurveda. They may be either individual preparations or mixtures. Required only in small doses, they act quickly. They are employed in treating several diseases and are also used for rejuvenation (Valiathan, 2006).

Bhasmas have not only aroused extraordinary interest but also some concern because in addition to herbs they generally contain a metal or mineral also. Mercury, gold, silver and lead and sulphur and arsenic sulphide are common ingredients of several *bhasmas*. These substances are processed in several stages and require special procedures lasting over days or weeks.

Health authorities generally dislike the use of *bhasmas* in therapeutics but practitioners of *Siddha* and Ayurveda have always claimed that they are no more unsafe or toxic than other traditional formulations. Most studies conducted till now to test this have used destructive methods for analysis. What we really need is a careful physico-chemical analysis of the microstructure of the *bhasmas* by using the tools of nanotechnology. This can provide new and interesting data on *bhasmas* and possibly give clues to their reported nontoxicity.

With modern science exploring different dimensions of Ayurveda, a new edifice of Ayurvedic biology can be created. This goal can materialize by taking the following seven routes:

1. Modern biology discovers a molecular identity of *doshas*;
2. Plant sciences find a biological basis for the anti-*dosha* effects of herbs;
3. Biochemistry and immunology discover a sequence of chemical and immunological changes caused by *pancakarma*;
4. Human and *Drosophila* genetics demonstrate the anti-aging power of *rasayanas*;
5. Chemistry reveals the existence of metals in nanoform in *bhasmas*;
6. Physiology vindicates the concept of *ritucarya*; and
7. Archeo-epidemiology lifts the curtain on the ancient canvas of diseases and suffering.

Even if all the above 7 projects were successfully completed, collated and worked into a comprehensive survey, they would still fail to constitute the wholeness of Ayurveda. The whole truth would still elude us because Ayurveda is more than the sum total of scientific studies. The philosophical tradition of Ayurveda warrants that we perceive the reality of

Ayurveda as a whole, which expresses itself not only in scientific insights, but also in innate disposition, beneficence, time, chance and destiny (Valiathan, 2006).

Herbal Management of Cancer: Medicinal Plants

Nature is a rich source of many potential therapeutic agents. Ethnobotany and Ethnopharmacology look specifically at the empirical knowledge of indigenous peoples concerning medicinal substances, their potential health benefits and the health risks associated with such remedies. Many of the plant-derived pharmaceuticals and phytomedicines currently in use have been widely used by native people around the world. Many of the secondary plant metabolites used in modern medicine were first discovered through ethnobotanical investigation. Majority of the pure chemical compounds extracted from higher plants used in medicine have the same or related use as the plants from which they are extracted.

The rosy periwinkle (*Catharanthus roseus*, Apocynaceae) is a classical example of the importance of plants used by local peoples. This herb is native to southeastern Madagascar and is the source of numerous alkaloids, two of which are used to treat childhood leukaemia and Hodgkin's disease. Like the rosy periwinkle, many drugs commonly used today, such as aspirin, ephedrine, ergometrine, tubocurarine, digoxin, reserpine and atropine came through the use of indigenous medicine. Table 9.2 lists selected examples of modern drugs derived from plants.

Catharanthus roseus (Apocynaceae). *Vinca Rosea*

The periwinkle has a long history of treating a wide variety of diseases and has also been used for centuries in Europe, West Indies and Indian Ocean Islands, against diabetes.

Table 9.2 Some botanical drugs used in traditional medicine.

Botanical name	Indigenous use	Uses in biomedicine	Biologically active compounds
Adhatoda vasica	Antispasmodic, antiseptic, insecticide	Antispasmodic, oxytocic, cough suppressant	Vasicin (lead molecule for Bromhexin and Ambroxol)
Catharanthus roseus	Diabetes, fever	Cancer chemotherapy	Vincristine, vinblastine
Condrodendron tomentosum	Arrow poison	Muscular relaxation	D-Tubocurarine
Ginkgo biloba	Asthma, anthelmintic	Dementia, cerebral deficiencies	Ginkgolides
Podophyllum peltatum	Laxative, skin infections	Warts, cancer chemotherapy	Podophyllotoxin and lignans
Prunus africana	Laxative	Prostate hyperplasia	Sitosterol
Papaver somniferum	Headache, arthritis, inducing sleep	Narcotic analgesic, antitussives	Codeine, morphine
Atropa belladonna, Hyoscyamus niger	—	Anticholinergic	Atropine, Hyoscyamine
Ephedra indica	Respiratory ailments	Bronchodilator	Ephedrine
Cinchona officinalis	Fever	Antimalaria	Quinine

Its use as a source of anti-cancer alkaloids originated from its reputation as a cure for diabetes.

Some of the alkaloids isolated from the periwinkle are indole alkaloids. Vincristine and vinblastine are effective against childhood leukaemia, breast cancer and Hodgkin's disease / choriocarcinoma, respectively.

The concentration of vincristine in the plant is extremely low (0.0002%); this is why its cost is very high.

Podophyllum peltatum (Berberidaceae)

The rhizome of *Podophyllum peltatum* is toxic and contains podophyllotoxin and α- and β-peltatin. Podophyllotoxin has a 5-membered lactone ring, a 3,4,5,-trimethoxyphenyl group and a methylene-dioxyphenyl group. This natural compound has been used to generate semi-synthetic derivatives—Etoposide and Teniposide. Etoposide is marketed as a drug for small cell lung cancer, testicular cancer and lymphomas. Teniposide is used in treating brain tumours.

Taxus brevifolia (Taxaceae)

Taxus brevifolia tree is the source of paclitaxel, more commonly known by its trademark name Taxol. Taxol is a complex terpene-based molecule. Extracts of the Pacific Yew were found to stop the growth of several mouse tumours. This represented a case in which ethnobotany provided no clues.

Table 9.3 Some selected Ayurvedic cytostatic plants.

Botanical name	Family	Property
Acorus calamus	Araceae	Light, sharp
Argemone mexicana	Papaveraceae	Light, dry
Bauhinia variegata	Caesalpiniaceae	
Calotropis procera	Asclepiadaceae	Light, dry, sharp
Carica papaya	Caricaceae	Light, dry, sharp
Carum roxburghianum	Apiaceae	Light, dry, sharp
Commiphora mukul	Burseraceae	
Curcuma longa	Zingiberaceae	Dry, light
Euphorbia neriifolia	Euphorbiaceae	
Melia azadirach	Meliaceae	Light, dry
Nerium indicum	Apocyanaceae	Sharp, dry, light
Piper betle	Piperaceae	
Podophyllum hexandrum	Berberidaceae	Light, dry, sharp
Polyalthia longifolia	Annonaceae	Light, dry
Semecarpus anacardium	Anacardiaceae	
Solanum indicum	Solanaceae	Light, dry, sharp
Solanum xanthocarpum	Solanaceae	Light, dry
Vitex negundo	Verbenaceae	Light, dry

Since paclitaxel occurs in the leaves (in very low yields: 0.004% from 12 kg of plant material) of various *Taxus* species, semi-synthetic conversions of the relatively abundant baccatins to paclitaxel and active paclitaxel analogs, such as docetaxel are major renewable natural sources of the drug.

Combretum caffrum **(Combretaceae)**

The roots of this plant are used in traditional medicine against body pain. Screening of the plant extracts yielded stilbene compounds—combrestatins, among which A-4 (CA4) is one of the most potent anti-mitotic agents. Combrestatins act as anti-angionic agents causing vascular shut down in tumours and necrosis in solid tumours. CA4 shows strong cytotoxicity against a variety of cancer cells including multi-drug resistant cancer cell lines. It exerts highly selective effect on proliferating endothelial cells. Two other notable sources of anti-cancer drugs are *Camptotheca acuminata* (Nyssaceae) and *Brucea antidysenterica* (Simaroubaceae). Camptothecin from *C. acuminata* particularly has attracted increasing market demand. It is extracted mainly from the bark and the seeds. The development of hairy root cultures and the cloning and characterization of genes encoding key enzymes of the pathway leading to camptothecin production in plants has opened new alternatives and more sustainable production systems for this important alkaloid.

Herbal Decoctions

Many ethnobotanical studies have been undertaken on herbs. Ayurveda has been successful from ancient times in using these natural drugs and in preventing or suppressing various tumours. Herbal decoctions consisting of multiple herbs are commonly used in Ayurveda. These formulations appear to work on several biochemical pathways and can influence several organ systems simultaneously. A herbal decoction nourishes the body as a whole by supporting various organ systems. Many herbs show anti-cancerous properties and are used for the treatment of various cancers. Some of these are listed below.

Andrographis paniculata

The extract and isolated diterpenes (andrographiside and neoandrographolide) of *Andropgrphis paniculata* are effective against tumourigenesis by their anti-lipoperoxidative action and by enhanced carcinogen detoxification action.

Phyllanthus niruri; P. amarus

An active alkaloid (piperine) extracted from this plant is used in anti-cancer formulations because of its antioxidative potency both *in vitro* and *in vivo*.

Podophyllum hexandrum

Podophyllum hexandrum provides a powerful anti-cancer drug against various sarcomas, adenocarcinoma and melanoma. Podophyllin and its active principle, podophyllotoxin, are cytotoxic by mitotic inhibition, nuclear fragmentation, impaired spindle formation and are also karyoplastic.

Tinospora cordifolia

The active principles from this plant improve host immune system by increasing immunoglobulin and blood leukocyte levels and by the stimulation of stem cell proliferation. Solid tumour volume can be reduced by over 55 per cent, comparable to the chemotherapeutic cyclophosphamide. Its immunostimulating properties prevent tumour mediated immunosuppression.

Semecarpus anacardium

Chloroform extract of *S. anacardium* nuts has antitumour action and prolongs the life of patients suffering from leukaemia, melanoma or glioma.

Some widely used Ayurvedic herbs scientifically proven for their anti-cancer properties are listed in Table 9.4.

Some of these herbs enhance therapeutic efficacy and/or reduce the toxicity of chemotherapeutic drugs. Also, some possess radiosensitising effect.

Withania somnifera, Sida cordifolia, Asparagus racemosa, Vitis vinifera, Plumbago zeylanica, Tinospora cordifolia, Zingiber officinale and *Coptidis rhizoma* are effective in managing weight loss.

Aegle marmelos, Holarrhena antidysenterica, Punica granatum, Cyperus rotundus, Emblica officinalis and *Plumbago zeylanica* act as antidiarrhoeals when diarrhoea becomes one of the complications of cancer cachexia. *Terminalia chebula* is effective against chronic constipation and digestive disorders which are common in cancer patients resulting in loss of appetite.

Eclipta prostrata, Emblica officinalis, Withania somnifera, Piper longum help in controlling nausea and vomiting. *Withania somnifera* and *Tinospora cordifolia* are immunostimulatory and increase body resistance power during cancer associated immunosuppression.

Some Popular Indian Herbal Remedies

Cancer treatment with herbal medicines is quite common in India. Ayurveda emphasizes the promotion of health through various approaches such as diet, lifestyle, exercise, personal hygiene and practising the concept of *Rasayana* or rejuvenation in daily life (see Shukla and Pal, 2004; Pal et al., 2006).

Rasayana is generally used to rejuvenate the general health of the body or aims at achieving the body's maximum potential.

Rasayana medicines (medical rejuvenation) utilize a group of individual herbs or medicinal drug preparations that are customarily complex mixtures based mostly on herbal products (Pal, 2002, 2002a).

Laboratory and clinical studies conducted with various *Rasayanas* have led to the development of: (i) *Brahma Rasayana*; (ii) *Narasimha Rasayana*; (iii) *Amruthaprasham*; and (iv) *Ashwagandha Rasayana*. These seem to be effective myeloprotective agents in cancer patients undergoing chemotherapy and/or radiotherapy. *Rasayanas* also protect tissues from cytotoxic injury associated with reduced serum and liver lipid peroxides, alkaline phosphatase and glutamate pyruvate transaminase in cyclophosphamide—and radiation-treated animals (Vayalil et al., 2002).

Table 9.4 Therapeutic enhancement potential of a few Ayurvedic herbs on cancer chemotherapy/radiation (condensed from *Pharmacological Research*, p. 51, 2005).

Herb	Chemotherapy/herbal intervention studies
Allium sativum	Water-soluble derivative of garlic, S-allylmercaptocysteine (SAMC), inhibited proliferation and cell cycle progression in two human colon cancer cell lines, like the effects of SS, a well-known colon cancer chemopreventive agent. Co-administration of SS with SAMC enhanced the growth inhibitory and apoptotic effects of SS, suggesting the usefulness of SAMC alone or in combination with SS.
Aloe vera	In a randomized double-blind clinical trial, comparing mild soap and *Aloe Vera* gel against incidence of radiation therapy induced skin reactions, the median time of five weeks revealed skin changes in the aloe/soap treatment as against three weeks in the 'soap only' treatment. The protective effect of adding aloe to the soap regimen increases during long time radiation exposure. In another trial involving patients with advanced solid tumours, for whom no other standard effective therapy was available, combination of pineal indole melatonin (MLT) plus *A. Vera* extracts was beneficial in stabilization of disease and survival when compared to 'MLT alone' treatment.
Alstonia scholaris	Pre-treatment with its extract increased the effect of radiation like the enhancement of cell-killing in HeLa and KB cells, followed by HL60, MCF7 and HePG2 cells. In *in vivo* studies with Ehrlich ascites carcinoma bearing mice, the pre-treatment of extract prolonged the life span of animals when compared with the untreated, irradiated group. Combined treatment of *A. scholaris* extract with cyclophosphamide was most effective against Ehrlich ascites carcinoma.
Curcuma longa	When radiation and curcuma were given together as synergical therapy, curcuma showed a radiation sensitizing effect in HeLa, K-562 and IM-9 cell lines. Curcumin, the active constituent, enhances the anti-cancer potential of cisplatin and reduces its nephrotoxicity in fibrosarcoma bearing rats.
Moringa oleifera	Pre-treatment with its leaf extract protects the bone marrow chromosomes in mice against radiation and overcomes the side effects of radiation therapy.
Ocimum sanctum	Orientin and vicenin, two water-soluble flavonoids isolated from its leaves protect human lymphocytes against the clastogenic effect of radiation, radiation lethality and chromosomal aberrations *in vivo*. This radioprotection associated with their antioxidant activity may have clinical potential in cancer therapy.
Withania somnifera	When administered for 4 days before paclitaxel treatment and continued for 12 days, *W. somnifera* caused significant reversal of neutropenia of paclitaxel in mice. It is used as an adjuvant during cancer chemotherapy for the prevention of bone marrow depression associated with anti-cancer drugs. The active component, withaferin A has significant anti-tumour and radiosensitising effects in experimental tumours *in vivo*, without systemic toxicity. In Ehrlich ascites carcinoma mice, the extract showed dose dependent inhibition of tumour growth and increased survival rate. Combination of radiation therapy with the extract increased tumour cure and tumour-free survival. It also reduces cyclophosphamide induced myelosuppression and leucopenia and is useful in combination chemotherapy.

Herbs Used in Various *Rasayanas*

Some herbs used in various *Rasayanas* are listed below:

Brahma Rasayana *Embelia officinalis, Terminalia chebula, Desmodium gangeticum, Gmelina arborea, Solanum nigrum, Tribulus terrestris, Aegle marmelos, Premna tomentosa, Stereospermum suaveolens, Oroxylon indicum, Sida rhombifolia, Boerhaavia diffusa, Ricinus communis, Vigna vexilata, Phaseolus adenanthus, Asparagus racemosus, Holostemma annulare, Leptadenia reticulata, Desmostachya bipinnata, Saccharum officinarum, Oryza malampuzhensis, Cinnamomum sp., Elettaria cardamomum, Cyperus rotundus, Curcuma longa, Piper longum, Aquilaria agallocha, Santalum album, Centella asiatica, Mesua ferrea, Clitoria ternatia, Acorus calamus, Scirpus crossus, Glycyrrhiza glabra* and *Embelia ribes.*

Amruthaprasham *Withania somnifera, Pureria tuberosa, Hemidesmus indicus, Cuminum cyminum, Aloe barbedensis, Vitis vinifera, Elettaria cardamomum, Zingiber officinale, Piper nigrum* and *P. longum.*

Narasimha Rasayana *Acacia catechu, Plumbago zeylanica, Xylia dolabriformis, Pterocarpus marsupium, Embelia ribes, Semecarpus anacardium, Eclipta alba, Terminalia chebula, Embelia officinalis* and *Terminalia belerica.*

Ashwagandha Rasayana *Holstemma annulare, Vigna vexilata, Phaseolus adenanthus, Glycyrrhiza glabra, Zingiber officinale, Asparagus racemosus, Boerhaavia diffusa, Sida retusa, Clerodendron serratum, Mucuna pruriens, Hedychium spicatum, Phyllanthus amarus, Piper longum, Vitis vinifera, Embelia officinalis, Pureria tuberosa, Saccharum officinalum, Piper nigrum, Cinnamomum zeylanica, Elettaria cardamomum, Garcinia morella* and *Mesua ferrea.*

Cancer Complementary and Alternative Therapies

Many have become popular as Cancer Complementary and Alternative Therapies (CCAT) in India. Hundreds of patients try these alternatives every year and their popularity is increasing. One reason behind this popularity could be the effectiveness of these therapies. Some prominent poly-herbal based therapies are *Maharishi Amrit Kalash, HUMA, Sarvapisti* and CARCTOL.

Maharishi Amrit Kalash (MAK)

Maharishi Amrit Kalash is produced by 'Maharishi Ayurveda Products'. It contains many important herbs and is processed in the extract of *Aegle marmelos, Oroxylum indicum, Gmelina arborea, Stereospermum suaveolens, Clerodendrum phlomides, Desmodium gangeticum, Uraria picta, Solanum indicum, S. xanthocarpum, Tribulus terrestris, Pedalium murex, Phaseolus trilobus, Teramnus labialis* (Leguminosae), *Ricinus communis, Sida cordifolia, Saccharum spontaneum, S. officinarum, Eragrostis cynosuroides, Asparagus racemosus, Boerhaavia diffusa, Leptadenia reticulata, Gymnema aurantiacum, Ipomoea digitata* and *Pueraria tuberosa.*

MAK-4 (Paste) It contains *Phyllanthus emblica, Terminalia chebula, Santalum album, Mesua ferrea, Convolvulus pluricaulis, Cinnamomum zeylanicum, Elettaria cardamomum, Centella asiatica, Curcuma longa, Piper longum, Glycyrrhiza glabra, Embelia ribes, Cyperus rotundus* and *C. scariosus.*

MAK-5 (Tablet) It contains *Withania somnifera, Glycyrrhiza glabra, Ipomoea digitata, Asparagus adscendens, Emblica officinalis, Tinospora cordifolia, Asparagus racemosus, Vitex trifolia, Convolvulus pluricaulis, Argyreia speciosa, Curculigo orchioides, Capparis aphyla* and *Acacia arabica.*

Patients using MAK show much reduction of side effects like loss of appetite, weight loss and nausea, while there is a lowering of the incidence of fever, pain and ulceration of the mouth.

HUMA

HUMA was advocated by a Lucknow-based Ayurvedacharya Dr SM Atiq in the 1980s. It contains important herbs viz., *Azadirachta indica, Acacia catechu, Asparagus racemosus, Curcuma longa, Calotropis procera, Catharanthus roseus, Emblica officinalis, Ocimum sanctum, Plumbago zeylanica, Semecarpus anacardium, Tinospora cordifolia, Tiliacora racemosa, Withania somnifera,* etc. When tested in the Central Drug Research Institute, Lucknow, *HUMA* was found to be non-toxic in animals. Hundreds of cancer patient all over the country now try this therapy every year. It has cured many advanced-stage patients without adverse side effects. Pal et al. (2006) published objective evidence for the effectiveness of *HUMA* in regression of oral cancer.

Sarvapisti

Sarvapisti is a dietary regimen and was developed by the DS Research Centre Varanasi, in 1983, by using hundreds of medicinal herbs and plants. A book published from the center recently, 'Cancer is Curable Now', provides evidence of many patients where marked remission of the cancer/tumour was observed along with substantial increase in the disease free survival (see Pal, 2006).

CARCTOL

CARCTOL was developed by Dr NL Tiwari from Rajasthan, who has been giving it to patients for the last many years. It consists of the seeds, roots and leaves of eight herbs: *Blepharis edulis, Piper cubeba, Smilax china, Ammannia vesicatoria (Lythraceae), Hemidesmus indicus, Lepidium sativum, Rheum emodi* and *Tribulus terrestris*. It is effective when used along with radiotherapy and chemotherapy, as it prevents patients from becoming neutropenic (i.e., there is no compromise of white cells). This gives the patient more of a 'fighting chance'.

10 Drugs and Treatment Options

Introduction

Combating cancer can be frustrating with final victory sometimes looking like a bridge too far. Understanding of the disease and the crushing blow that the medical fraternity has been hoping for has still not been delivered and the problem seems to have become more and more complicated.

The concept of cancer as a single disease has in recent years been replaced by a view of it as many different ones, each involving its own molecular process and each requiring its own therapeutic approach.

Advances in molecular biology are inspiring the development of therapies targeted at specific disease processes. But the therapies may only bring down the cancer mortality figures gradually rather than making quick or dramatic impact.

Certainly, possibilities exist not only for tangible progress in saving lives in the near future but also for developing novel approaches to stubborn problems. Science could certainly improve survival rates by finding new ways to detect cancers early. Even currently available treatments are much more effective when delivered early; and innovative technologies to detect disease earlier than ever before are looming large on the horizon. The major challenge is how to choose the right signs and understand what they mean. But even if we can detect cancers early, can the drugs target them correctly? It seems that they could be missing something—a small number of cancer stem cells could re-seed tumours after treatment.

Researchers are attempting to develop drugs aimed at cancer stem cells in the hope to prevent the recurrence of tumours—the leading cause of cancer deaths. Unfortunately, about nine out of ten drugs that look promising in preclinical tests fail to fulfil that promise when tried on humans. The mouse, the stalwart animal model of cancer, may not be an appropriate model for humans. But that may be changing—researchers are finding ever-more ingenious ways to engineer mice to be more like humans (see *Nature* 439: 735, 2006).

While anybody can be afflicted by cancer at any age, some 75 per cent of all cancers manifest in older people (over 55 years). Successful cancer management depends upon early detection and adequate treatment.

The first step is to eradicate the cancer. If this cannot be accomplished, then the treatment shifts to palliation. Treatments can be categorized into four chief types: surgery, radiation therapy, chemotherapy and biologic therapy.

Surgery

This is used in prevention, diagnosis, staging and treatment of cancer for both localized and metastatic disease, palliation and rehabilitation.

Radiation Therapy

This employs high-energy particles or waves, e.g., X-rays, gamma rays, electrons, or protons to destroy or damage cancer cells. It represents one of the commonest treatments and constitutes an important part of the main treatment for cancers of the head and neck, bladder, lung and Hodgkin's disease. Whereas all cells (cancerous or healthy) grow and divide to form new cells, cancer cells grow and divide more quickly than the healthy cells around them.

Special equipment delivers high doses of radiation to cancerous cells, killing or damaging them so much that they cannot grow or spread. It breaks the DNA strands of the cancer cell, so preventing it from growing and dividing. Some normal cells are also affected by radiation, but most of them recover. Unlike chemotherapy, which exposes the entire body to cancer-fighting chemicals, radiation therapy is more localized and affects only some specific part. Radiation can also generate indirect effects by interacting with water which makes up over 80 per cent of a cell volume, to release free radicals; these radicals often damage cell membranes, proteins and other organelles. Most X-ray induced damage is due to the formation of hydroxyl radicals as follows:

$$H_2O \rightarrow H_2O^+ + e^-$$
$$H_2O^+ + H_2O \rightarrow H_3O^+ + OH^*$$

Therapeutic radiation It can be administered in three ways:

1. Teletherapy, with beams of radiation generated at a distance and focused at the tumour inside the patient;
2. Brachytherapy, with encapsulated radiation in the form of a wire or pellet implanted directly into or adjacent to tumour tissues; and
3. Systemic therapy, with radionuclides targeted to a site of the tumour.

Among the three, teletherapy is the most commonly employed in practice.

Chemotherapy

In this, medicines are used to treat the cancer. Medicine is either given alone or in combination with, for instance, surgery and radiation therapy. Chemotherapy kills rapidly dividing cells. These cells include cancer cells and quickly dividing healthy cells of bone marrow, gastrointestinal tract, reproductive system and hair follicle. Often chemotherapy is given as a combination of drugs that work together to kill cancer cells. Combining drugs that have different actions at the cellular level can destroy a larger number of cancer cells and also reduce the chances of cancer developing resistance. The drugs used for chemotherapy are usually grouped into various categories (Table 10.1). New therapeutic entities introduced in the last five years are included in Table 10.2.

Targeted therapy half a century ago, cancer chemotherapy initially used antifolate drugs and nitrogen mustards. The clinical use of these cytotoxic (cell-killing) chemother-

Table 10.1 Some chemotherapeutic agents useful in neoplastic disease (after Goodman and Gillman's *The Pharmacological Basis of Therapeutics*, 10th Ed., p. 1383, 2001).

Class/Type of agent	Drugs
Alkylating agents	
Nitrogen mustards	Cyclophosphamide ifosfamide, Melphalan (L-sarcolysin), Chlorambucil
Ethylenimines, Methylmelamines	Hexamethylamelamine, Thiotepa
Alkyl sulfonates	Busulfan
Nitrosoureas	Carmustine (BCNU), Streptozocin (streptozotocin)
Triazenes	Dacarbazine (DTIC; dimethyltriazenoimid-azolecarbo- xamide), temozolomide
Antimetabolites	
Folic acid analogues	Methotrexate (amethopterin), Fluorouracil
Pyrimidine analogues	(5-fluorouracil; 5-FU), Floxuridine (fluorodeoxyuridine; FudR); Cytarabine (cytosine arabinoside), Gemcitabine
Purine analogues and related inhibitors	Mercaptopurine; Thioguanine (6-thioguanine; TG); Pentostatin (2'-deoxycoformycin); Cladribine; Fludarabine; Vinblastine (VLB)
Natural products	
Vinca alkaloids	Vincristine
Taxanes	Paclitaxel, Docetaxel
Epipodophyllotoxins	Etoposide, Teniposide
Camptothecins	Topotecan, Irinotecan
Antibiotics	Dactinomycin (actinomycin D); Daunorubicin, Doxorubicin, Bleomycin; Mitomycin (mitomycin C)
Enzymes	L-Asparaginase, Interferon alfa
Biological Response Modifiers	Interleukin 2
Miscellaneous agents	
Platinum coordination complexes	Cisplatin (cis-DDP), Carboplatin
Anthracenedione	Mitoxantrone
Substituted urea	Hydroxyurea
Methyl-hydrazine derivative	Procarbazine (N-methylhydrazine, MIH)
Adrenocortical suppressant	Mitotane (o;p'-ODD), Aminoglutethimide
Tyrosine kinase inhibitor	Imatinib
Hormones and antagonists	
Adrenocortico steroids	Prednisone
Progestins	Hydroxyprogesterone caproate, medroxyprogesterone acetate, megestrol acetate
Oestrogens	Diethylstilbestrol
Androgens	Testosterone propionate
Antiandrogen	Flutamide
Gonadotropin-releasing hormone analogue	Leuprolide

Table 10.2 Some new and recent therapeutic entities for cancer treatment.

Drug	Type of drug	Therapeutic use
Bexarotene	Retinoid X receptor agonist	Cutaneous T cell lymphoma
Exemestane	Steroidal	Oestrogen dependent tumours
Gemtuzumab ozogamicin	Antibody targeted recombinant protein	Antibody targeted antineoplastic agent
Alemtuzumab	Humanized monoclonal antibody	B-cell chronic lymphocytic leukaemia
Imatinib mesilate	Tyrosine kinase inhibitor	Chronic myelogenous leukaemia
Ambrubicin hydrochloride	Synthetic anthracycline	Normal-sized cell and small cell lung cancer
Fluvestrant	7-Oestrogen antagonist	Hormone receptor positive metastatic breast cancer
Ibritumomab tiuxetan	Monoclonal antibody murine anti(human CD20) radio-immunoconjugate	B-cell non-Hodgkin's lymphoma
Temoporfin	Porphyrin derivatie	Photodynamic therapy of advanced head and neck cancer 2002
Brotezomib	N-acyl pseudodipeptidyl boronic acid as mannitol ester	Ubiquitin proteosome (26S) inhibitor for multiple myeloma
Ceftuximab	Human/mouse chimeric monoclonal antibody that blocks EGFR	Colorectal cancer
Tositumomab	Murine anti-CD20 radio-immunoconjugate	Radioimmunotherapeutic antibody for treating B-cell non Hodgkin's lymphoma

apeutic agents against malignant tumours does succeed in many cases, but has several drawbacks such as the lack of selectivity, severe side effects and limited efficacy; and the emergence/selection of drug resistance. Traditional chemotherapy usually weakens the patients with nausea, diarrhoea and/or opportunistic infections. Cytotoxic chemotherapy also creates several long-term health problems in survivors, including hearing loss, heart damage, joint problems and memory impairment. Despite these limitations and the emergence of targeting agents with high tumour selectivity, many specialists feel that these traditional agents will continue to be used for some years.

Cancer drug therapy has now moved from the pregenomic cytotoxic era to the current postgenomic targeted era. New cancer drugs that target tumour cells but do not affect normal healthy cells are changing the practise of treatment. Our current knowledge of the regulation of cell growth and biochemical changes that lead to malignancy has generated novel opportunities for targeted cancer drug discovery. Even if specialists cannot cure some tumours, they can at least use the new targeted therapies to turn the tumours into chronic illnesses that can be managed, for instance, like diabetes.

Table 10.3 Examples of approved targeted drugs in cancer (after *Progress in Drug Research, Advances in Targeted Cancer Therapy*, vol. 63, p. 5, 2005).

Drug	Company	Mechanism	Indications	Toxicities
Trastuzumab (Herceptin)	Genentech	Humanized monoclonal antibody against HER2	Metastatic breast cancer expressing HER2	Cardiotoxicity
Imatinib (Gleevec)	Novartis	Small molecule inhibitor of Bcr-Abl and c-kit tyrosine kinases	Chronic myelogenous leukaemia and gastro-intestinal stromal tumours	Nausea, diarrhoea, myalgia, edema
Gefitinib (Iressa)	AstraZeneca	Small molecule tyrosine kinase inhibitor of EGFR	Third line treat-ment of non-small cell lung cancer	Diarrhoea, nausea, rash, pulmonary toxicity
Cetuximab (Erbitux)	Imclone/Bristol-Myers, Squibb	Chimeric monoclonal antibody against EGFR	EGFR-positive, irinotecan- refractory metastatic colorectal carcinoma	Acneiform rash, folliculitis, hypersensitivity reactions
Bevacizumab (Avastin)	Genentech	Humanized monoclonal antibody against vascular endothelial growth factor (VEGF)	First line treatment for metastatic colorectal cancer	Hypertension, intestinal perforation
Bortezomib (Velcade)	Johnson and Johnson	Small molecule proteasome inhibitor	Multiple myeloma relapsed after two prior treatments	Gastrointestinal symptoms, fatigue, thrombocytopenia; sensory neuropathy
Rituximab (Rituxan)	IDEC Pharmaceuticals	Chimeric monoclonal antibody against CD20 antigen (expressed on mature B-cells)	Refractory low-grade and follicular B-cell non-Hodgkin's lymphoma	Fever, chills, nausea, urticaria

Work is also underway toward tailoring cancer care to suit a particular patient's genetic make-up. Selected examples of currently marketed/targeted drugs are shown in Table 10.3. A great diversity of targets is available for potential cancer therapeutics. There exist over 100 distinct types of cancers and tumour subtypes. Tumourigenesis, being a multistep process, involves a series of premalignant changes. The complex signalling pathways in tumour progression, the multiple stages in tumour growth; the dependence on the tumour microenvironment, the development of tumour cell invasion and metastasis formulation and the interaction of the tumour with complex cell types offer many targets for therapeutic intervention in cancer.

Biologic Therapy

Biologic therapy prepares the immune system of the body to fight against the cancer or weaken any side effects of treatments. Biological response modifiers (BRMs) are found naturally in the body and can also be produced in the laboratory. They modify the interaction between the body's immune defenses and cancer cells to boost, direct, or enhance one's ability to fight the disease. Examples of biological therapies are interferons, interleukins, colony-stimulating factors, monoclonal antibodies, vaccines, gene therapy and nonspecific immunomodulating agents. The immune system functions against diseases, including cancer, in various ways. It may differentiate between healthy cells and cancer cells in the body and remove cancerous cells. However, the system does not always recognize cancer cells as 'foreign'. Also, cancer can appear if the immune system breaks down or does not function properly. The aim of biological therapies is to repair, stimulate, or improve the immune system's responses. Immune system cells include lymphocytes (B and T cells) (which are a type of white blood cells found in the blood and many other parts of the body) and natural killer (NK) cells.

Biological Response Modifiers

Some antibodies, cytokines and other immune system substances are produced in the laboratory for use in cancer treatment. These substances are called biological response modifiers (BRMs). They modify the interaction between the body's immune defenses and cancer cells to boost, direct, or restore the body's ability to fight the disease. BRMs include interferons, interleukins, colony-stimulating factors, monoclonal antibodies, vaccines, gene therapy and nonspecific immunomodulating agents.

Biological therapies They are employed to stop, control or suppress processes that permit cancer growth. They:

- Improve recognition of cancer cells therapy, enhancing their destruction by the immune system.
- Boost the killing power of T cells, NK cells and macrophages.
- Alter the growth patterns of cancer cells to make them behave more like healthy cells.
- Block or reverse the process that changes a normal cell or a precancerous cell into a cancerous cell.
- Enhance the body's ability to repair or replace normal cells that have been damaged or destroyed by chemotherapy or radiation.
- Prevent cancer cells from spreading to other parts of the body.

Some BRMs constitute a standard part of treatment for certain types of cancer, while others are undergoing clinical trials (research studies). BRMs are used individually, in combination, or with radiation or chemotherapy.

Drugs from the Seabed

The sea may be hiding a treasure of extremely valuable chemicals and useful organisms such as corals, sponges, microbes and other biota which contain useful chemicals in their cells (see Blunt et al., 2006). Natural products from these organisms have considerable pharmaceutical potential.

Oceans cover two-thirds of Earth's surface and harbour many marine creatures. Notable medicines are derived from the following three marine creatures (see Blunt et al., 2006).

1. *Conus magus* is a cone snail that paralyses its prey by using a poison-tipped barb. The poison is a painkiller far more potent than morphine and is being marketed as Prialt.
2. *Ecteinascidia turbinata* is a sea squirt, produces an antitumour compound for soft-tissue sarcomas, brand-named Yondelis by PharmaMar. Marketing approval is still awaited.
3. *Aplidium albicans*. This anti-cancer drug has also been isolated from a squirt. PharmaMar calls it Aplidin.

Marine natural products are valuable sources for novel antibiotics because they are mostly secondary metabolites—not essential to an organism's growth and development, but represent compounds that do something else, such as deter predators—and could be re-engineered to aid our fight against infectious disease (Marris, 2006).

Work is underway to determine how organisms make natural products. Surprisingly, many compounds are in fact produced by an associated microbe, rather than by the organism itself. This means that either the microbes may be grown in pure cultures in the laboratory or their genes responsible for generating the secondary metabolite might be identified so as to insert them into some other organism which may be easier to work with, such as *Escherichia coli*. Moreover, many more natural products can be made from scratch by chemists (Nicolaou and Snyder, 2004).

With some effort, many marine microbes can be fermented and grown in large flasks by including the right ingredients in the culture medium. Mincer et al. (2002) explored a deep-ocean sediment and discovered many species of actinomycetes—in sharp contrast to the hitherto popular and widely held view that the sea lacked any such microbes! The first genus of these actinomycetes was named *Salinospora*. From one of these microbes came salinosporamide A, a compound that binds extremely selectively to the proteasome in tumour cells (Feling et al., 2003). This compound is now undergoing clinical trials for multiple myeloma, a cancer of the blood (Marris, 2006).

Another new genus, *Marinispora* has been discovered by Kwon et al. (2006). It produces compounds with promising antibiotic and anticancer properties. The limiting factor in this kind of research is the difficulty in collecting samples from deep-sea mud. Sampling probes have been developed that fall to the sea floor; drive a corer into the mud, release weights and rise to the surface. Recent technical advances are also benefiting the field. Nuclear magnetic resonance imaging work needs only tiny quantities of compounds, making the work easier. Assays are also becoming better. Use of specific enzymes is replacing some outdated cytotoxic and antibiotic assays. This means that instead of finding out whether a compound has any biological activity, researchers determine whether it binds to a particular target (Marris, 2006).

Cancer Cells, High Throughput Screening and Drug Discovery

Spectacular advances in our knowledge of the genetic basis of human cancer have brought to light the potential for developing therapeutics aimed at targeting the genetic differences that exist between tumour cells and normal cells in the body (see Harris and Ford,

2000; Gibbs, 2000). However, this potential has so far only been realized in a few tumour types that contain overexpressed or deregulated cellular oncogenes such as ST1571, an inhibitor of the c-abl/c-kit tyrosine kinases and trastuzumab (Herceptin), a humanized monoclonal antibody that inhibits the human epidermal growth factor receptor-2 (HER-2/neu) (see Pegram et al., 2000).

Although tissue culture cell-based screening for anticancer drugs has been used for decades; a major problem with such cell-based screening lies in the nature of the control cells. While many compounds are toxic to cancer cells, most are also toxic to all growing cells. Normal cells corresponding to the cell types represented by common tumours are generally not available or do not show growth properties similar to those of the tumours. This has hindered the design of rational screens for drugs with specific activity toward cancer-related genetic and phenotypic variations (Torrance et al., 2001). To address this issue, Torrance et al. described a strategy for drug screening based on isogenic human cancer cell lines in which key tumourigenic genes were deleted by targeted homologous recombination (see Kain, 1999). As a test case, a yellow fluorescent protein (YFP) expression vector was introduced into the colon cancer cell line DLD-1 and a blue fluorescent protein (BFP) expression vector was introduced into an isogenic derivative in which the mutant *K-Ras* allele had been deleted. Co-culture of both cell lines allowed facile screening for compounds with selective toxicity toward the mutant Ras genotype. Among 30,000 compounds screened, a novel cytidine nucleoside analogue was identified that displayed selective activity *in vitro* and inhibited tumour xenografts containing mutant *Ras*. These data demonstrate a broadly applicable approach for mining therapeutic agents targeted to the specific genetic alterations responsible for cancer development (Torrance et al., 2001).

Enhancement of Release and Efficacy of Liposomal Cancer Drugs

While many drugs can kill cancer cells, the tricky problem is how to kill the cancer cells selectively while sparing the normal cells. Three basic strategies have been used to achieve this specificity. One (selective toxicity) uses drugs that have stronger growth-inhibitory effects on tumour cells than on normal cells (Sawyers, 2004). It is this approach that underlies the success of conventional chemotherapeutic agents as well as those of modern targeted therapies such as imatinib (Gleevec).

The second strategy (delivery) makes use of such agents as antibodies which specifically react with those molecules which are mostly expressed in tumour cells (Yamamoto and Curiel, 2005). The third (angiogenic) strategy focuses on abnormal aspects of the tumour vasculature either with agents such as bevacizumab (Avastin) (Kerbel and Folkman, 2002), or drugs incorporated into liposomes (Thurston et al., 1998). Liposomes are fairly large particles capable of penetrating through the fenestrated endothelium in tumours and in some other organs (Hashizume et al., 2000). Upon reaching tumours, they persist and later unload their contents. This raises local drug concentrations through the enhanced permeabilization and retention effect (see Cheong et al., 2006).

Unfortunately, the specificity achieved with any of the above strategies is not cent per cent; this limits the amount of drug that can be safely administered without causing systemic toxicity. To address this challenge, Cheong et al. (2006) combined all three strategies. They investigated *Clostridium novyi-NT*, an anaerobic bacterium that can infect hypoxic regions within experimental tumours. Since *C. novyi-NT* lyses red blood cells, it was thought that its membrane-disrupting properties might be exploited to enhance the release of liposome-encapsulated drugs within tumours. *C. novyi-NT* can selectively infect and partially destroy experimental cancers because of the hypoxic nature of the tumour environment (Ryan et al., 2006).

Cheong et al. tested this hypothesis and showed that treatment of mice bearing large, established tumours with *C. novyi-NT* plus a single dose of liposomal doxorubicin often led to eradication of the tumours. The bacterial factor responsible for the enhanced drug release was identified as a previously unrecognized protein termed liposomase. This protein might potentially be incorporated into diverse experimental approaches for the specific delivery of chemotherapeutic agents to tumours (Cheong et al., 2006).

Iron Sandwich Compounds and DNA Cleavage

Understanding how iron sandwich compounds cleave DNA may help development of anticancer drugs, according to Kowalski et al. (2007). Ferrocene compounds contain two aromatic rings that sandwich a central iron cation (Fig. 10.1). These compounds are attracting interest as possible anticancer agents. Ferrocenium salts kill cancer cells by cleaving their DNA. This fact aroused interest in discovering the mechanism behind this process, to help scientists in designing ferrocene-based drugs.

The iron cations in ferrocenes can have either a 2+ or 3+ oxidation state. Classically, Fe^{3+} has been regarded as triggering the DNA scission but the latest research has shown that Fe^{2+}-containing azaferrocenes, which have a nitrogen atom in one of the aromatic rings, can also cleave DNA. It appears that the bonding strength between the metal ion and the aromatic rings is more relevant to DNA cleavage than the ion's oxidation state.

The researchers also found that azaferrocenes with positively-charged nitrogens had higher DNA cleavage activity than the neutral compounds tested. Conceivably, an electrostatic interaction with the negatively-charged DNA is important for DNA cleavage (see Kowalski et al., 2007).

Some potentially 'smart' cancer drugs act by inhibiting specific tyrosine kinases associated with uncontrolled growth. Gefitinib and erlotinib target the kinase activity of the epidermal growth factor receptor (EGFR); these prove effective when initially admin-

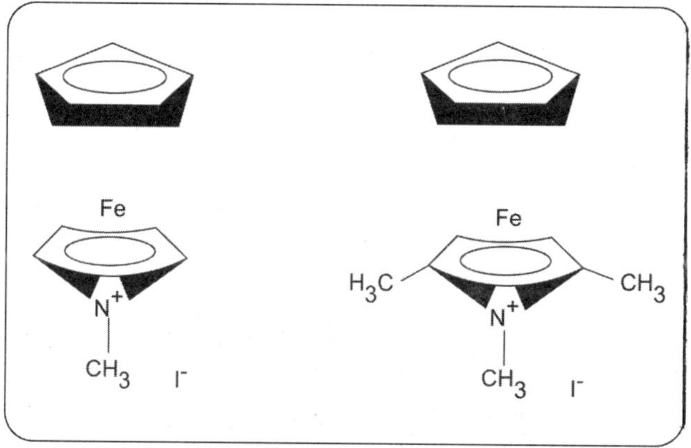

Fig. 10.1 Fe^{2+} sandwich compounds with positively-charged nitrogen atoms that can cleave DNA (after Kowalski et al., 2007).

istered to lung cancer patients whose tumours contain activating mutations in the EGFR gene. Most often, however, these tumours become resistant to the drugs and re-grow. It appears that drug resistance in a subset of these tumours is caused by amplification of the MET oncogene. This in turn activates, via a different pathway, the same cellular signalling route that is originally activated by the mutant EGFR.

Antisense Therapy

Much recent work has led to identifying, cloning, sequencing and characterizing some genes involved in cancer development. Genetic therapy involves two general approaches: one; termed gene therapy, means the introduction of a vector that can insert a gene into the patient's genome to restore normal function or to correct an abnormal function; the second, termed RNA-based therapy includes antisense technology. It delivers RNA silencing molecules that hybridize with and inhibit the expression of pathogenic genes in target cells.

In general, antisense nucleic acids (DNA, RNA and DNA/RNA chimeras) are single-stranded oligonucleotides (oligos) complementary to the sequence of a target RNA or DNA. Antisense RNA is really a natural mode of regulation of gene expression in most living cells. Recent advances in automated oligo synthesis and better understanding of gene regulation have greatly stimulated work on developing antisense techniques. Antisense technology such as RNA silencing approach is useful in many areas such as: (i) identification of gene function and of novel targets for therapy; (ii) pharmacogenetics and pharmacogenomics; and (iii) novel therapeutic agents.

Vitravene, the first antisense drug has already been approved for the treatment of patients with cytomegalovirus-induced retinitis. Several other antisense oligos are undergoing clinical trials as anticancer agents (Table 10.4) and several are in preclinical development.

Laser Therapy

Lasers are very often being used to treat superficial cancers (i.e., cancers on the surface of the body or the lining of internal organs) such as basal cell skin cancer and early stages of cervical, penile, vaginal, vulvar and non-small cell lung cancers. Lasers are also used to relieve certain symptoms of cancer, such as bleeding or obstruction. They can shrink or destroy a tumour blocking a patient's trachea or oesophagus, or remove any colon polyps or tumours that block the colon or stomach.

Although laser therapy can be used alone, most often it is combined with surgery, chemotherapy, or radiation therapy. Also, lasers can seal nerve endings to reduce pain after surgery, or seal lymph vessels to reduce swelling and limit the spread of tumour cells. Three types of lasers being used to treat cancer are the carbon dioxide (CO_2) laser; argon laser and Nd:YAG.

Photodynamic Therapy

Photodynamic therapy (PDT) also uses lasers. In PDT, a photo-sensitizer or photosensitizing agent is injected into a patient and absorbed by the patient's cells. Laser light is then used to activate the agent and destroy cancer cells. Since the photo-sensitizer makes the

Table 10.4 Antisense anti-cancer drugs in clinical trials since 1995 (Source: *Progress in Drug Research, Advances in Targeted Cancer Therapy*, vol. 63, p. 229).

Drug	Target	Chemical modification(s)	Company
Affinitakl/ISIS3521/ Aprinocarsen	PKC-alpha	PS	Lilly/ISIS
Oblimersen, G3139	Bcl-2	PS	Aventis/Genta
ISIS2503	H-ras	PS	ISIS
GTI-2040	RR R2 subunit	PS	Lorus Therapeutics
GTI-2501	RR R1 subunit	PS	Lorus Therapeutics
GEM-231	PKA	MBO (PS/2/-O-Me)	Hybridon
MG98	DNA methyl-transferase	MBO (PS/2/-O-Me)	MethyGene, MGI Pharma, British Biotech
Oncomyc-NGI/AVI 4126	*c-myc*	Morpholino	AVI BioPharma
AVI 4557	Cyp3A4	Phosphorodiamidate Morpholino	AVI BioPharma
AP12009	TGF-B2	PS	Antisense Pharma
ISIS5132	c-raf	PS	ISIS
LErafAON	c-raf	PS (liposome)	NeoPharm
OGX-011	Clusterin	MBO (PS/2/-O-Me)	Oncogenix ISIS
LR-3001	c-myb	PS	Lynx Therapeutics/ Inex/ Temple Univ.
OL(1)p531/EL-625	P53	PS	Lynx Therapeutics/ Elos Inc.

skin and eyes sensitive to light for approximately 6 weeks, the patient must avoid direct sunlight and bright indoor light during that period.

PDT is usually used in combination with radiation therapy, hyperthermia or chemotherapy. Magnetic fluid hyperthermia (MFH) uses magnetic particles to offer the thermal effect biologically in living cells.

Gene Therapy

Scientists today can alter genetic material of patients to fight or prevent disease by introducing DNA or RNA into a patient's cells. It is undergoing clinical trials for many different types of cancers, but no gene therapy has yet been approved for routine clinical use.

Some approaches to treat cancer by using gene therapy include:

- Replacing missing or altered genes with healthy genes. Some of the missing or altered genes (e.g., *p53*) can lead to cancer.
- Stimulating the body's immune response.
- Injecting cancer cells with genes that make them more sensitive to chemotherapy, radiation therapy, or other treatments.
- Placing genes into healthy blood-forming stem cells to make them more resistant to the side effects of high doses of anticancer drugs.

- Injecting cancer cells with genes ('suicide genes') that destroy the cells. This is followed by administering a pro-drug (an inactive form of a toxic drug) to the patient. The pro-drug is activated in cancer cells containing these 'suicide genes'. This leads to the destruction of those cancer cells.
- Preventing cancer cells from developing new blood vessels (angiogenesis).

Hyperthermia

In hyperthermia (thermotherapy), body tissue is exposed to high temperatures (up to 113°F) which can damage and kill cancer cells, usually with minimal injury to normal tissues by: (a) killing cancer cells and damaging proteins and structures within cells; and (b) shrinking tumours. It is always used with other therapies such as radiation and chemotherapy. Hyperthermia also enhances the effects of certain anticancer drugs.

Monoclonal Antibodies for Cancer Treatment

Monoclonal antibodies (MAbs) achieve their therapeutic effect through the following mechanisms:

- Direct induction of apoptosis or programmed cell death. They can block growth factor receptors and so arrest proliferation of tumour cells. In cells that do express MAbs, they induce anti-idiotype antibody formation.
- 'Indirect effect' involves recruitment of cytotoxic cells such as monocytes and macrophages. This type of antibody-mediated cell killing is termed 'antibody dependent cell-mediated cytotoxicity' (ADCC).

MAbs also bind complement, leading to direct cell toxicity, known as 'Complement Dependent Cytotoxicity' (CDC).

The MAb binds to the receptor and initiates the 'complement cascade'. The end result is a membrane attack complex that creates a hole within the cell membrane, cell lysis and death.

An antibody fragment can hit a cancer target that has previously been thought to be undruggable. Mutations that activate Ras proteins manifested in as many as 30 per cent of cancers, but the difficulty of blocking their protein-protein interactions inside the cell had rendered them intractable targets. T. Rabbits (Leeds Institute of Molecular Medicine) and his associates have shown that an antibody fragment, termed iDab#6, jams mutant Ras by blocking a key interaction site. In mice injected with human tumour cells, tumour growth ceased if the cells expressed the antibody fragment. While delivering the genetic material to express iDab#6 in human patients could be difficult, the team's characterization of the Ras-antibody interaction may at least help small-molecule drug development (see *EMBO J.* doi: 10.1038/sj.emboj.7601744, 2007).

Antibody Direct Enzyme Prodrug Therapy (ADEPT)

This involves a two-step treatment for cancer. An antibody enzyme conjugate is administered first. The antibody is raised against tumour specific antigens and localizes to the tumour, carrying an exogenous enzyme with it. This is followed by administration of a prodrug, which is activated by the exogenous enzyme at the tumour site.

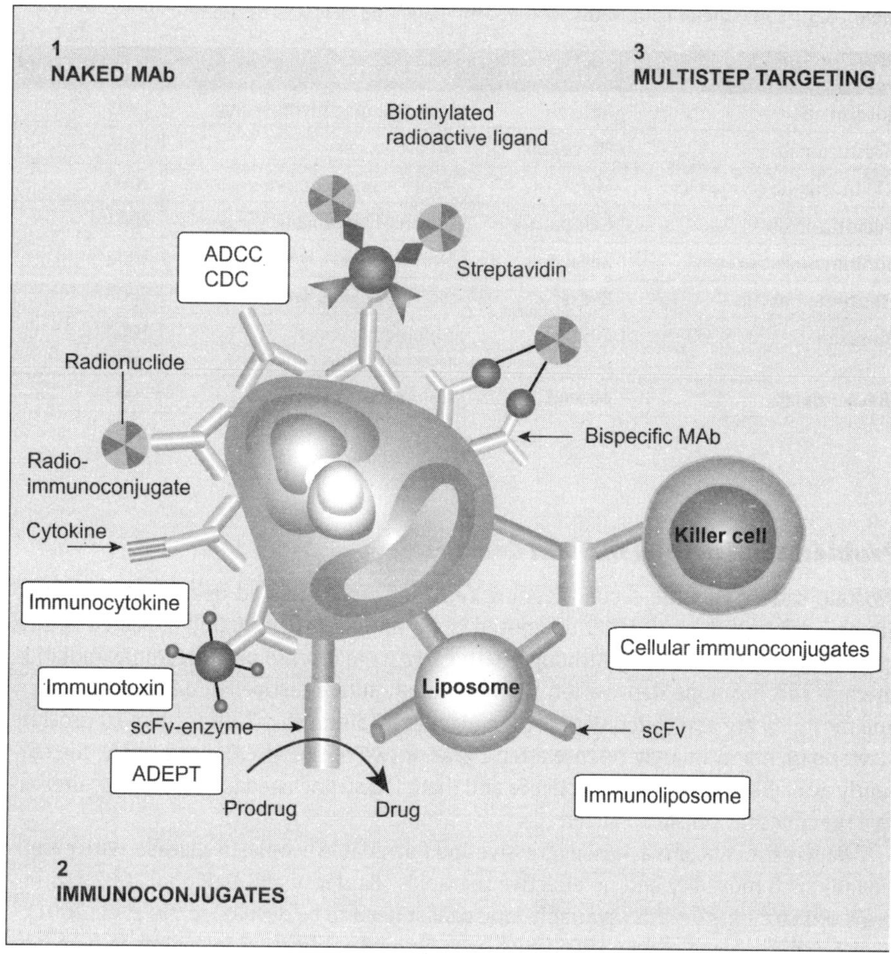

Fig. 10.2 MONOCLONAL ANTIBODIES FOR CANCER. ADEPT, antibody directed enzyme prodrug therapy; ADCC, antibody dependent cell-mediated cytotoxicity; CDC, complement dependent cytotoxicity; MAb, monoclonal antibody; scFv, single-chain Fv Fragment. Modified from Carter, P. Improving the efficacy of antibody-based cancer therapies *Nature Rev. Cancer* 1: 118-129 (2001).

Types

Two types of MAbs are usually employed.

- Naked MAbs are those without any drug or radioactive material attached to them.
- Conjugated MAbs are those joined to a chemotherapy drug, radioactive particle or a toxin (a substance that poisons cells).

Bispecific MAbs. 'Bispecific MAbs' are developed by fusing two hybridoma cells together to generate a hybrid; these hybridomas secrete MAbs with two different sets of binding sites, the areas where they attach to antigen receptors. One binding site may recognize a tumour cell and the other site may recognize a cell or toxin that can be recruited to kill the tumour cell. Some MAbs marketed for therapeutic applications in the USA are listed in Table 10.5.

Table 10.5 Some therapeutic MAbs approved for marketing by FDA in the USA.

MAb	Trade Name	Used to Treat	Approved in
Rituximab	Rituxan	Non-Hodgkin's lymphoma	1997
Trastuzumab	Herceptin	Breast cancer	1998
Gemtuzumab ozogamicin	Mylotarg	Acute myelogenous leukaemia	2000
Alemtuzumab	Campath	Chronic lymphocyticleukaemia	2001
Ibritumomab tiuxetan	Zevalin	Non-Hodgkin's lymphoma	2002
Tositumomab	Bexxar	Non-Hodgkin's lymphoma	2003
Cetuximab	Erbitus	Colorectal cancer; Head and neck cancers	2004 2006
Bevacizumab	Avastin	Colorectal cancer	2004

Problems in Therapy of Solid Cancers

Prostate cancer was the second-leading cause of cancer-related deaths in the United States, with less than 200,000 diagnosed cases and less than 30,000 expected deaths in 2007 (Jemal et al., 2007). Although with early stage disease prostatectomy, radiation therapy and hormone deprivation therapy being quite effective; significant morbidity and mortality are associated with these procedures (Simoneau, 2006) and most prostate cancer patients ultimately relapse after a year or two of therapy. Consequently, the currently available treatments do not cure and there is a strong need for developing alternative therapies for prostate cancer.

Pancreatic cancer is a most aggressive and formidable neoplastic disease, with exceptionally high mortality and no effective therapies (Bardeesy and DePinho, 2002), so improved treatments for this invariably fatal cancer need to be developed (Su et al., 2001).

Reactive oxygen species (ROS) such as superoxide radical anion, hydrogen peroxide, singlet oxygen and the hydroxyl radical and ion modify cellular functions affecting development, growth, aging and survival (Thannickal and Fanburg, 2000). Overproduction of ROS or disturbance in the critical balance between ROS and biochemical antioxidants initiates a lethal chain of reactions resulting in damaged cellular integrity and cell death. This toxicity can be utilized as an effective strategy for treatment of various cancers (Hileman et al., 2004). D-amino acid oxidase, glucose oxidase, xanthine oxidase, arsenic trioxide, hydrogen peroxide and dithiophene generate ROS inside or around cancerous tissues.

Singlet oxygen is a virtually active ROS whose toxicity exceeds that of oxygen radicals in inducing apoptosis in certain cells (Godar, 2000). Endoperoxides (EPXs) can store and transport oxygen, which is then released thermally as singlet oxygen (Fig. 10.3) (Schweitzer and Schmidt, 2003). The flux of singlet oxygen from the decomposition of EPXs can be tuned over several orders of magnitude to create the desired biological effect. Singlet oxygen generated *in vitro* in this way has effectively inactivated enveloped viruses and bacteria, including herpes simplex 1, vesicular stomatitis virus, HIV and *Escherichia coli* (see Peflieux et al., 2000).

The *mda*-7/IL-24 (melanoma differentiation associated gene-7/interleukin-24) seems to promote cancer-specific apoptosis through ROS induction, mitochondrial de-

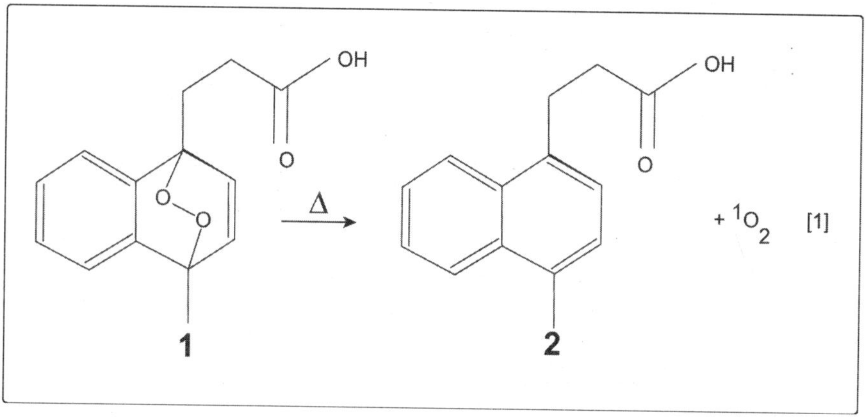

$$\text{EPX } (\mathbf{1}) \xrightarrow{\Delta} \mathbf{2} + {}^1O_2 \quad [1]$$

Fig. 10.3 STRUCTURE AND SYNTHESIS Of EPX. EPX (1) has a half-life of 25–30 min at 37°C in PBS (see Mueller and Ziereis, 1992 for details). The thermal decomposition to yield the propionic acid (2) may follow two paths; roughly 45 per cent follows a concerted path generating 2 and singlet oxygen, whereas the rest follows a diradical path generating 2 and ground-state oxygen (after Turro et al., 1979; Turro and Chow, 1981; Lebedeva et al., 2007).

stabilization and modulation of the ratio between pro- and antiapoptotic proteins of the *bcl* gene family (Fisher, 2005). Now, Lebedeva et al. have shown that Ad.*mda-7*, in combination with a new targeted ROS-inducer EPX (potent endoperoxide) that generates singlet oxygen; specifically kills prostate and pancreatic carcinoma cells. This combinatorial treatment selectively induces *in vitro* apoptosis in those prostate cancer cells which are sensitive to *mda-7*/IL-24 or chemotherapy, as well as tumour cells that are naturally resistant to chemotherapy or engineered resistance to *mda-7*/IL-24. Additionally, the combination of Ad.*mda-7* + EPX induces apoptosis in pancreatic carcinoma cells that are inherently resistant to any current treatment modality, including *mda-7*/IL-24. In contrast, normal prostate and pancreatic cells remain unaffected by these agents at doses eliciting negative effects in cancer cells. These findings point to their potential in developing and exploiting this anticancer therapeutic approach for therapy-resistant tumours (Lebedeva et al., 2007).

Although further studies are warranted to identify and understand mechanism of action of this combinatorial approach, in principle, this strategy could help in inducing cell death in other cancer subtypes and might therefore be a general approach for selectively treating both therapy-sensitive and therapy-resistant cancers (Lebedeva et al., 2007).

Cell's Own Guardian for Cancer Therapy (*p53*)

New drugs that improve survival of cancer patients are being developed. Some, for example, Herceptin, specifically block the oncogenic proteins that drive tumour growth. But oncogenes are only one part of the equation. Many human cancers also have defects in so-called tumour-suppressor genes that would normally prevent cancer development. Researchers are focusing on the tumour- suppressor genes to explore whether therapies that work by restoring their activity could be developed (Marx, 2007).

Transcription factors such as the oestrogen receptor and *p53* have a crucial role in the development of breast cancer. Genomic technologies allow mapping the exact control mechanisms of these factors and potentially direct precise changes by using special drugs. Hopefully, targeted therapeutics will soon become a reality.

Several novel cloning technologies have been developed that allow for remarkable speed and precision in identifying not only all the transcripts in a cell system but also all the binding sites of any transcription factor. This breakthrough technology has enabled researchers to explore the underlying control mechanisms, especially in cancer (*p53*, *myc* and oestrogen receptor) and stem cells (*Oct4*, *Sox2*, *Sal4*, *Nanog*).

The tumour-suppressor gene *p53* has attracted the most attention. Recent studies show that restoring *p53* activity halts the growth of cancerous tumours in mice and, in some cases, even causes tumours to disappear. Restoration of *p53* function in every cell may effectively suppress tumours. Work is also underway on the development of small molecule drugs that reactivate the *p53* protein. A drug called nutlin which showed promise in preclinical testing is being followed by several additional drugs now in the pipeline.

Why are drug developers so interested in *p53*?

Mutations in the gene contribute to the development of about 50 per cent of all human cancers. In addition, tumours lacking mutations in *p53* itself, often carry mutations in other genes that produce proteins which interact with and regulate *p53* pathway that may be inactivated in all human cancers. This pathway probably evolved as a protection against cancer, helping cells to cope with stresses such as DNA damage triggered by exposure to environmental toxins or radiation. Upon being activated, the *p53* protein turns on genes that halt cell division until the DNA damage is repaired, or it can set off cell suicide (apoptosis). In this way, *p53* prevents the accumulation of potentially cancer-causing mutations and also stops abnormal cell growth. This is what prompted *p53* pioneer David Lane to christen *p53* 'the guardian of the genome'.

Three independent research teams at University of California, San Francisco and Cold Springer Harbor Lab., New York, have reported that *p53* reactivation can indeed halt tumour growth (see Marx, 2007). Both teams used mice that had been genetically engineered so that the *p53* gene could be turned on and off at will in the animals' cells. The mice also carried oncogene mutations to allow the development of cancers—lymphoma alone or lymphomas as well as sarcomas.

Researchers genetically engineered liver tumour cells so as to turn the cells' *p53* gene on and off. These cells were then transplanted into the mice livers. In all cases, the researchers kept the *p53* gene "off" until the tumours grew to an advanced stage. Then, they turned the gene back on. It emerged that when *p53* is restored to the system, cancer cells respond. Depending on the tumour type, the exact mode of the responses differed, however.

The lymphoma cells in the other team's mice died by apoptosis, with the tumours beginning to shrink in about 12 hours. The effect on the tumour was quite catastrophic but not permanent. Eventually, the tumours grew back in all the animals and this time *p53* could not be reactivated, either because that gene or the one for a protein called MDM2 known to inhibit *p53* had been lost. This warrants some cautionary note in efforts to treat human cancers by activating *p53*. Assuming that can be done, it is not known how long a remission will last. The Cold Spring Harbor group also noted that the changes that occurred in the senescent cells not only triggered a strong inflammatory attack on but also destruction of the tumour cells.

The above results showed that *p53* activity can squelch tumour growth at least temporarily—a possibility hinted at by early gene therapy efforts to restore *p53* in human cancers. Clinical trials conducted a decade ago also had used adenovirus to carry a normal copy of *p53* into the tumours of patients with head and neck cancer or non-small cell cancer of the lung; tumour growth was reduced in some patients and there was even tumour shrinkage in a few.

Another approach using adenovirus does not attempt to reactivate *p53* but instead exploits the virus's ability to kill the cells it infects. For this cell-killing, the virus must replicate. Normally, *p53* can inhibit that replication, but adenovirus has a defense: a gene that makes a protein that stops *p53* from doing that.

In the mid-1990s, Frank McCormick et al. of Onyx Pharmaceuticals in Richmond, California, had identified a natural adenovirus mutant that cannot inhibit *p53*. They reasoned that this virus should only be able to replicate in and kill cancer cells that lack *p53*, whereas the active *p53* of normal cells should block the mutant virus's replication, thus sparing the cells from its lethal effects (see Marx, 2007). In another study, the liver tumours of seven of the 17 patients with metastatic colorectal cancer who were treated with the virus either stopped growing or shrank and there were few signs of liver toxicity (see online paper by Tony Read in *Cancer Gene Therapy* of Dec. 1, 2006).

But, these viral-based therapies are by no means ideal, chiefly because the agents have to be injected directly into the tumours or, for the liver tumours, into the hepatic artery. One problem with this approach is that it is not possible to get sufficient quantities of the virus into every cell of every tumour a patient might carry. There is a pressing need for more effective delivery systems.

To avoid drug-delivery problems, the focus now is on the development of small-molecule drugs to be administered by mouth and transported by the bloodstream to the entire body. One aim is to block the natural *p53* inhibitor, MDM2. Small peptides that bind to MDM2 prevent its interaction with *p53* and turn up the activity of the tumour-suppressor protein. The biggest boost came a few years ago with the discovery of nutlins by Lyubomir Vassilev and associates at Hoffmann-LaRoche's labs in Nutley, New Jersey.

These compounds, called imidazolines, fit well into the small pocket where MDM2 contacts *p53* and prevent the interaction between the two proteins. The Roche team found that nutlins inhibited the growth of human tumours transplanted into mice by 90 per cent, apparently without causing adverse side effects. But more recently, other researchers reported that activating *p53* in mice lacking a functional MDM2 gene kills the animals. It seems that in the absence of this natural brake on *p53* activities, the tumour-suppressor triggered massive apoptosis and growth arrest.

Any drug that completely took out MDM2 might be fatal to the patient. However, a drug is unlikely to be that efficient and it may be possible to adjust the dose of a nutlin or other MDM2 inhibitor in such a way that it acts in the tumour without causing strong side effects.

As the nutlins are directed at MDM2, they will only work on tumours that still retain functional *p53*. That, of course, is not the case for the 50 per cent of cancers in which the *p53* gene itself is mutated, but researchers are also identifying small-molecule drugs that do restore *p53* activity in such cells. Mutated *p53* proteins tend to undergo abnormal folding and so cannot regulate their target genes. Some of the new *p53* activators probably function partly by helping the *p53* fold into a more normal configuration (Marx, 2007). Several early successes in identifying activators of the *p53* pathway have inspired others to contribute their might. Some are searching for drugs that mimic *p53*'s effects in activating gene transcription. The screen turned up many candidates, some of which worked even in cells that lack *p53* expression altogether because they increase production or stabilization of a *p53* relative called *p73*, which also has tumour-suppressive effects.

In fact, researchers now have several *p53* activators available and more are on the way. But not everyone intends to activate *p53* to help fight cancer. In some conditions, inhibiting its ability to induce apoptosis might prove beneficial. The side effects of gene-damaging cancer therapies, including radiation and some types of chemotherapy, accrue largely from cell death triggered in normal tissue by *p53* activation. It has been reported that tumour-suppression by *p53* does not depend on this response to gene damage but is rather due to its activation by a different path triggered by oncogene activity (see Marx, 2007). This points to the possibility of splitting the bad effects of *p53* away from tumour-suppression and to protect cancer patients during therapy by temporarily shutting down *p53*. A drug called pifithrin can inhibit *p53*-induced apoptosis without changing its effects on gene transcription.

Of course, much more work will be needed before cancer therapies targeting the *p53* pathway make it to the clinic.

Resurrecting the *p53* Pathway

A cell's chief guardian against cancer is the *p53* tumour-suppressor protein. While most cancers get rid of *p53*, the *p53* pathway is not completely damaged. The implication: resurrecting it could possibly help cancer therapy.

As discussed by Felsher and Bishop (1999) and Chin et al. (1999), when fully established, many cancers depend for their maintenance on the persistent activation of certain cancer-promoting oncogenes. Drug companies are interested in exploiting this dependency, as it renders tumours susceptible to inhibitors of the associated oncogenic proteins. Some such inhibitors are proving effective in cancer treatments.

Ventura et al. (2007) and Xue et al. (2007) have confirmed an analogous idea for a tumour-suppressor protein that limits cancer growth. Persistent inactivation of the *p53* tumour-suppressor route is similarly required for tumour maintenance and so opens new therapeutic windows against cancer (Sharpless and DePinho, 2007).

Cancer results as a consequence of many mutations. The presence of so many genetic aberrations in each cancer makes it difficult to distinguish the primary 'driver' events that trigger the cancer from secondary 'passenger' alterations. But even if the primary mutations are known, an understanding of how these lesions interact to cause cancer is extremely difficult.

Indeed, identification of the key 'targets' needed for tumour maintenance has been a major challenge in drug development (Kola and Landis, 2004).

The work of Ventura et al., Xue et al. and Martins et al. (2006) focuses on the *p53* protein. This tumour-suppressor is a strong player in cancer biology, as direct inactivation of the gene that encodes it is the commonest mutation in human cancer and the route that it controls is probably compromised to some extent in all human cancers. The *p53* route normally helps the cell to address any DNA damage caused by radiation or carcinogenic chemicals. This damage activates *p53* which in turn induces the expression of proteins that stop the cell-division cycle to allow for repair. Activation of *p53* can also initiate apoptosis or permanent growth arrest (senescence) if the DNA damage happens to be persistent and severe (Sharpless and DePinho, 2007).

Ventura et al., Xue et al. and Martins et al., described three distinct genetic approaches to producing mice that lack *p53* function, either by inactivating the gene encoding *p53*, or by interfering with production of the protein. Mice lacking *p53* are highly prone to spontaneous and carcinogen-induced tumours. The new contribution is that these mice are engineered so that the dormant *p53* gene is reawakened in tumours by treating the animals with a particular chemical.

Notably, despite the different technical approaches and tumour types in the three studies; the reinstatement of *p53* expression always promptly regressed when established *in situ* tumours. It should, however, be borne in mind that the mere synthesis of *p53* in a cell is not by itself sufficient to suppress tumours—the protein also needs to be stabilized and switched on—this does not generally occur in normal cells.

All three groups reported that restoring expression of *p53* caused tumour regression, suggesting that there is some aspect of a cancer that suffices to activate *p53* and that such a reinstatement of physiological *p53* function is enough to stop tumour growth. Tumour cells contain the signals that can trigger the destructive power of *p53* if it is present. The most significant finding of the work of the three teams may be that established tumours are persistently vulnerable to *p53* tumour-suppressor function.

The manner in which *p53* performs its anticancer act may differ according to the tumour type and context. Reinstating *p53* function in *p53*-deficient lymphomas (blood cancers) rapidly induces apoptosis. In contrast, *p53* reactivation in soft tissue sarcoma and hepatocellular carcinoma induces a strong growth arrest featuring hallmarks of cellular senescence (Ventura et al., 2007; Xue et al., 2007).

Senescence is involved in suppressing the early steps of cancer development in several tissues (Narita and Lowe, 2005) and both Ventura et al. and Xue et al. have established that ongoing resistance to senescence is also required to maintain established tumours. What is not clear is which features of a cancer determine whether its response to *p53* activation is apoptosis or senescence. But both outcomes are associated with tumour regression and hence could be therapeutically beneficial.

The tumour regression reported in the sarcomas and hepatocellular carcinomas was associated with senescence without apoptosis—but if there is no cell death, how does the tumour become smaller?

Xue et al. point to an unexpected cause of tumour shrinkage—a rapid, non-apoptotic clearance of senescent tumour cells by a robust immune-mediated mechanism. As this tumour clearance occurs in 'nude' mice, which lack functional B and T cells, Xue et al. suggest that it represents activation of an innate immune response as a result of the production of certain proinflammatory molecules by the senescent cells.

As pointed out by Sharpless and DePinho (2007), however, markers of senescence accumulate in many tissues with age (Herbig et al., 2006) and senescent cells in precancerous tissue can persist for decades or longer in humans (Michaloglou et al., 2005). Thus, some senescent cells may be impervious to this clearance mechanism. A deeper understanding of how this phenomenon operates may allow unleashing the process on cancerous cells, while sparing normal ageing tissues. The three recent papers point to the possibility that reactivation of *p53* and of other tumour-suppressor genes might prove useful in treating certain cancers. Reinstating *p53* will be difficult in practise, but not so

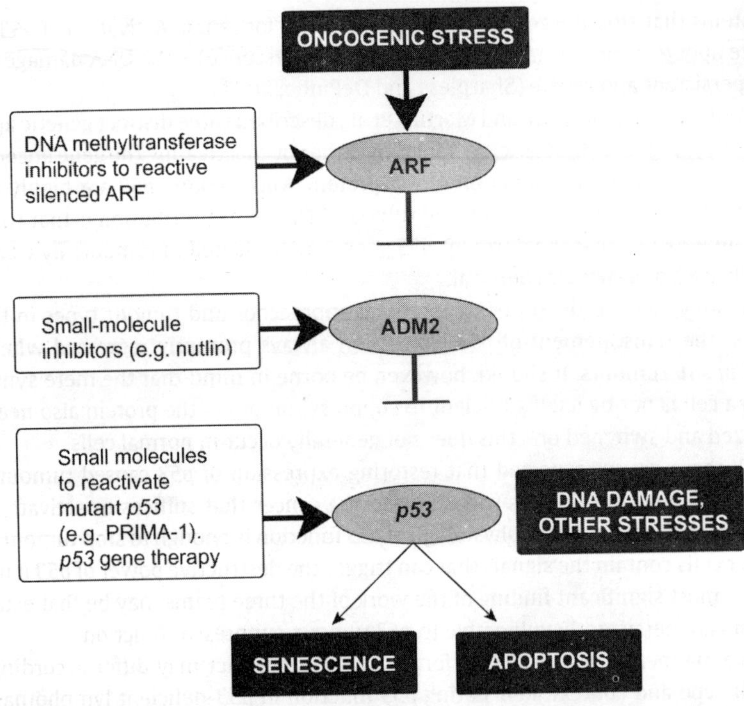

Fig. 10.4 SOME APPROACHES TO REACTIVATING THE *p53* PATHWAY. In the cell, *p53* is usually degraded by the MDM2 protein. Some cellular stresses, including DNA damage, can activate *p53*. Once triggered, *p53* can initiate either apoptosis or senescence. The pathway is probably compromised to some extent in all human cancers. Several potential approaches to reactivating the pathway in human cancers depend on the type of lesion in the *p53* pathway. Mutant *p53* could be targeted directly with drugs or gene therapy. Or *p53* signalling could be reactivated in tumours that overexpress MDM2 by using MDM2 inhibitors such as the nutlin molecules (see Vassilev et al., 2004). Likewise, the ARF tumour-suppressor, which inhibits MDM2, is sometimes switched off in cancer by 'epigenetic' silencing and agents that reverse such silencing are now being tested in humans (e.g., DNA methyltransferase inhibitors) (after Sharpless and DePinho, 2007).

difficult in tumours with normal *p53* that lack tumour-suppressor activity because of other mutations in the *p53* route (Fig. 10.4). A rigorous identification of which factors are involved in tumour maintenance and the precise genetic and biological context in which they function can create better therapeutic possibilities (Sharpless and DePinho, 2007).

The depressing finding in human patients, however, has been that although therapies that target tumour-maintaining oncogenes are initially quite effective, secondary genetic events can render the tumours resistant to such treatment.

11 Nanoscience and Nanotechnology for Therapy

Introduction

Nanotechnology is the science of very small matter and material that deals with the particle size in nanometres. It aims at understanding the world at the atomic level, manipulating material on the scale of atoms and molecules. Nanoparticles can successfully achieve tissue-targeting of many things. Nanoparticles are extremely small colloidal particles made of non-biodegradable and biodegradable polymers, and their diameter is less than around 200 nm.

Nanodevices can be up to 10,000 times smaller than human cells. In size, they are like biological macromolecules such as enzymes and receptors. They facilitate study of normal and cancer cells at the molecular and cellular scales and in the earliest stages of the cancer process. Small size allows nanoscale devices to interact with biomolecules on both the surface and inside of the cells. By gaining access to so many areas of the body, they can potentially detect disease and deliver treatment.

Nanoscience and nanotechnology are not only poised to revolutionize cancer diagnostics, imaging and treatment, but also to herald the golden era of personalized medicine, especially in cancer care.

There are more than 200 types and numerous variants of cancers. Some of these are aggressive and some docile. Some are easily treated whereas others are almost always fatal. Diagnosing, treating and following the progress of therapy for each type of cancer has long been a cherished desire of oncologists and one that may soon materialize as a result of parallel revolutions in genomics, proteomics and cell biology. A new revolution in nanotechnology is bringing personalized cancer treatment closer than ever before (Service, 2005).

Nanotechnology allows manipulating molecules and has opened the door to a new generation of diagnostics, imaging agents and drugs for detecting and treating cancer at its earliest stages. It enables researchers to make nano-sized particles loaded with drugs to kill tumours. It allows targeting of drugs to home in on malignancies. Imaging agents can be designed to light up even the earliest stage cancers. Some nanoparticle-based imaging agents and therapeutics are already in the market, others are in clinical trials or awaiting (Table 11.1).

Nanotechnologists hope to create new tools for tracking and targeting cell surface receptors and other molecules specific to cancer cells. Already, the drug Herceptin, which

Table 11.1 Some nanoproducts being marketed or undergoing trials (from Service, 2005, Table 1; reproduced with permission from AAAS).

Product	Type of nanomaterial	Indication	Phase	Company
VivaGel	Dendrimer	Topical microbicide for HIV	Phase 1	StarPharma
MRX-952	Branching block copolymer self-assembled nanoparticulate formulation of irinotecan metabolite	Oncology	Preclinical	ImaRx Therapeutics
Abraxane	Nanoparticle albumin	Non-small cell lung cancer, breast cancer, others	NDA filed	American Pharmaceutical Partners
Cyclosert-camptothecin	Cyclodextrin nanoparticle	Metastatic solid tumours	IND filed	Insert Therapeutics
TNT AntiEpCAM	Polymer-coated iron oxide	Solid tumours	Preclinical	Triton BioSystems
Verigene platform	DNA-functionalized gold nanoparticles	Diagnostics	On market	Nanosphere
INGN-401	Liposome	Metastatic lung cancer	Phase 1	Introgen
Combidex	Iron oxide nanoparticle	Tumour imaging	NDA filed	Advanced Magnetics

homes in on a receptor called Her-2 that is overexpressed in certain cancer cells, is administered only to those patients whose diagnostic tests show that they carry Her-2 positive cells. Nanotechnologists wish to extend this approach to many diagnostics, imaging agents and medicines.

Nanoelectrode arrays capable of electrically detecting single mutations in the *BRCA1* gene have been created (see Service, 2005). This gene predisposes patients to several cancers, e.g., breast and ovarian cancers. Strands of DNA complementary to *BRCA1* DNA were first taken and bound to electrodes made from carbon nanotubes. A solution containing *BRCA1* was then poured over the arrays, which latched on to the target. By oxidizing nucleotides on the target, researchers could change the conductivity of the nanotubes, which produced a signal that could be detected electronically.

Attempts are underway to use tiny gold nanoparticles to help detect protein and DNA signatures for several diseases, including cancer. A new protein-detecting technique that is about a million times more sensitive than ELISA assays was reported in *Science* (26 Sept. 2003, p. 1884).

Antibodies that specifically bind to proteins of interest are attached to gold nanoparticles which are tagged with readily identifiable DNA strands. If the target protein is in a test sample, the protein binds to the antibody on the nanoparticle. Then another target-seeking antibody tethered to a magnetic bead is attached. A magnet is used to pull the beads—and everything bound to them—away from the rest of the sample. Their target protein is then identified by sequencing the DNA strands. Multifunctional nanoparticles have been made that can combine tumour-seeking sensors, imaging agents and toxins that kill cancer cells.

Finding cancer cells is only the first step. Nanotechnologists are developing particles that may destroy tumours as well. Chemotherapeutic-containing nanoparticles can be linked to an antibody that homes in on the surface of human cancer cells. This slows down the growth of a variety of tumours in part because the nanoparticles can ferry large amounts of the chemotherapeutic drugs to the tumour (Service, 2005).

Nanotechnology's strongest merit over conventional therapies is probably the ability to combine more than one function. Even the tiny nanoparticles are larger than molecules; this enables decorating them with various kinds of materials to perform multiple functions.

Raoul Kopelman of the University of Michigan, Ann Arbor, for example, has produced three-component nanoparticles that target, image, and destroy tumours in the brains of rats. These particles consist of an iron oxide core that acts as an MRI contrast agent. Copies of a cancer-targeting peptide called F3, as well as a light-absorbing compound called photofrin that kills cells when hit with red light can be attached to the nanoparticles. Combination particles were used to treat rats previously injected with cancer cells inside their brains—animals receiving the combination nanoparticles survived more than twice as long as control animals receiving the non-targeted photofrin compound (see Service, 2005).

Targeting tumbleweed-like organic molecules called dendrimers designed to ferry large concentrations of traditional chemotherapeutic drugs and imaging agents inside cancer cells has also been successful. Unfortunately, nanotechnology products also face hurdles in entering clinical practice. Ways need to be found to prevent immune cells from clearing nanoparticles before they reach their targets. Tumours' acquired ability to 'spit out' cancer drugs that get inside cells must also be overcome. The toxicity of nanoparticles is also not very clear and biosafety aspects need critical scrutiny.

Development of Cancer

When a mutation occurs, the cell produces the wrong proteins that alter the cell's function, sometimes leading to cancer.

The gene mutation may be identified by the modified functions, extra growth, being not replaceable by new cells, and the genetic markers producing the biomarkers that can be identified, and in this way, cancer cells can be accurately located and eliminated.

Preparation of Nanoparticles

Polymer nanoparticles, including nanospheres and nanocapsules, are generally prepared by the following methods—polymerization, supramolecular biovector and surface-modification.

Nanotechnologies in Diagnosis and Treatment

Nanowires

Man-made constructs made with carbon, silicon and other materials that can monitor the complexity of biological phenomenon and can detect the presence of altered genes associated with cancer and help researchers pinpoint the exact location of those changes.

Nanoscale cantilevers

Microscopic flexible beams resembling a row of dividing boards—built using semiconductor lithographic techniques—are coated with molecules that can bind to the biomarkers of cancer like prostate-specific membrane antibody (PSMA). Cantilevers, made as part of a larger diagnostic device, provide rapid and sensitive detection of cancer-related molecules. As a cancer cell secretes its molecular products, the antibodies coated on the cantilever fingers selectively bind to these secreted proteins, change the physical properties of the cantilever and point to cancer. This change is read in real time. It informs about the presence or absence as well as about the concentration of different molecular expression markers (Satyakumar and Babu, 2006).

Nanoshells

They have a core of silica and a metallic outer layer. They can be linked to antibodies that recognize tumour cells (PSMA). Once the cancer cells take them up and applying a near infrared light that is absorbed by the nanoshells, it generates intense heat that selectively kills the tumour cells but not the healthy cells. This increases efficacy of the therapeutic treatment and significantly reduces the side effects.

Combidex (ferumoxtran-10) It is a prospective imaging agent, made of iron oxide nanoparticles, for use along with MRI (Magnetic Resonance Imaging) to aid in distinguishing cancerous nodes from normal lymph nodes. Administered via a 30-minute infusion, it accumulates preferentially in normal lymph nodes. It facilitates differentiation between malignant and non-malignant lymph nodes. Lymph nodes are a common site for different cancers, e.g., of breast and prostate.

Lymph node imaging has a role in staging patients and determining appropriate patient management. The cross-sectional imaging modalities used currently for imaging lymph nodes are computed tomography (CT) and MRI without contrast. But CT and MRI without contrast fail to distinguish between enlarged nodes due to inflammation and enlarged cancerous nodes and those that are not enlarged. The current practice is based on the assumption that enlarged nodes (larger than 10 mm) are cancerous; biopsy is then performed to establish their true status. In contrast, Combidex accumulates in macrophage cells associated with normal lymph node tissue and so facilitates differentiation between cancerous and other nodes.

Polysaccharide-coated nanoparticles show long blood residence time, which depends not only on their size, but also on the properties of their coating layer. These particles allow targeting to specific tissue, such as lymph nodes or brain tumours. The direct targeting of solid tumours is also possible by taking advantage of the uptake by tumour cells and tumour-associated macrophages. These properties were mainly obtained with carriers loaded with contrast agents like ferro fluids for magnetic resonance imaging *in vivo*. They show very promising results in tumour delineation.

Dendrimers

Man-made tree-like polymer molecules with many branches to which various molecules including drugs can be attached.

Methotrexate It is a powerful anti-cancer drug, which attached to the dendrimer branches on which are also attached fluorescent imaging agents along with the vitamin—folic acid. While folic acid is required for the healthy functioning of all cells, cancer cells need more than average amounts. To soak up as much folate as possible, some cancer cells display more docking sites (folate receptors) on their membranes. Exploiting a cancer cell's appetite for folate, we can prevent the cells from developing resistance to chemotherapeutic drugs.

Folate molecules on nanoparticles bind to receptors on tumour cell membranes and the cell immediately internalizes it, mistaking it for the vitamin it needs. But while it brings folate across the cell membrane, the cell also draws in the methotrexate that will poison it. In conventional chemotherapy, drugs like methotrexate must diffuse across a cell membrane to get inside a cancer cell; this occurs very slowly and requires a high concentration of the drug in the extracellular fluid, which can damage normal cells and tissues.

Quantum dots Tiny crystals which glow when stimulated by ultraviolet light. The wavelength of the light depends on the size of the crystal. Latex beads filled with these nanoscale semiconductor dots can be designed to bind to specific DNA sequences. By combining different-sized quantum dots within a single bead, probes are created that release distinct colours and intensities of light. When the crystals are stimulated by UV light, each bead emits light that serves as a sort of spectral bar code (nano bar code), identifying a particular region of DNA (Satyakumar and Babu, 2006).

To detect cancer, quantum dots can be designed that bind to sequences of DNA that are associated with the disease. When the quantum dots are stimulated with light, they emit their unique bar codes, or labels, making the critical cancer associated DNA sequences visible. The diversity of quantum dots can help to create many unique labels that can identify numerous regions of DNA simultaneously—important in the detection of cancer, which results from the accumulation of many different changes within a cell. Another merit of quantum dots—they can be used in the body, eliminating the need for biopsy.

Development of CORE Technology

Nanogen Company utilizes the natural positive or negative charge of biological molecules. Applying an electric current to individual test sites on the nanochip micro-array rapidly moves and concentrates the molecules. Molecular binding on nanochip micro-array can be 1,000 times faster than by traditional passive methods. It involves electronically addressing biotinylated DNA samples, hybridizing complementary DNA reporter probes or removing unbound and non-specifically bound DNA after hybridization.

Analysis of Cells

Immunicon

Immunicon has developed this technology in the following parts.

Kits and marker reagents Magnetic nanoparticles (ferro fluids) conjugated to antibodies directed against tumour and endothelial cells are used in cellular analysis kits and associated marker reagents for counting and characterizing circulating tumour or endothelial cells. Ferro fluid consists of a magnetic core coated with basic stabilization agents and conjugated with antibodies for capturing cells. Ferro fluid particles, being colloidal, prevent settling even after long incubations.

Automated and standardized sample processing Ferro fluid and staining reagents are added to each specimen and magnetic incubations are precisely timed to obtain the final enriched sample.

Cell presentation A magnetic field causes the magnetically labelled cells to form a monolayer on one focal plane inside the reaction cartridge. Essentially all of the cells from the starting samples (7.5 ml) can be analysed with minimal loss.

Counting and characterization The reaction cartridge scans and displays a gallery of images of candidate targets to the user for classification.

Advantages of Nanotechnology

1. Imaging agents and diagnostics allow clinicians to detect cancer in its early stages.
2. Multifunctional, targeted devices can cross or bypass biological barriers and deliver multiple therapeutic agents directly to cancer cells.
3. Can monitor predictive molecular changes and prevent precancerous cells from becoming malignant.
4. Enables effective management of cancer symptoms that adversely impact quality of life.
5. Enables rapid identification of new targets for clinical development and for predicting drug resistance.

Nanocarriers and Cancer-targeting Therapy

Chemotherapy involving the use of nanocarriers has been designed for effective clinical treatment of solid tumours by effecting high accumulation of drugs in tumour tissues but limited accumulation in normal organs. Doxil, a liposomal adriamycin (ADR), has already been used clinically (see Muggia, 2001; Ferrari, 2005). It shows therapeutic effects on some cancers with hypervascular characteristics (Hassan et al., 2004), including Kaposi sarcoma and ovarian cancers. Nanocarriers (polymeric micelles) are also being used in clinical trials (see Duncan, 2006; Hamaguchi et al., 2005).

Despite the urgent need for effective chemotherapy for various intractable solid tumours, nanocarriers have not shown any significant therapeutic effects on such cancers. Pancreatic cancer, for instance, is the fifth leading cause of cancer-related death in Japan. The median survival period of patients who suffer from advanced pancreatic adenocarcinoma is only about six months, despite considerable progress in conventional chemotherapies (see Kano et al., 2007).

Although these tumour cells are sensitive *in vitro* to conventional anti-cancer agents such as ADR (Watanabe et al., 1996), most of these agents are ineffective therapeutically *in vivo*, regardless of formulation, whether encapsulated in nanocarriers or not. Nanocarriers seem to specifically accumulate in tumour tissue by the leakiness of tumour vessels to the macromolecular agents; this is termed the 'enhanced permeability and retention (EPR) effect'; it was shown and named by Maeda and Matsumura (1989). The major hurdles in treating these cancer cells may thus be insufficient EPR effect because of certain characteristics of their cancer microenvironment, including hypovascularity and thick fibrosis (Sofuni et al., 2005).

Transforming growth factor (TGF)-β has a crucial role in regulating progression of cancer through effects on tumour microenvironment as well as on cancer cells (Roberts and Wakefield, 2003). TGF-β inhibitors can prevent the growth and metastasis of certain cancers. However, adverse effects can be caused by TGF-β signalling inhibition, including the induction of cancers by the repression of TGF-β-mediated growth inhibition.

Kano et al. (2007) reported that administration of the small-molecule TβR-I inhibitor (LY36947) (Sawyer et al., 2003) at a low dose, which could minimize the potential side effects of TβR-I inhibitor, can change the tumour microenvironment and enhance the EPR effect. This effect of low-dose TβR-I inhibitor was shown with two recently developed nanocarriers—Doxil and a polymeric micelle incorporating ADR (micelle ADR) (Bae et al., 2005).

An application of the short-acting TβR-I inhibitor at a low dose proved successful in treating several experimental intractable solid tumours; including pancreatic adenocarcinoma and diffuse-type gastric cancer, characterized by hypovascularity and thick fibrosis in tumour microenvironments. Low-dose TβR-I inhibitor altered neither TGF-β signalling in cancer cells nor the amount of fibrotic components; but it decreased pericyte coverage of the endothelium without reducing endothelial area, specifically in tumour neovasculature, and promoted accumulation of macromolecules, including anticancer nanocarriers in the tumours. As compared with the absence of TβR-I inhibitor, anticancer nanocarriers showed potent growth-inhibitory effects on these cancers in the presence of TβR-I inhibitor. The use of TβR-I inhibitor combined with nanocarriers may thus be clinically and practically important in treating intractable solid cancers (see Kano et al., 2007).

Since low-dose TβR-I inhibitor does not affect cancer cells, it may reduce the potential side effects of TGF-β inhibitors. Also, its enhancing effect is independent of the reactivity of cancer cells to TGF-β signalling. Use of TGF-β inhibitors should therefore enable reduction of the systemic doses of nanocarriers and thereby decrease the adverse effects of anti-cancer drugs (Kano et al., 2007).

Colorectal Cancer

Colorectal cancer (CRC) happens to be the third commonest neoplasm and the second leading cause of cancer-related mortality in the US (Table 11.2) (Meyerhardt and Mayer, 2005). Surgery has a major role in survival in early-stage disease, by removing detectable tumour; but residual micrometastases sometimes cause a relapse. Recurrence rates can vary from 3 per cent in stage I to >50 per cent for tumours that have spread to regional lymph nodes (stage III). About half of surgically treated patients have a relapse, with 30 per cent recurring locally or regionally and 70 per cent recurring at distant sites—primarily the liver and lung (O'Connell et al., 2004). There is a strong clinical need for image-based detection, targeted delivery, and ablation of metastases, to improve survival in this disease (Fortina et al., 2007). Guanylyl cyclase C (GCC), which is selectively expressed in the apical membranes of intestinal mucosa cells in normal adults and in colon cancer cells, might be the 'magic bullet' for targeted ablation of CRC micrometastases (Frick et al., 2005). In recent years, nanotechnology has been gainfully applied in clini-

Table 11.2 Causes of some cancers prevalent among men and women, and associated mortality by site (source: American Cancer Society, 2006; http://www.cancer. org/docroot/PRO/content/PRO_1_1_Cancer_Statistics_2006_ Presentation.asp).

Estimated US cancer cases*			
	Men (%)	Women (%)	
New cancers anticipated	720,280	679,510	
Prostate	33	31	Breast
Lung and bronchus	13	12	Lung and bronchus
Colon and rectum	10	11	Colon and rectum
Urinary bladder	6	6	Uterine corpus
Melanoma of skin	5	4	Melanoma of skin
Leukaemia	3	2	Urinary bladder
Pancreas	2	2	Pancreas
Estimated US cancer deaths			
	Men (%)	Women (%)	
	291,270	273,560	
Lung and bronchus	31	26	Lung and bronchus
Colon and rectum	10	15	Breast
Prostate	9	10	Colon and rectum
Pancreas	6	6	Pancreas
Leukaemia	4	6	Leukaemia
Urinary bladder	3	2	Multiple myeloma

*Excludes basal and squamous cell skin cancers and *in situ* carcinoma except urinary bladder.

cal laboratory analysis, imaging and therapeutics (Ferrari, 2005; Couvreur and Vauthier, 2006). Nanotechnology shows great potential in the detection, staging and treatment of cancer and other diseases (see Tables 11.2 and 11.3). Fortina et al. outlined one promising application—the use of nanostructures with surface-bound ligands for the targeted delivery and ablation of CRC. Normal colonic epithelial cells as well as primary CRC and metastatic tumours all express a unique surface-bound GCC which binds the diarrheagenic bacterial 'heat-stable' peptide, enterotoxin ST. This makes GCC a suitable target for metastatic tumour ablation using ST-bound nanoparticles in combination with thermal ablation with near-infrared or radiofrequency energy absorption. The incorporation of iron or iron oxide into such structures facilitates MRI. Nanotechnology may also prove advantageous for attacking other types of cancer.

Nanobiotechnology

Nanobiotechnology uses biological materials, biological principles or applications and deals with the study, creation, or manufacture of ultra-small structures made up of a sin-

Table 11.3 Some applications of nanostructures in diagnostics (after Fortina et al., 2007).

In vitro diagnostic	
Nanostructures	**Application**
Nanocrystal CdS, CuS, PbS	Single nucleotide polymorphism
Nanoparticles EuIII-chelate-doped polystyrene	PSA
Au	Prion protein
Polystyrene	Single-base mutation
Silica	Calf thymus DNA
Ag on Au	IgG
Nanopores Silicon nitride	DNA sequencing
Nanorods Au/Ag/Ni/Pd/Pt	IgG
Nanotubes Carbon	DNA
Nanowires Si	Influenza A
Au	*E. coli*
Polypyrrole	DNA
***In vivo* diagnostic**	
Nanostructures	**Application**
Liposomes Gadolinium	MRI imaging
Dual-fluorescence or iron oxide	Optical and MRI imaging
Dendrimers Gadolinium	MRI imaging
Nanoparticles Dextran-coated iron oxide	MRI imaging
Quantum dots	Near-infrared imaging
Gold	Optical detection
Nanoshells Gold	Optical detection
Nanotubes Ultrashort Gd packed nanotubes	MRI imaging

gle molecule. It derives help from molecular biologists to understand the nanostructure and nanomachines designed by nature's four billion years of engineering. It accomplishes several goals that are otherwise impossible to achieve by other means. For example, the DNA, as a biological information storage molecule, may form a basis for the next generation computer chips, thereby converting microprocessors and microcircuits to nanoprocessors and nanocircuits. The structure of the DNA is being exploited for 2D and 3D constructions like DNA-based shape shifting structures to gears and walkers (Seeman, 2005). Forthcoming applications of nanobiotechnology include creation of bionanostructures, miniaturizing biosensors, speeding up disease diagnostics and improving the specificity and timing of drug delivery. Application of nanotechnology to medicine could significantly improve the diagnosis and treatment of cancer (Vicent and Duncan, 2006). Highly innovative approaches of this technology promise early detection and diagnosis; these include nanostructured surfaces for proteomics, the bio-bar code method for the amplification of protein signatures via the use of two-particle sandwich assay, nanowires as biologically gated transistors, to transduce molecular-binding events into real-time electrical signals and silicon cantilevers for the mechanics-based recognition of biomolecular populations (Cheng et al., 2006).

Future applications include development of *in vivo* sensors. Nano devices could potentially be injected into the body where they act as reporters and transmit data to an external data-capturing system. Some nano objects having important analytical applications are exemplified by nanotubes, nanochannels, nanoparticles, nanopores, nanocapacitors, nanocantilevers, quantum dots, nanorods and nanoprisms. To automate molecular manufacturing, engineering of molecular products needs to be performed by robotic devices (nanorobots). The nanorobot is a handy machine at the nanometre or molecular scale which is composed of nanoscale components (Ummat et al., 2006). These materials advance our ability to develop more sensitive analytical systems and future diagnostics (Fortina et al., 2005). To eliminate death and suffering from cancer by 2015, the National Cancer Institute, USA is intensifying research to exploit the power of nanotechnology to drastically change the way of diagnosing and treating cancer.

Semiconductor Nanocolloids

Applications in Biomedicine and Cancer Control

Novel semiconductor nanocolloids have unique optical, catalytic, magnetic and electrical properties (see Bruchez et al., 1998; Daniel and Astruc, 2004; Hicks et al., 2002) of interest to biologists and biomedical engineers for applications such as biolabels, biosensors and image-contrast agents. Nanosemiconductors are also used to fabricate devices used in drug delivery and medical therapeutics. Wang et al. (2005) reviewed some semiconducting nanostructures that have been gainfully employed to address various problems in biotechnology, especially biosensing and bioimaging.

The diversity in composition (inorganic or organic, metals or semiconductors), shape (particles, rods, wires, tubes, cubes, tetrapods, or triangles), and the propensity for surface functionalization (physical, chemical, or biological) has made possible the fabrication of a wide variety of functional nanoscale devices (Gangopadhyay and De, 2000; Daniel and Astruc, 2004). Biologists are now using these nanotools and applying them for applications ranging from diagnosis of disease to gene therapies. Integration of such biomaterials as proteins, peptides, or DNA (Wang et al., 2002; Patolsky et al., 2003) with semiconductor quantum dots (QDs) and metal nanoparticles (NPs) greatly increases the impact of biophotonics and bioelectronics, particularly in optical imaging and biosensing; as well as therapeutic interventions (Elghanian et al., 1997; Xiao et al., 2003).

The combination of magnetic nanocolloids and biomaterials has prompted the development of useful biological separation and purification, hyperthermia, and magnetic resonance imaging techniques. The similarity of size scales between nanomaterials and many biomolecules enhances the utility of these nanostructures for intracellular tagging and for bioconjugation, such as antibody targeting of contrast agents (Wang et al., 2005).

Effective methods of synthesizing one-dimensional nanowires (NWs) and carbon nanotubes (CNTs) have been developed. These should promote applications of one-dimensional nanostructures in the designing of novel nanoscale devices such as biosensors that integrate the conductive or semiconductive properties of nanomaterials with the recognition or catalytic properties of biomaterials. A special kind of sensor system, based on the concept of field effect transistors, has attracted considerable attention. Sensing devices made of semiconductor nanostructures, such as semiconductor SWNTs and Si,

SnO_2, ZnO, and In_2O_3 NWs are proving useful (Kong et al., 2000; Cui et al., 2001). Some one-dimensional nanostructures may be sensitive enough to allow single-molecule detection of surface species (Wang et al., 2005).

Applications of 1-, 2- or 3-D nanostructures stand to gain much from bioconjugation techniques. The field of bioconjugation chemistry and the richness in surface chemistry of nanomaterials enables effective merger of biological and nonbiological systems at the nanoscale.

Semiconductor QDs have been widely used as fluorescence labels in bioimaging and biosensing. These QDs, also called semiconductor nanocrystals, are generally made of atoms from groups II and VI or III and V of the periodic table. Their nanoscale size generates the quantum-confinement effect, resulting in interesting optical and electronic properties. Unique photo-physical properties of inorganic nanomaterials provide a novel class of biological labels that are not affected by the limitations of conventional organic fluorophores.

Good examples of application of QDs as luminescence labels in bioimaging are CdSe/ZnS QDs coated with a silica shell, biotinylated QDs with red photoluminescence, green-emitting QDs with trimethoxysilylpropyl urea and acetate groups showing high affinity to the cell nucleus; as well as water-soluble CdSe QDs prepared by surface exchange of the organic ligands for mercaptoacetic acid, which offer pendant carboxylic acid groups for further coupling (see Chan and Nie, 1998; Tang et al., 2002).

Imaging of live cells by using semiconductor QDs as labels boosted the popularity of using QDs in biological systems (Dahan et al., 2003; Lidke et al, 2004). Good cancer imaging has been achieved by using semiconductor nanocrystals. Wu et al. (2003) conjugated immunoglobulin G (IgG) and streptavidin to CdSe QDs with different emission spectra for labelling the breast cancer marker Her-2 on the surface of fixed and live cancer cells. Conjugated nanoparticles were also used to stain cytoplasmic actin and microtubule fibres, and to detect nuclear antigen inside the nucleus. The idea was to identify tumours that might respond to an anticancer drug. Success has been recorded for some but not all tumours.

Among cancer cell lines that move around or spread in the body, even those that cannot be detected by a membrane can be trapped by QDs (see Wang et al., 2005). The increasing demand for imaging structures deep inside the body is directing attention to QDs that emit in the near-infrared region (NIR, 650–1000 nm), where transmission of light through tissues and blood is maximal. NIR QDs have been produced with tunable photoemission, such as HgTe, CdHgTe, PbSe, InP, and InAs for biological applications. Kim et al. (2004) have used CdTe/CdSe core/shell QDs in cancer imaging.

Besides bioimaging involving the use of luminescent semiconductor QDs, high-contrast, high-resolution images with molecular specificity to cancer can also be produced by using metal NPs (Elghanian et al., 1997).

Quantum Dots for Immunoassays

The construction of biosensors for immunoassays using nanomaterials also involves bioconjugates. In fact, immunoassay biosensors may be a logical extension of the imaging applications of nanostructures, where both make use of the dependence of nanomaterial properties on the attached biological ligands. The large difference comes from the properties of biosensors, which need to be highly sensitive to external stimuli. Integrating the functionality of biological molecules with the unique characteristics of nanostructures generates a novel hybrid design for nanoscale devices (Wang et al., 2005).

Current nanoscale biosensors are of two kinds: light-driven or electron-driven. For optical nanosensing, semiconductor-QDs are particularly useful in view of their long-term photo-stability which allows continuous real-time monitoring.

QDs can be used for sensing by making a donor/acceptor complex that shows switching capability via fluorescence resonance energy transfer (FRET). QDs seem to be suitable FRET donors or acceptors in view of their tunable absorption/emission. High FRET efficiency has been reported for QDs connected to various acceptors (Willard et al., 2001). Complexes can be created by grafting complementary bioconjugates, i.e., antibody-antigen pairs, onto the surfaces of different luminescent CdTe NPs. Their interactions can then be gainfully exploited (Wang et al., 2002, 2005).

Medintz et al. (2004) have designed a biosensor showing reversible FRET connecting CdSe/ZnS core/shell QDs with a photo-activatable species that function as the reversible FRET acceptor. Well-controlled, reversible switching events could be demonstrated by alternating the illumination light source between white and UV light. Incorporation of an emission unit that can be modulated through a biological stimulus facilitates the creation of photochromically switched devices or sensors, in which QD emission modulation presets the device below a predetermined critical threshold (Wang et al., 2005).

Field Effect Transistors (FETs)

Nanowires (NWs) and CNTs may be used for direct, label-free, real-time detection of biomolecule binding by exploiting their electrical properties. FETs have been made from semiconductor NWs and SWNTs and show good potential for high sensitivity, since the depletion or accumulation of charge carriers caused by the binding of charged biological macromolecules on the surface of NWs or SWNTs, affect the entire cross-sectional conduction pathway of these nanostructures (Wang et al., 2005). In this context, semiconducting Si NWs are quite promising, since the doping type and concentration can be controlled, and so sensitivity can be tuned in the absence of an external gate.

Patolsky et al. (2004) have successfully fabricated Si NW FETs for electrical detection of single virus. The principle underlying this is that when a virus particle binds to the antibody receptor on a NW device, the conductance should change from the baseline value, and when the virus unbinds, the conductance should return to the baseline value. Indeed, a valuable and crucial achievement of this work has been the multiplexed detection of different viruses at the single particle level by modifying NWs in an array with antibody receptors specific either for influenza A (nanowire 1) or adenovirus (nanowire 2) (Patolsky et al., 2004). Simultaneous conductance measurements could be recorded when adenovirus, influenza A and a mixture of both viruses were delivered to the devices. As the charged viruses pass over the Si NWs, the specific binding/unbinding behaviour of the viruses can be easily distinguished from rapid diffusion processes by the duration of the conductance change. Diffusion gives a much shorter duration of 0.4 s as compared to 16 ± 6 s in specific, controlled assembly.

Chen et al. (2003) used biomodified SWNTs and showed the selective detection of proteins in solution via specific antigen and antibody interactions.

Exploiting the twin advantage of the specificity of interaction between biological molecules and the flexibility to functionalize CNT surfaces has enabled fabrication of

SWNT-FETs. The CNTs are assembled in contact with Au electrodes via a three-strand homologous recombination reaction between a double-stranded DNA (dsDNA) molecule serving as a scaffold and an auxiliary single-stranded DNA (ssDNA) (Keren et al., 2003). RecA proteins are at first polymerized on the auxiliary ssDNA molecules having an identical sequence to the dsDNA; these bind to the scaffold dsDNA molecules. A streptavidin-functionalized SWNT is guided and immobilized on the dsDNA molecule by means of antibodies bound to RecA and biotin-streptavidin-specific binding. Ag wires are formed by reduction of Ag salts and subsequent electroless Au plating covers the ends of the CNT to form two contact electrodes. Keren et al. also suggested a self-assembly strategy to scale up one-dimensional nanomaterials into conventional sensor devices.

Besides their electronic properties, the desirable optical properties of semiconductor NWs and CNTs can be gainfully utilized for biosensors. Barone et al. (2005) made optical biosensors based on SWNTs that were first noncovalently functionalized with glucose oxide (GOD) enzyme. Electro-active mediators, such as potassium ferricyanide, $K_3Fe(CN)_6$, irreversibly adsorb on the CNT surface, and quench the CNT emission after photoexcitation. Such absorbed electro-active species can react selectively with a target analyte to modulate the fluorescence of CNTs. Based on this concept, the assembled system has been tested for the reaction of β-D-glucose to D-glucono-1,5-lactone with a H_2O_2 co-product catalysed by GOD. The fluorescence emission of the CNTs (λmax = 944 nm) responds to the local glucose concentration and has a detection limit of 34.7 μM. The NIR signalling from this device makes it suitable for implantation into thick tissue or whole-blood media.

Recent researches have demonstrated that the application of QDs in biotechnology is compelling; yet, they may not entirely replace traditional organic dyes as biological labels because of their much higher cost and large size. Another emerging possibility is to use QDs together with some metal nanomaterials for combining nanocrystal imaging agents with therapeutic agents. This would allow tracking of pharmacokinetics; and diseased tissue could be treated and monitored simultaneously and in real time.

It is also clear that a careful combination of the electrical and optical properties of one-dimensional nanostructures with the recognition features of biomolecules can open the door for scientists and engineers to bridge nanobiotechnology and nanomedicine (Wang et al., 2005).

12 Nanoparticles, Nanomagnetism and Nanomedicine for Therapy

Introduction

The use of nanoparticles (NPs) in nanomedicine has great potential in diagnostics as well as therapeutics of various diseases. Multiple functions can be built into these NPs. The most striking function is the ability to home to specific sites in the body. Simberg et al. (2007) described biomimetic particles that not only home to tumours, but also promote their own homing. In this system, a peptide recognizes clotted plasma proteins and selectively homes to tumours, where it binds to vessel walls and tumour stroma. Iron oxide NPs and liposomes coated with this tumour-homing peptide accumulate in tumour vessels, where they induce additional local clotting; creating new binding sites for more particles.

The system mimics platelets, which also circulate freely but accumulate at a diseased site and amplify their own accumulation there. The self-amplifying homing is a novel function for NPs. The clotting-based amplification greatly enhances tumour imaging and the addition of a drug carrier function to the particles is conceivable.

Although specific targeting of NPs to tumours has been reported in several experimental systems (Akerman et al., 2002; Cai et al., 2006), the delivery is not very efficient. In nature, amplified homing ensures sufficient platelet accumulation at sites of vascular injury. Amplified homing involves target binding, activation, platelet-platelet binding and formation of a blood clot. This idea prompted Simberg et al. to design a NP delivery system in which the particles amplify their own homing in a manner that resembles platelets.

The NP system designed by Simberg et al., conducive to effective accumulation of the particles in tumours, is based on four elements.

First, coating of the NPs with a tumour-homing peptide that binds to clotted plasma proteins endows the particles with a specific affinity for tumour vessels (and tumour stroma). Second, decoy NP pretreatment prolongs the blood half-life of the particles and increases tumour targeting. Third, the tumour-targeted NPs induce intravascular clotting in tumour blood vessels. Fourth, the intravascular clots attract more NPs into the tumour and so amplify the targeting.

Besides the self-amplifying tumour-homing enabled by NP-induced clotting in tumour vessels and the binding of additional NPs to the clots, this NP system combines several other functions into one particle: specific tumour- homing, avoidance of the reticuloendothelial system tissues and effective tumour imaging.

Another appropriately useful function of the targeted NPs may be the physical blockade of tumour vessels caused by local embolism. Blood vessel occlusion by embolism or clotting reduces tumour growth (Huang et al., 1997).

Monolayer-protected Nanoparticles

The ability to engineer the surface properties of different core materials makes monolayer-protected nanoparticles (MPNPs) excellent scaffolds for targeting biomacromolecules. You et al. (2007) highlighted the control of biomacromolecule structure and function through engineered interactions with NP surfaces. Recognition of biomacromolecule surfaces by artificial receptors allows for regulating biomacromolecular interactions such as protein-carbohydrate, protein-protein and protein-nucleic acid interactions. This facilitates controlling cellular and extracellular processes for therapeutic applications. It also offers new directions for biosensing and clinical diagnostics (Fig. 12.1).

The recognition of biomacromolecule surfaces is difficult in view of their size and complexity. Two difficulties need to be removed before specific/selective NP-biomacromolecule surface recognition can be realized. First, need for a large surface area for high-affinity binding; protein-protein interactions suggest that surface areas less than 6 nm^2 per protein are typically buried in these interactions. Another difficulty is preorganization, where a structurally well-defined surface is required for efficient and selective interaction.

Scaffolds with large surfaces are particularly useful for biomolecular recognition. Monolayer-protected clusters (MPCs) and mixed MPCs (MMPCs), where polyhedral metal cores are immediately surrounded by a self-assembled monolayer, have potential for generating biomacromolecular receptors. NPs are readily fabricated with sizes from 1.5 nm to less than 10 nm, comparable to proteins and other biomacromolecules; they provide large surface areas for interaction with biomacromolecules. The self-assembled monolayer on the particle surface confers preorganization to the appended recognition elements. The variety of readily available metal and semiconductor core materials provides access to exciting optical, electronic and magnetic properties.

You et al. (2007) described some recent advances in the use of NP surfaces for DNA and protein recognition with particular reference to the use of MPNPs as multivalent receptors.

Fabrication of MPNPs

The introduction of organic ligands onto NPs enhances their usefulness by avoiding aggregation and agglomeration. These ligands also impart NPs important recognition, transportation and catalytic properties. MPCs are fabricated with a diverse array of metal, alloy, oxide and semiconductor materials, but there is no common procedure for all materials. The core materials provide a scaffold for anchoring organized organic layers and also feature unique physical properties, for example, the unique optical properties of Au and Ag NPs because of their surface plasmon-resonance. Some other good core materials are highly luminescent semiconductor quantum dots (QDs) and magnetically active metallic and oxide particles. Table 12.1 summarizes the properties of some representative core materials and corresponding possible ligands.

Outlook

MPNPs make a versatile scaffold for creating biomacromolecular receptors whose surface properties can be engineered through the introduction of functional ligands. One

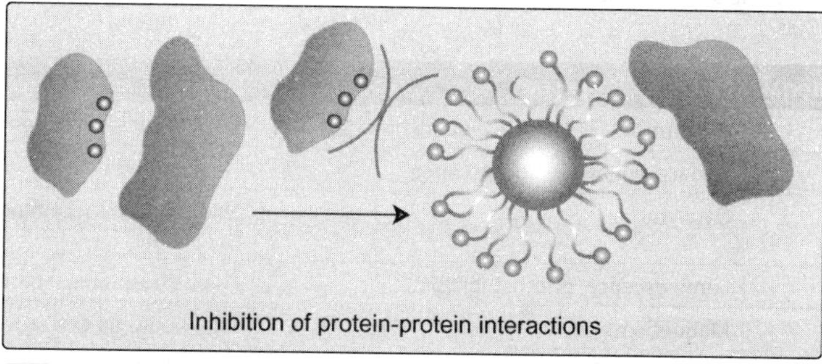

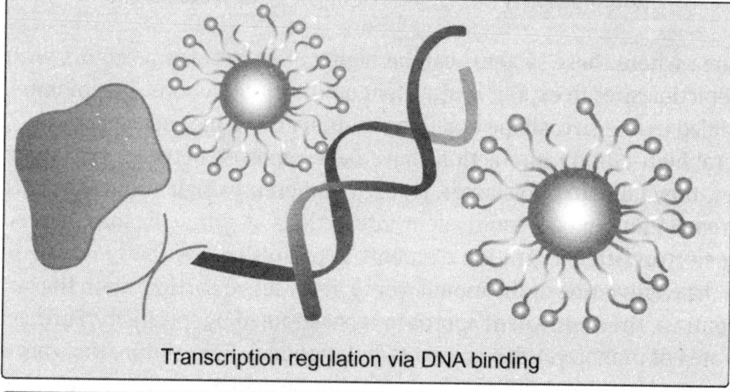

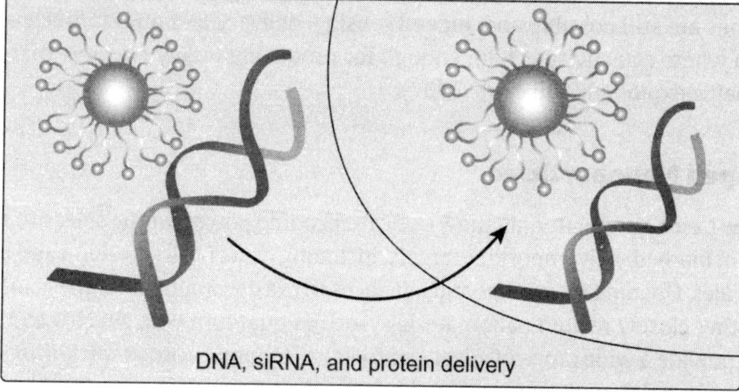

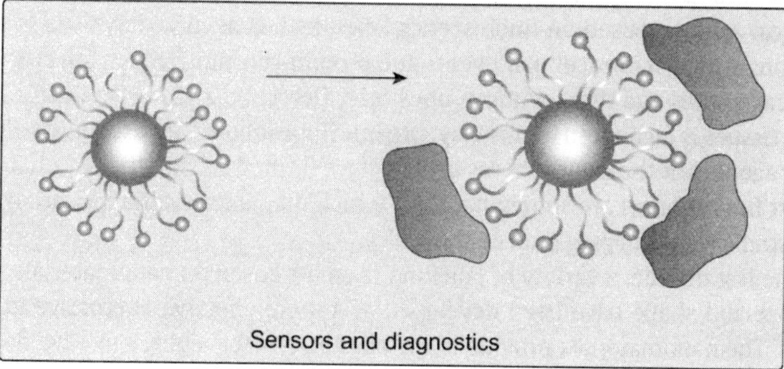

Fig. 12.1 Some applications made possible through controlled biomolecule-NP interactions (after You et al., 2007).

Table 12.1 Some selected metal and semiconductor materials as nanometer-sized scaffolds (after You et al., 2007).

Core material	Property/Properties	Ligand
Au	Absorption, fluorescence quenching, stability	Thiol, disulfide, phosphine
Ag	Surface-enhanced fluorescence	Thiol, amine
Pt	Catalytic	Thiol, phosphine, amine, isocyanide
CdSe	Luminescence, photostability	Thiol, phosphine, pyridine
Fe_2O_3	Magnetisms	Diol, dopmine derivative, amine
SiO_2	Biocompatibility	Alkoxysilane

notable area where these systems can be highly effective uses receptors with multiple weak interaction sites to exploit multivalent binding interactions. This biomimetic binding is enabled by the size, shape and templatability of NP monolayers.

Several high-affinity interactions have been reported between NPs and biomacromolecules; they fall into two classes: (i) use of inherently high affinity interactions, e.g., biotin-streptavidin; and (ii) multivalent interactions of simple ligands, especially those featuring electrostatic recognition elements. A promising possibility for the former approach is the engineering of the monolayer to be an active participant in the binding process. In contrast, the multivalent approach is constrained by specificity. Further researches in the area of monolayer design and templation may help eliminating this limitation. However, even if true and full specificity cannot be achieved with these systems, some applications are still possible and, indeed sensing, delivery and protein/nucleic acid stabilization where selectivity is high enough for producing highly effective materials, are already being exploited (You et al., 2007).

Dye-doped Nanoparticles

New silica-based nanomaterials show optical-encoding power for the selective tagging of a variety of biomedically important targets, including cancer cells, bacteria and individual biomolecules. Ongoing researches and advances in the development of these materials as well as other closely related nanomaterials, such as quantum dots, Au NPs and magnetic NPs may provide a wide range of advanced tools for genomics, proteomics, drug discovery and diagnosis and therapy of cancer and infectious diseases (Yan et al., 2007).

Optical analysis based on fluorescence labelling has been widely used to study the interactions amongst intracellular events and protein-receptors which are crucial for basic medical studies and therapeutic applications. Detection and *in vivo* imaging of living cells and tissues is facilitated in this way. Organic fluorophores are used most often as the labelling agents but the fluorophores usually have limited sensitivity and photostability. Also most fluorophores are somewhat toxic which precludes their application in *in vivo* cellular studies and imaging (Yan et al., 2007).

In the last decade, a variety of labelling reagents based on nanomaterials with controlled size and shape have been developed as a more effective alternative to the fluorophores. The nanomaterials provide many possibilities for highly sensitive detection of various targets under different conditions, from the single-molecule level to human body applications, from *in vitro* diagnosis to *in vivo* real-time imaging (Tansil and Gao, 2006).

Some NPs currently used for bioanalysis include metallic (Au and Ag) NPs, quantum dots (QDs), magnetic NPs, lanthanide NPs and silica NPs (see Huhtinen et al., 2005; Pinaud et al., 2006).

Au NPs (commonly known as Au colloid or colloidal Au) are suitable as colorimetric probes and have been used to develop highly sensitive detection schemes for many targets (Chah et al., 2005). They are also employed as biomarkers. Oh et al. (2006) have developed the lateral flow strip for fast pathogen detection and point-of-care diagnosis.

Quantum dots (QDs) are semiconductor crystals (i.e., CdSe, CdTe, CdS, ZnSe, PbS and PbTe) with typical diameters ranging between 2 nm and 10 nm (without outside coating). They provide bright fluorescence and a higher photostability against photobleaching than organic dyes. Their narrow emission bands can be precisely tuned from blue (usually CdSe) to near-infrared (PbS and PbSe) by varying the QD size and components. Their near-infrared emission greatly expands their application, e.g., deep-tissue imaging in clinical and life science studies. The wide absorption spectra of QDs facilitate simultaneous excitation of different QDs (see Bruchez et al., 1998).

Magnetic NPs with superparamagnetic properties are ideal agents for the manipulation of biological materials, targeting delivery of therapeutic compounds and hyperthermia treatment. They can also act as a contrast reagent in magnetic resonance imaging (MRI) for diagnosis (Atanasijevic et al., 2006; Gould, 2006).

Lanthanide (Ln^{3+}) NPs These and other NPs prepared from Eu^{3+}, Sm^{3+}, Tb^{3+}, Gd^{3+}, etc. are photostable and usually provide sharp emission spectra (<10 nm) and long fluorescence lifetimes. Their surface can be modified without altering their properties significantly. This makes them suitable for use as biolabels. These NPs also show excellent up-conversion fluorescence and do not suffer from blinking. Lanthanide NPs are used in the development of immunoassays, time-resolved fluorescence imaging for quantitative histochemistry, specific targeting and DNA detection (see Nichkova et al., 2005; Chen et al., 2007).

Dye-doped Silica NPs

Silica-based NPs are widely used in bioanalysis and show less aggregation and little dye leakage (Chah et al., 2005). A large number of organic or inorganic dye molecules can be incorporated inside a single silica particle. Dye-doped NPs produce a highly amplified optical signal compared with a single dye molecule. Silica NPs can also confer much improvement in analytical sensitivity. Excellent photostability makes these NPs suitable for applications where high intensity or prolonged excitations are needed. The flexible silica chemistry also provides versatile routes for surface modification (Yan et al., 2007). It is possible to introduce different types of functional groups onto the NPs for conjugation with biomolecules. Also, the silica surface renders the NPs chemically inert and physically stable (Smith et al., 2005). Silica NPs are indeed excellent labelling reagents for bioanalysis and bioimaging (Bagwe et al., 2006).

Synthesis of Fluorescent Silica NPs

There are two main methods for the synthesis of dye-doped silica particles. The Stöber method involves the hydrolysis of a silica alkoxide precursor (such as tetraethyl orthosilicate, TEOS) in an ethanol and aqueous ammonium hydroxide mixture. The silicic acid is produced during hydrolysis and, when its concentration is above its solubility in ethanol, nucleates homogeneously to form nm-sized silica particles.

Both organic and inorganic dyes can be incorporated using this method but, because of the hydrolysis procedure the NPs tend to have a relatively large size distribution. To avoid this, more hydrophobic dyes have been incorporated inside the silica NPs. One modification is based on the combination of both hydrophobic and hydrophilic precursors which makes the NPs, such as phenyltriethoxysilane (PTES), hydrophobic and TEOS hydrophilic. Rhodamine 6G (R6G) can also be incorporated into silica NPs. The hydrophobic component keeps the organic dye in the silica matrix while the hydrophilic component disperses the resulting NP in aqueous solutions.

The second method is the reverse microemulsion method, based on the formation of a water-in-oil reverse microemulsion. Water, surfactant and oil make up the reaction mixture. The stabilized water nanodroplets formed in the oil solution act as mini microreactors, where silane hydrolysis and the formation of NPs with dye trapped inside take place.

The NPs produced are highly uniform and well dispersed in water. However, in most cases, the method can only be used to incorporate inorganic dyes, some of which have lower quantum yields than those of organic fluorophores. Organic-dye-doped silica NPs are more difficult to prepare because of the hydrophobic properties of the organic dye compared with the hydrophilic surface of the NPs. Coupling of organic dyes to hydrophilic dextran group can help keep the linked dye molecule within the silica. Fluorescein has been successfully doped into the silica NPs without leakage (Yan et al., 2007).

Besides single-dye doping, multiple-dye incorporation into the silica matrix can also be achieved. Simultaneous doping of NPs with two inorganic dyes, tris(2'2-bipyridyl)dichlororuthenium(II) (Rubpy) and tris(2'2-bipyridyl)dichloro-osmium (II) (Osbpy) is also possible.

Surface Functionalization

Silica NPs can be further modified with silane reagents. Si chemistry is highly versatile so various functional groups can be easily introduced onto the particle surface. The process requires an additional coating of the silica surface with the alkoxysilane reagent, such as carboxyethylsilanetriol for introduction of carboxylic acid groups, 3-aminopropyltriethoxysilane for amino groups, or 3-mercaptopropyl trimethoxysilane for thiol groups (Bagwe et al., 2006).

Another approach, based on the formation of noncovalent interactions, is the attachment of avidin (which has an overall positive charge) to the negatively charged NP surface through electrostatic interactions. After modifying the silica surface; proteins, enzymes, antibodies, oligonucleotides, etc. can be linked to the NP by standard conjugation protocols (Niemeyer, 2004). Some conjugation procedures are illustrated in Figure 12.2.

Applications

Extremely high optical intensity, high photostability and easy bioconjugation of silica NPs have made them highly useful in bioanalysis.

Immunoassays The affinity and specificity of the antigen-antibody recognition process is exploited in developing immunochemical techniques. Silica NPs are used as a

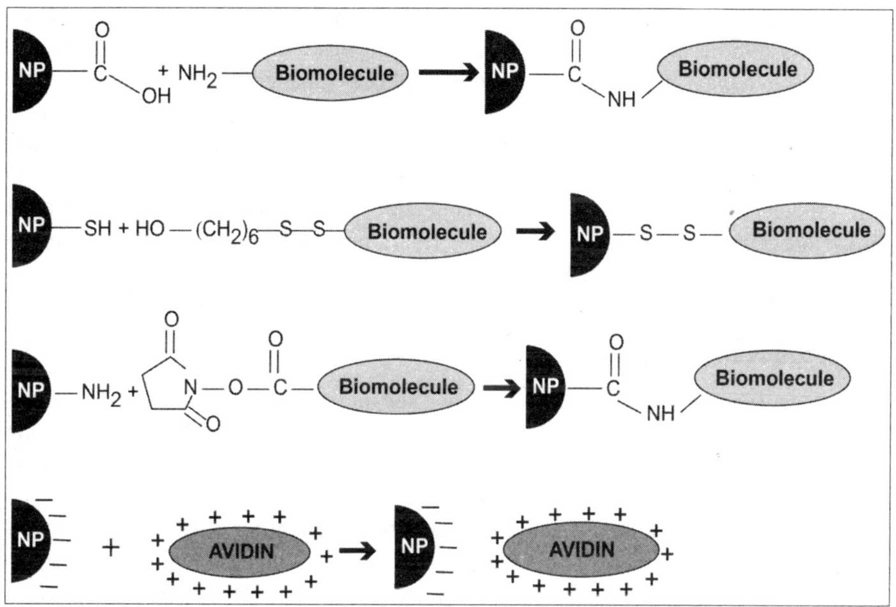

Fig. 12.2 Some bioconjugation protocols for attaching biomolecules to the surface of silica NPs (after Wang et al., 2006).

superior signalling element in an immunoassay by conjugating them to an antibody. Proteins, cells and bacteria can be detected by these NPs (Zhao et al., 2004).

Zhao et al. (2004) developed a method for the detection of a single bacterium. The silica NPs were doped with Rubpy and surface-modified with a specific antibody against *E. coli* O157:H7. A single pathogenic *E. coli* O157:H7 bacterium could be detected within 20 minutes in a complex matrix, e.g., as spiked beef sample. High-throughput and multiple-sample bacterial detection was demonstrated by using a 384-plate format.

Cellular imaging He et al. (2004) produced FITC-doped silica NPs labelled with anti-human liver cancer monoclonal antibody HAb18. Liver cancer cells can be easily distinguished from other cells with this labelling scheme.

Nucleic acid analysis Molecular recognition based on the hybridization of nucleic acid strands is widely employed in disease diagnosis, drug development and other biotechnology applications (Golub et al., 1999). Dye-doped NPs are used as labels for increased sensitivity and throughput in this approach.

A sandwich-assay setup for silica NP-based DNA detection was devised by Zhao et al. (2003). Three different DNA species were present in the assay: capture DNA, immobilized on a glass surface as probe sequence attached to TMR-doped silica NPs; and the unlabelled target sequence, complementary to both the capture sequence and the probe sequence through different parts of the sequence (Yan et al., 2007). In this assay, there is no need to label the target and the hybridization of target DNA also brings one dye-doped silica NP to the surface, providing many dye molecules on the surface for signalling. By monitoring the luminescent intensity from the surface-bound NPs, DNA target molecules are detected. NPs containing over 10000 TMR dye molecules have been successfully used with an Affymetrix GeneChip (Yan et al., 2007).

Aptamers are a novel, promising alternative to antibodies as affinity probes. Commonly, the aptamer is a single DNA or RNA strand evolved from systematic evolution of ligands by exponential enrichment procedure (SELEX) (Shangguan et al., 2006). It binds to the target with a specific steric conformation. Herr et al. (2006) modified two types of silica NP with an aptamer selected toward a specific type of leukaemia cell. One of these was doped with Rubpy dye for fluorescence sensing and the other contained a magnetic core for selective capture and magnetic collection. The two-particle assay could catch leukaemia cells from a spiked blood sample. This approach has great potential for clinical diagnostic applications (Yan et al., 2007).

Targeted Nanoparticles

The past few years have witnessed impressive advances in cancer diagnostics and therapeutics and yet cancer is still the second leading cause of death in the USA, second only to heart disease. An estimated 1450000 new cases of cancer may be diagnosed in 2007 (ACS, 2007).

Although chemotherapy is an integral part of treatment for most cancers, conventional chemotherapeutic agents are not very specific in reaching tumour tissue. They are also often restricted by dose-limiting toxicity. The combination of developing controlled-release technology and targeted drug delivery may provide a better, less harmful solution to address the drawbacks of conventional chemotherapy. For this purpose, nanoscale delivery vehicles that can control the release of chemotherapeutic agents directly inside cancer cells is attracting interest (see Farokhzad et al., 2006; Gu et al., 2007). Controlled release is achieved by attaching a natural or synthetic polymer to a drug in such a way that the drug is encapsulated within the polymer system for subsequent release in a predetermined manner. Polymeric drug delivery particles range in size from 50 nm to over 10 μm; they release their encapsulated drug through surface or bulk erosion, diffusion, or swelling followed by diffusion, in a time- or condition-dependent manner. The release of the active agent can be triggered by some external stimulus or action (Langer and Tirrell, 2004). Controlled-release polymer systems provide optimum drug levels longer than other drug delivery methods and so increase the efficacy of the drug as well as maximize patient compliance. This mode of drug delivery achieves more effective therapies while minimizing or avoiding under- or over-dosing. Controlled-release delivery systems also maintain drug levels within a desired range, require fewer administrations and use the drug optimally (Gu et al., 2007).

Passive versus Active Targeting

Strategies for delivering drug-encapsulated NPs to cancerous tissue may involve passive or active targeting. The former exploits the unique properties of the tumour microenvironment, notably: (i) leaky tumour vasculature that is highly permeable to macromolecules relative to normal tissue; and (ii) a dysfunctional lymphatic drainage system that leads to greater fluid retention in the tumour interstitial space.

Consequently, the concentration of polymeric NPs and macromolecular assemblies found in tumour tissues can be up to 100 times greater than those in normal tissue. The tumour-specific deposition termed 'enhanced permeability and retention (EPR)' effect, takes place as NPs extravasate out of tumour microvasculature, resulting in drug accumulation in the tumour interstitium. Particles of diameter less than 200 nm are the most effective in extravasating tumour microvasculature. But passive tumour targeting cannot achieve a high enough level of drug concentration at the tumour site and hence results in low therapeutic efficacy; it can elicit undesirable systemic adverse effects (Ferrari, 2005).

Active targeting can be accomplished by delivering drug-encapsulated NPs to uniquely identified sites while minimizing undesirable effect elsewhere. It is achieved by both local and systemic administration of NPs with targeting molecules conjugated on the particle surface—molecules that recognize and bind to specific ligands unique to cancer cells. In local delivery, the cytotoxic NP-encapsulated drug is delivered directly to cancer cells with minimal toxicity to non-cancerous cells near the targeted tissue. This approach is applicable to primary tumours which have not yet spread to other areas.

NP Carriers

Active targeting is enabled by functionalizing NPs with ligands such as antibodies, peptides, nucleic acid aptamers, carbohydrates and small molecules. Most success has been limited to ligand-drug conjugates. Researches are on to enhance these systems by encapsulating the therapeutic agents in NPs. Biodegradable polymers, dendrimers, nanoshells, nucleic-acid-based NPs and liposomes have been developed for targeted NPs (see Gref et al., 1994; Langer, 1998).

Liposomes are made of amphiphilic unilamellar/multilamellar membranes of natural or synthetic lipids. Lipids have a hydrophilic head group and a hydrophobic tail. Hydrophobic and hydrophilic molecules have been successfully encapsulated into liposome NPs. Doxorubicin-encapsulated liposome (Doxil) shows potent antineoplastic activity against a wide range of human cancers including Kaposi's sarcoma and ovarian cancer (Mrozek et al., 2005). However, liposomes as nanocarriers suffer from suboptimal stability and drug release profiles *in vivo* (Slepushkin et al., 2004).

Dendrimers are synthetic, highly branched, spherical, monodispersed macromolecules with an average diameter of 1.5–14.5 nm. They represent an important class of drug-encapsulating NPs. A typical dendrimer molecule has an initiator core, highly branched layers made of repeating units and multiple active terminal groups—a design that allows good control over the dendrimer size, shape, branching length and surface functionality. Biodegradable polyester dendrimers have been developed for intracellular release of doxorubicin after hydrolysis of their hydrazone linkage (Padilla De Jesus et al., 2002).

Some NPs for developing therapeutic and imaging nanocarriers use DNA and RNA as substrates. Li et al. (2004) used a multivalent DNA delivery vehicle, (average size, 100 nm) for simultaneous targeted drug delivery, imaging and gene therapy. Targeted multifunctional 25–40 nm RNA NPs have been developed with a trivalent RNA core, RNA aptamers for targeting and siRNAs for therapeutic effect (Khaled et al., 2005).

Polymeric nanoshells consist of diblock copolymers assembled into a core/shell structure. In these, the drug release rate can be regulated by the chemistry of the polymers and the diffusion coefficient through the polymeric layer. Metallic nanoshells, approximately 20 nm in diameter, have a dielectric core covered with a thin metallic shell to improve their biocompatibility and optical absorption. These particles possess a highly tunable plasmon resonance mediated by the size of the core and the thickness of the shell, which in turn determines their absorbing and scattering properties over a broad range of the spectrum from the near-ultraviolet to the mid-infrared (Hirsch et al., 2006). Gold nanoshells have also been developed for *in vivo* photothermal therapy using near-infrared light. Combining magnetic nanoshells with a drug-encapsulated biodegradable polymer enables particle targeting to specific sites of the body in response to externally applied magnetic field.

Targeting Molecules for Developing Targeted NPs

Monoclonal antibodies These are used in cancer therapy (Adams and Weiner, 2005). Monoclonal antibodies (mAb) are the preferred class of targeting molecules. Chimeric, humanized and fully humanized derivatives of antibodies are used to decrease their immunogenicity. Some antibody-based drugs have already entered clinical practice, e.g., rituximab, trastuzumab, cetuximab and bevacizumab (Gu et al., 2007; Kay, 2004, 2007). Yet, mAb-conjugated NPs do have limitations. Since mAb molecules are very large and complex, they have to be engineered at the molecular level to be effective (Brennan et al., 2004). Also, antibodies are more expensive than small-molecule drugs.

Aptamer targeting molecules Certain nucleic acid ligands (aptamers) potentially rival antibodies for therapeutic and diagnostic applications (Gold, 1995). Aptamers are DNA or RNA oligonucleotides or modified DNA or RNA oligonucleotides that fold by intramolecular forces into unique conformations with ligand-binding characteristics. Like antibodies, they can bind target antigens with high specificity and affinity (Gu et al, 2007).

As targeting molecules aptamers offer some potential merits over antibodies. Aptamers with high affinity for a target can be prepared through *in vitro* selection—a process termed systemic evolution of ligands by exponential enrichment (SELEX) (Schneider et al., 1992). Aptamers isolated using this process are smaller than antibodies, lack immunogenicity and seem to have better tumour/plasma distribution and tumour-penetration properties than antibodies (Ellington and Szostak, 1992).

SELEX being a chemical process that does not involve animals; nucleic acid ligands can be prepared to bind to any target regardless of the toxicity or immunogenicity of the latter. Another merit: nucleic acid ligands identified through the SELEX can be synthesized by using chemical oligonucleotide synthesis, which scales-up well, with little or no variation from batch to batch in binding affinity. This contrasts with antibodies, which usually show batch-to-batch variation in quality during scaled-up production.

Binding aptamers to NPs provides more efficient targeted therapeutics or selective diagnostics than nontargeted NPs. Gu et al. developed NP-aptamer (NP-Apt) conjugates that target the prostate specific membrane antigen (PSMA), a transmembrane protein that is upregulated in various cancers, by using an aptamer first isolated by Lupold et al. (2002). Aptamers have even been conjugated to liposomes to prolong their circulation lifetime and effect *in vivo*.

Oligopeptide-based targeting molecules Combinatorial libraries have led to the discovery of short peptides (10-15 amino acids) that specifically bind to targeted proteins, cells, or tissues (Newton et al., 2006). Peptides are a suitable alternative to antibodies because of their small size, lower immunogenicity, higher stability and ease of manufacture.

Cilengitide is a cyclic arginine-glycine-aspartic acid (RGD) peptide that binds to integrins and is undergoing clinical trials for the treatment of non-small cell lung cancer and pancreatic cancer (Burke et al., 2002). RGD-targeted therapy also faces some challenges, such as the limitation associated with the nonspecific adhesive nature of the RGD-integrin targeting system. Integrins are non cancer specific.

Folate Folic acid (folate), a high-affinity vitamin, is a widely employed ligand for cancer targeting because folate receptors (FRs) are frequently overexpressed in a range of tumour cells (Antony, 1992). Folate specifically binds to FRs, enabling folate derivatives and conjugates to deliver molecular complexes to cancer cells without harming normal cells. It has been used as a targeting moiety combined with a wide array of vehicles such as liposomes, protein toxins, polymeric NPs, linear polymers and dendrimers to deliver drugs selectively into cancer cells by using FR-mediated endocytosis. Dendrimer-based targeted anti-cancer therapeutics using folate also show good *in vivo* efficacy in terms of targeting and specific killing of cancer cells via multivalent interaction (Hong et al., 2007). However, because FRs are expressed not only in tumour tissue but also in normal epithelia in the choroids plexus, placenta, lung, intestine and kidney, an FR-targeted NP delivery system needs to be further refined and tuned to enhance tumour selectivity.

Other Novel Targeting Molecules

Some antibody fragments can improve tumour penetration but retain high antigen binding specificity. Affibody molecules (small polypeptides derived from an antibody binding domain of staphylococcal protein A; Nord et al., 1997) have been used as a scaffold for the construction of combinatorial phage libraries from which affibody variants that target a specific cell marker are selected by means of phage display technology.

Nanobodies are the smallest fully functional antigen-binding fragments evolved from the variable domain of heavy-chain antibodies. Nanobodies are low molecular weight polypeptides with antigen binding affinity like that of the traditional mAb. They evolved from single-domain antibodies carrying only a functional heavy chain without the light chain. Compared to their parent antibodies, these smaller molecules improve tumour penetration and weaken immunogenicity (Willuda et al., 1999).

A-domain proteins are 40-amino-acid oligopeptides that attach to the cell surface at many points. Other novel targeting molecules, named avimers, have been made from A-domain proteins (Silverman et al., 2005). An avimer is a single protein chain containing multiple domains, each with a distinct function. Silverman et al. (2005) isolated an avimer that binds to interleukin-6 and shows higher affinity and specificity than A-domain proteins.

AdNectins represent another class of targeting molecules. They are thermostable, protease-resistant oligopeptides initially derived from a domain of human fibronectin (Xu et al., 2003). Each AdNectin typically has three distinct loop structures. A library of AdNectins has been made by introducing diversity into these loops. These antibody fragments and oligopeptides are promising targeting molecules whose conjugation to drug-encapsulated NPs might further enhance targeted chemotherapy.

Microfluidics for Targeted Drug Delivery NPs

In microfluidics, nanoliter volumes can be handled in microscale fluidic channels. Labour-intensive, time-consuming steps such as sample preparation, purification, mixing, reactions, separations and detection can be performed on a single monolithic microfabricated device. Miniaturization in conjunction with integration of multiple functionalities has led to microfluidic systems that fare better than microscale systems, reduce labour input and may be mass produced at low cost (Gu et al., 2007).

Microfluidic systems are especially valuable for the synthesis of NPs (DeMello and DeMello, 2004). Millisecond timescale control of reaction conditions in a droplet-based microfluidic device has made it possible to synthesize highly monodisperse CdS NPs and CdS/CdSe core-shell NPs (Shestopalov et al., 2004). Microfluidic systems have also been used for the synthesis of high-quality CdS, CdSe, Ag, Pd, Cu and CdSe/ZnS core-shell NPs (DeMello, 2006).

While it seems doubtful that microfluidics can enable synthesis of NPs from start to finish at least in the near future, microfluidic synthesis can be useful for some critical processing steps—notably NP precipitation which usually involves dissolving NP precursors such as drugs and polymers in a water-miscible solvent and adding it to water—operations for which microfluidic devices are well suited. Microfluidics allow manipulating small volumes of fluid on even microsecond timescales. This opens up the possibility of controlling reaction conditions for NP synthesis on the timescale of NP formation itself, as has been demonstrated for CdS NPs. Rapid advances in two-phase microfluidics are expected to lead to novel techniques for emulsion- or droplet-based syntheses of NPs. Microfluidics may also prove useful in serial or parallel combinatorial synthesis of NPs (DeMello, 2006).

The ability to control reaction conditions precisely, understand the complex process of precipitation and potentially generate libraries of NPs can prove useful for targeted drug delivery of NPs. These advantages, when combined with high-throughput screening methods such as cell micro-arrays, will go a long way in tackling the critical issues of reproducible synthesis and selection of the best NPs for drug delivery (Gu et al., 2007).

Therapeutic Gold Nanoparticles

Electrons of gold nanoparticles (Nps) resonate in response to incoming radiation. This makes them both absorb and scatter light. This process is termed plasmon resonance and can be exploited to either destroy tissue by local heating or release therapeutically important payload molecules. Also gold NPs (10-100 nm) can be conjugated to biologically active moieties for their possible targeting to particular tissues (Pissuwan et al., 2006).

Two remarkable properties of gold NPs for therapeutic applications are: (1) antibodies and other biological molecules can be readily attached to their surface; and (2) the plasmon resonances of the NPs of certain shapes cause them to have photon capture cross-sections that are much greater than those of photothermal dyes (Loo et al., 2004). These attributes are utilized for the localized heating, or drug release in certain therapeutic applications (see Daniel and Astruc, 2004).

Relevant Properties

Resistance to oxidation and plasmon resonance with light are two therapeutically important characteristics of gold. The plasmon resonance for ordinary gold nanospheres occurs at approximately 520 nm but can be red-shifted into the near infrared (NIR), with excitation wavelengths of 800–1200 nm required for more complex shapes, such as nanorods. This is pertinent because body tissue is fairly transparent to NIR light (O'Neal et al., 2004); this exerts therapeutic effects in deep tissues.

Another route for the spectral control of both absorption and scattering of light is offered by gold or silver metallo-dielectric core-shell particles, particularly when the core is a dielectric (most commonly gold sulfide, silica or polystyrene) and the shell is a metal. The spectral properties of these shapes may be controlled by varying the relative dimensions of the core and the shell (West and Halas, 2000). Particles of these shapes have been synthesized and are finding valuable medical applications. For these particles, the term nanoshell is popular in North America whereas the term core-shell particle is commonly used in Europe (Caruso, 2001) for both metal-on-dielectric and dielectric-on-metal particles.

One commonly observed problem with many drug-based therapies (particularly when administered orally or intravenously) is that the compound does not localize to the target site but is widely dispersed. Treatments based on NPs facilitate accumulation of the therapeutic agent either by passive targeting - where the body concentrates inert NPs, or by active targeting; in the latter case, functional modification of the surface of the gold NP enhances the therapeutic delivery system and results in specific tissue targeting (Moghimi et al., 2005).

In passive targeting, nanoparticle colloids are designed in such a manner that the particles are large enough to be retained in the liver and spleen but can pass through the other organs. Such passive targeting is used in the radiotherapeutic treatment of liver cancers, where the sinus endothelium has openings of 150 nm in diameter. The spleen filters out particles larger than 250 nm. Also, as tumour vasculature is a little more permeable than that of healthy tissue, NPs can be concentrated. Nanoshells (130 nm) pass preferentially through the walls of vessels and concentrate in the surrounding tumourous tissue (O'Neal et al., 2004). This phenomenon is termed extravasation and constitutes another passive method of concentrating particles (up to 300 nm) in some tumours or inflamed tissues (Moghimi et al., 2005).

Since the dependence on size-specific filtration for the retention of NPs has some drawbacks, a better approach is to modify the NP surface by the addition of an antibody or ligand with affinity for the desired target; unfortunately, this also has limitations of non-specific binding and the potential activation of the normal host immune response. Recourse to "stealth" technologies can reduce the likelihood of an interaction between NPs and the immune system. These methods involve coating the nanoparticle with a self-assembled layer of a thiolated PEG (poly-ethyleneglycol) (McNeil, 2005).

Concentrating the gold NP at the desired site activates it through the absorption of radiation of an appropriate wavelength. This action delivers one of two therapeutic payloads: the localized generation of heat or the localized release of a chemical. Furthermore, the attached gold particles can be used to simultaneously track or image the cells (Loo et al., 2004).

In therapeutic medicine, heat is applied locally to treat cancer and other conditions. Energizing sources, such as infrared lamps, ultrasound or lasers are commonly used. By using gold NPs that absorb in the NIR spectrum, the resulting localized heating causes irreversible thermal cellular destruction (West and Halas, 2003). Dyes have generally been used for this purpose but gold nanoshells have much greater absorption efficiencies as compared to dyes and remain unaffected by photobleaching (O'Neal et al., 2004).

Gold-on-silica nanoshells can target breast carcinoma cells, actively, by using the HER-2 antibody (Loo et al., 2004). Extravasation is then harnessed to concentrate PEG-sheathed gold-on-silica nanoshells by passive targeting in an *in vivo* murine model

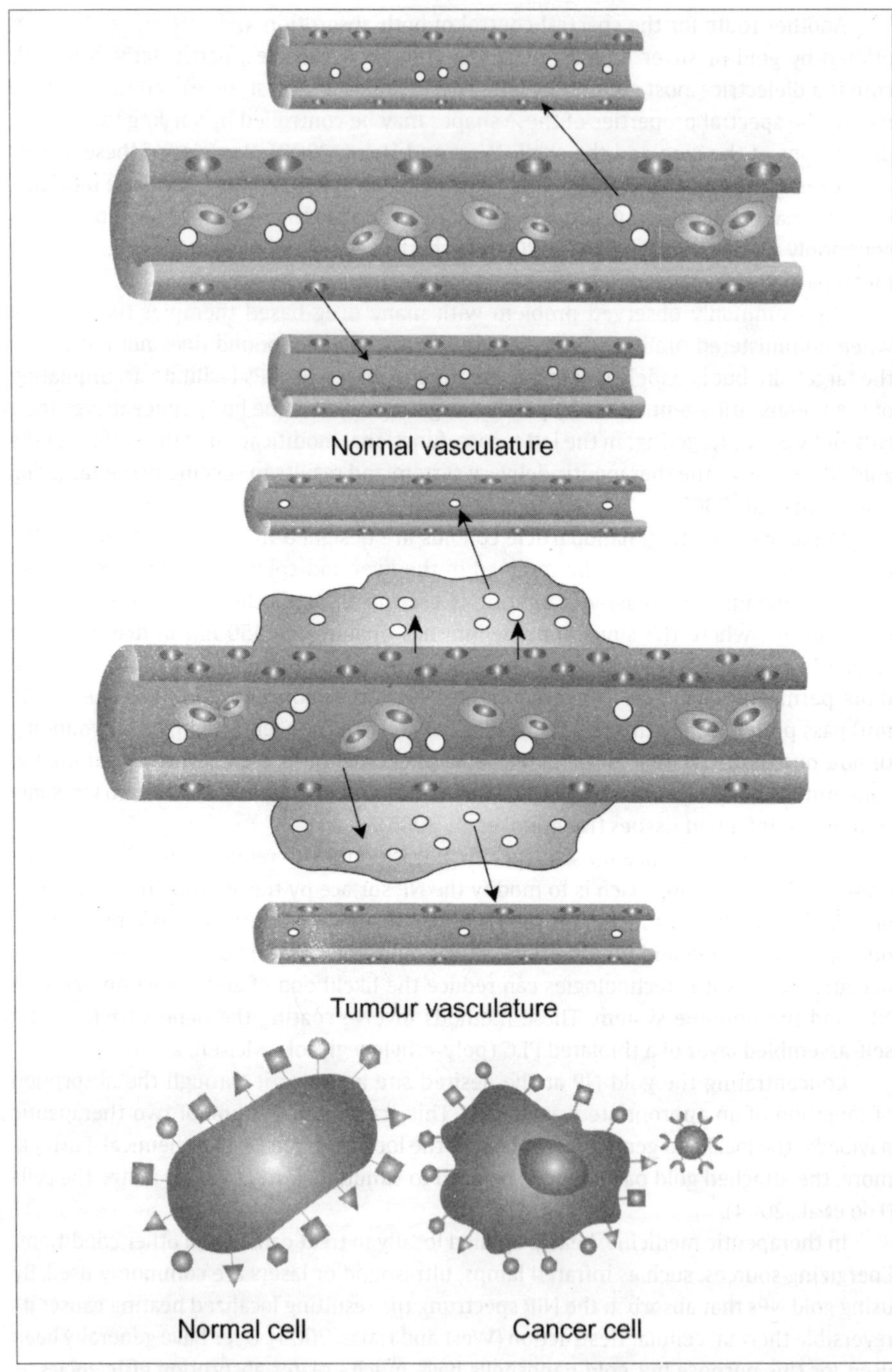

Fig. 12.3 PASSIVE AND ACTIVE TARGETING OF NANOPARTICLES: A. Passive, using the enhanced permeability and retention (EPR) effect, which exploits the increased permeability of the tumour vasculature (extravasation) to concentrate therapeutic agents. B. Active targeting of a carcinoma by an antibody-functionalized nanoparticle. Once concentrated at the target site, the therapeutic payload is released in response to light of a specific wavelength (after Liu et al., 2005 and Pissuwan et al., 2006).

(O'Neal et al., 2004). NIR irradiation raises the temperature of the target regions by 40 to 50°C, which selectively destroys the carcinomas. The survival rate of mice treated in this way was much better than in controls.

For effective drug delivery, some available options are encapsulating the payload inside a gold core-shell particle, impregnating a larger drug-containing nano- or microparticle with suitably designed gold NPs or binding the payload to the outer surface of a gold NP. Once the particle reaches the target tissue, the payload is released by plasmonic heating, preferably by using a laser. Gold NPs are small enough to deliver a payload of therapeutic agent, or heat, directly into the cytoplasm or nucleus of the target cell (Glomm, 2005).

Another option involves binding the drug to the outside of a gold NP by using a light-sensitive, conformation changing molecule, such as spyropyran (Thomas and Kamat, 2003), which holds it in place. Irradiating spyropyran by UV light (320 nm) changes its conformation from an open form to a closed one, where the former can form complexes with amino acids; these complexes are destroyed when the molecule reverts to the closed form, releasing the amino acids. Gold is an ideal substrate for this, with a convenient chemistry for attachment, but its optical properties were not exploited in this work. Such particles are targeted passively only but, again, the localization of the therapeutic effect can only be achieved with a light source (Pissuwan et al., 2006).

The chief limitation of the above drug delivery protocols is that the volume of payload that can be carried by individual nanoparticles is very small. In the absence of any external scheme to trigger release, the concentration of a therapeutic agent released by gradual diffusion, or owing to the breakdown of the packaging, is sometimes too low to be effective (Moghimi et al., 2005).

Magnetic Nanoparticles for Drug Delivery

Controlled release of drugs from nanoparticles (NPs) is attracting increasing attention in view of its many opportunities in cancer therapy and the treatment of other diseases. The potential of magnetic NPs emanates from the intrinsic properties of their magnetic cores combined with their drug loading capability and the biochemical properties that can be conferred on them by means of a suitable coating. Arruebo et al. (2007) have reviewed the problems and recent advances in the development of magnetic NPs for drug delivery, focusing particularly on the materials involved.

Most NPs are submicron moieties (1–100 nm) made of inorganic or organic (e.g., polymeric) materials, which may or may not be biodegradable. The properties of NPs differ from those of bulk materials of the same composition mainly because of size effects, the magnetic and electronic properties and the role played by surface phenomena as the size is reduced.

NPs are usually prepared by 'bottom-up' methods, where nanomaterials are fabricated from atoms or molecules in a controlled manner that is thermodynamically regulated by means such as self-assembly. Some biomedical applications require core-shell magnetic NPs which consist of a metal or metallic oxide core, encapsulated in an inorganic or a polymeric coating that renders the particles biocompatible, stable and may serve as a support for biomolecules.

The magnetic properties enable these particles to be used in many applications in one or more of the following groups (Arruebo et al., 2007):

1. Magnetic contrast agents in magnetic resonance imaging (MRI),
2. Hyperthermia agents, where the magnetic particles are heated selectively by application of a high frequency magnetic field (e.g., in thermal ablation/hyperthermia of tumours); and
3. Magnetic vectors that can be directed by means of a magnetic field gradient towards a certain location, such as for targeted drug delivery.

The most promising applications of magnetic NPs relate to the diagnosis and treatment of cancer. NPs can act at the tissue or cell level. The latter means that they can be endocytosed or phagocytosed (e.g., by dendritic cells or macrophages), resulting in internalization of the NP so that the NP can reach beyond the cytoplasmic membrane and, in some cases, even beyond the nuclear membrane (transfection applications).

Tumour targeting with magnetic NPs may involve passive or active strategies. Passive targeting occurs as a result of extravasation of the NPs at the diseased site (tumour) where the microvasculature is hyperpermeable and leaky, a process aided by tumour-limited lymphatic drainage. These factors lead to selective accumulation of NPs in tumour tissue, a phenomenon known as enhanced permeation and retention (EPR). Apart from tumours, size-dependent removal of NPs is common in healthy capillaries. The limitation is not the size of the NPs but their residence time in the bloodstream. This limits the use of conventional NPs for drug delivery by passive targeting to tumours in organs of the mononuclear phagocyte system (MPs) such as liver, spleen and bone marrow.

Active targeting is based on the over- or exclusive- expression of different epitopes or receptors in tumour cells and also on specific physical characteristics. Vectors sensi-

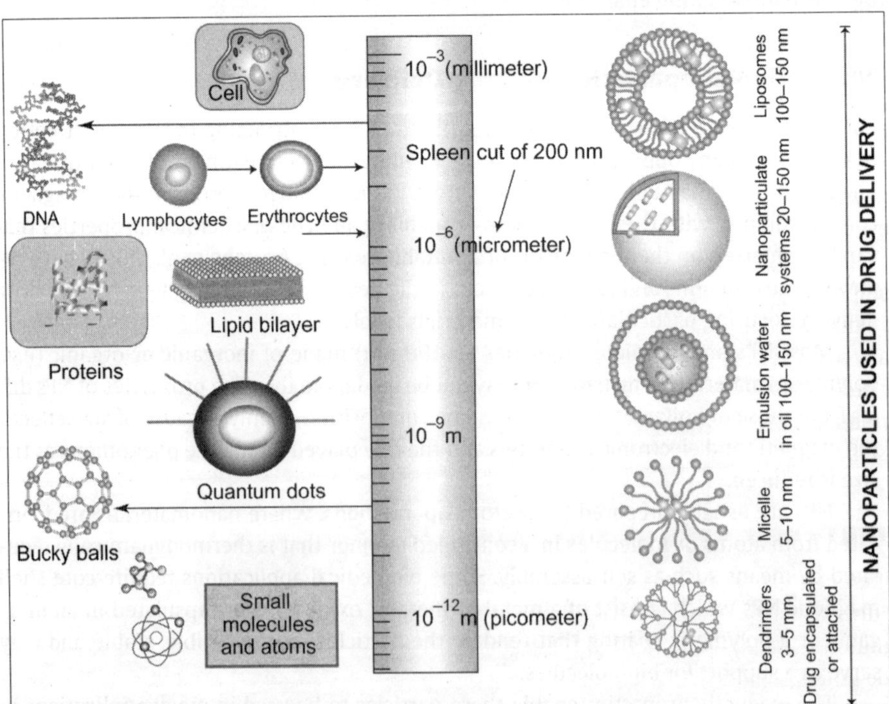

Fig. 12.4 Nanoparticle systems for drug delivery application (after Tomalia, 2005; Boyd, 2005; Arruebo et al., 2007).

tive to a variety of different physical stimuli have been developed and conjugated to drugs. It is also possible to base active targeting on overexpressed species such as low molecular weight ligands (folic acid, thiamine and sugars), peptides, proteins (transferring, antibodies, lectins), polysaccharides, polyunsaturated fatty acids and others.

Dendrimers, micelles, emulsions, nanoparticulate drugs and liposomes can be used to target specific areas in the body (Fig. 12.4) (Tomalia, 2005; Boyd, 2005; Arruebo, 2007). The NPs must possess the specific characteristics needed to reach a given target, such as a suitable combination of nature, size, manner of conjugating the drug to the NP (attached, adsorbed, encapsulated), surface chemistry, hydrophilicity/hydrophobicity, surface functionalization, biodegradability and physical response properties (temperature, pH, electric charge, light, sound, magnetism). Among these, size is the primary factor as it critically affects the fate of NPs in passive targeting processes depending on the permeability of the capillary vessel.

Freeman et al. (1960) first proposed that magnetic NPs could be transported through the vascular system and concentrated in a specific part of the body by means of a magnetic field. In 1976, Zimmermann and Pilwat used magnetic erythrocytes for the delivery of cytotoxic drugs. Widder et al. (1978) targeted magnetic albumin microspheres encapsulating an anti-cancer drug (doxorubicin) in animal models. Other authors have used magnetic microcapsules and microspheres to deliver different drugs (see Gupta et al., 1989). In 1994, Häfeli et al. successfully designed biodegradable poly (lactic acid) microspheres that incorporated magnetite as well as beta-emitter ^{90}Y for targeted radiotherapy; these were successfully applied to subcutaneous tumours (Häfeli et al., 1995).

However, all these early approaches were based on using microsized particles. Magnetic NPs were first used in animal models by Lübbe et al. (1996). The same year, the first clinical trial was done in patients with advanced cancers using magnetic NPs loaded within epirubicin. In that first trial, more than 50 per cent of the NPs ended up in the liver (see Arruebo et al., 2007). Since then, several groups have synthesized magnetic vectors with potential applications. Magnetic micro- and NPs are being manufactured and used in MRI, magnetic fluid hyperthermia, cell sorting and targeting, bioseparation, sensing, enzyme immobilization, immunoassays and gene transfection and detection systems. Several companies are marketing drug-loaded magnetic NPs.

For magnetic targeting, a drug or therapeutic radionuclide is bound to a magnetic compound, introduced in the body and then concentrated in the target area by means of a magnetic field (using either an internally implanted permanent magnet or an externally applied field). Depending on the application, the particles either release the drug or produce a local effect. Drug release can take place by simple diffusion or through enzymatic activity or changes in pH, osmolality, or temperature (Alexiou et al., 2000). It can also be magnetically triggered from the drug-conjugated magnetic NPs.

Drug Delivery with Magnetic NPs

Different organic materials (polymeric NPs, liposomes, micelles) have been investigated as drug delivery nanovectors by using passive targeting and active targeting with a recognition moiety (e.g., magnetism in magnetoliposomes). All these organic systems provide limited chemical and mechanical stability. They are also likely to cause swelling, are susceptible to microbiological attack, have inadequate control over the drug release rate and are very costly.

Polymer NPs suffer from high polydispersal. Synthesis produces particles with a broad size distribution and irregular branching, which can lead to heterogeneous pharmacological properties. A better alternative is to use dendrimers, but their visualization requires tagging with a specific moiety (i.e., a fluorophore or metal) and they are also very costly.

Passive targeting using drug-conjugated dendrimers and dendritic polymers has been examined by using the EPR effect. Therapies based on active targeting, such as antibody-conjugated dendrimers, may be better in view of the potential of antibodies for selective targeting. For the reasons of the disadvantages of organic NPs for drug delivery, inorganic vectors are the focus of intense research.

Magnetic (organic or inorganic) NPs can be: (i) visualized, (ii) guided or held in place by means of a magnetic field; and (iii) heated in a magnetic field to trigger drug release or to produce tissue hyperthermia/ablation. This latter is not restricted to magnetic NPs but is also true for other particles capable of absorbing near-infrared, microwave and ultrasound radiation.

In NPs, the drug is covalently bound to the surface or entrapped or adsorbed within the pores of the magnetic carrier (polymer, mesoporous silica, etc.). The term nanocapsules refers to magnetic vesicular systems where the drug is confined to an aqueous or oily cavity, commonly prepared by the reverse micelle procedure and either surrounded by an organic membrane (magnetoliposomes) or encapsulated within a hollow inorganic capsule. Depending on the synthesis procedure, either magnetic NPs or nanocapsules can be made.

The key parameters in the behaviour of magnetic NPs are surface chemistry, size and magnetic properties. The surface chemistry is critical for avoiding the action of the reticuloendothelial system (RES) (part of the immune system)—and to increase the half-life in the blood stream. Coating the NPs with a neutral and hydrophilic compound (e.g., polyethylene glycol) prolongs the circulatory half-life to hours or even days (see Neuberger et al., 2005). Besides cancer treatment, magnetic NPs may also be used in disorders associated with the musculoskeletal system (Fig. 12.5).

Limitations

Since the magnetic gradient decreases with the distance to the target, the chief limitation of magnetic drug delivery is related to the strength of the external field that can be applied to create the required magnetic gradient to control the residence time of NPs in the desired area. The geometry of the magnetic field is crucial in designing a magnetic targeting process.

To overcome the limitations of using external magnetic fields, internal magnets can located in the vicinity of the target by using minimally invasive surgery. Another limitation is the small size of NPs, a requisite for superparamagnetism, which is in turn needed to avoid magnetic agglomeration once the magnetic field is removed. Small size implies weak magnetic response which makes it difficult to direct particles and keep them in the proximity of the target while withstanding the drag of blood flow (Pankhurst et al., 2003). Targeting is more effective in regions of slower blood velocity, especially when the magnetic field source is close to the target site.

As for all biomedical applications, there are limitations in extrapolating from animal models to humans. Here, physiological parameters which need to be considered range from differences in weight, blood volume, cardiac output and circulation time to tumour volume/location/blood flow. All these complicate the extrapolation of data obtained in animal models.

Effective treatment of emerging tumours will depend on the development of a new generation of seek-and-destroy NPs that can specifically recognize small clusters of cancer cells and carry the needed elements (drugs or hyperthermia agents) for their destruction. Fortunately, NPs can access tumours in regions where conventional surgery is not applicable.

Tailoring of Magnetic NPs

The primary requirement for tailoring of magnetic NPs for biomedical applications is often superparamagnetism. This occurs in magnetic materials composed of very small crystallites (threshold size depends on the nature of the material; for instance, Fe-based NPs become superparamagnetic at sizes <25 nm). In a paramagnetic material, the thermal energy overcomes the coupling forces between neighbouring atoms above the Curie

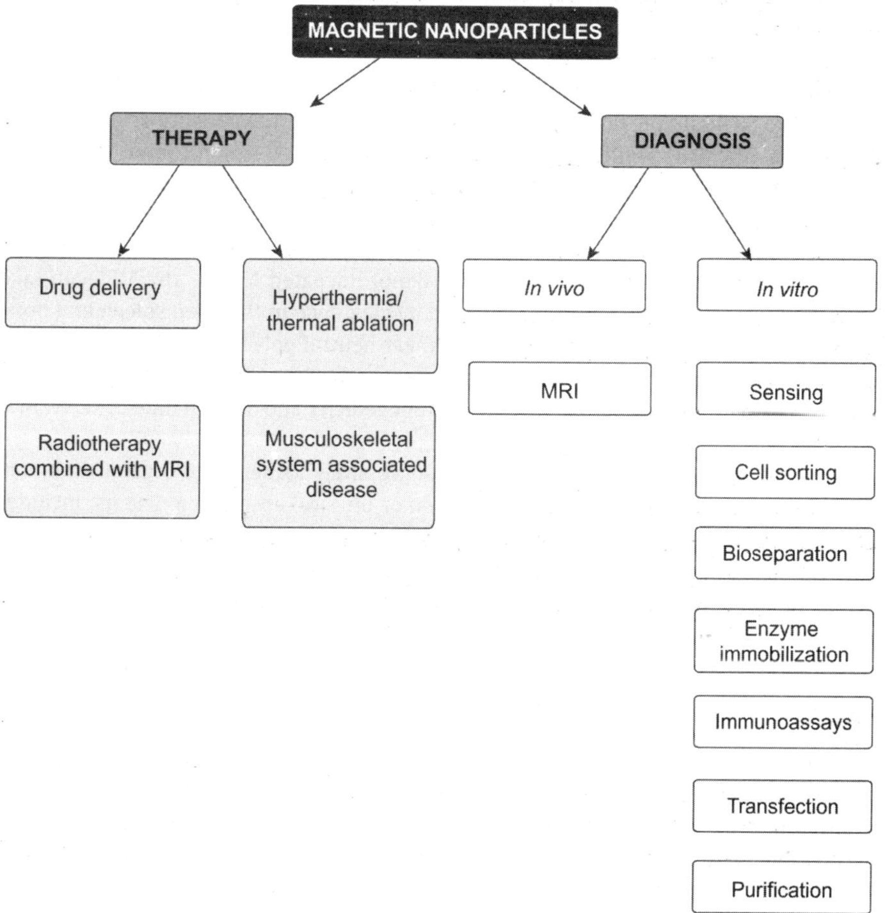

Fig. 12.5 Some biomedical applications of magnetic NPs (after Arruebo et al., 2007).

temperature, causing random fluctuations in the magnetization direction and result in a null overall magnetic moment. In contrast, in superparamagnetic materials, the fluctuations affect the direction of magnetization of entire crystallites. As the magnetic moments of individual crystallites compensate for each other, the overall magnetic moment becomes null.

In large NPs, energetic considerations favour the formation of domain walls. But, when the particle size decreases below a certain value, the formation of domain walls becomes unfavourable and each particle comprises a single domain. This is the case for superparamagnetic NPs. Superparamagnetism in drug delivery is desirable because once the external magnetic field is removed, magnetization disappears and so agglomeration (and the possible embolization of capillary vessels) is avoided (Arruebo et al., 2007).

Another crucial requirement is the biodegradability or intact excretion of the magnetic core. For nonbiodegradable cores, a specific coating is needed to avoid exposure and possible leaching of the magnetic core and to facilitate intact excretion through the kidneys, so that the half-life of the agent in the blood is determined by the glomerular filtration rate (see Saebo, 2004).

The coatings on magnetic NPs serve several purposes. They reduce leaching of the cores. The coating also often stabilizes NPs in an environment with a slightly alkaline pH or a significant salt concentration.

Silica coatings have additional merits. Their external surface coatings can be functionalized to facilitate the binding of biomolecules. The internal porosity of silica is used to host a specific drug while avoiding the unwanted physical adsorption of larger molecules. Finally, silica and other microporous inorganic materials are heat resistant, with high surface areas and good mechanical strength.

Coatings also retard clearance by the RES. Depending on their size, surface functionalization and hydrophilicity, a rapid uptake of uncoated NPs by the MPS can take place after systemic administration, followed by clearance to the liver, spleen and bone marrow. One widely used coating is PEG, a linear neutral polyether, whose attachment to NP surfaces provides a 'stealth' shielding effect and delays the action of the RES (Ferrari, 2005). PEG shows little toxicity and immunogenicity and as such intact excretion is possible.

A wide variety of molecules have been successfully loaded onto organic and inorganic shells, e.g., by chemical functionalization or physical absorption. The list includes many tumour-recognition moieties such as antibodies in 'smart' contrast agents and cell-penetrating peptides for MRI applications, enzymes, toxins, genes (transfection), growth factors, radionucleotides, folic acid and several drugs for drug delivery applications (see Arruebo et al., 2007).

Fate

The distribution of NPs and their loads throughout the body depends on numerous physicochemical factors, e.g., size of particles, toxicity, surface charge, capacity for protein adsorption, drug loading and release kinetics; stability and others. The fate (and also the possible toxicity) of magnetic NPs also depends greatly on the dose and administration route (oral or parenteral; including delivery routes such as intravenous, pulmonary, transdermal and ocular, in addition to less conventional routes, e.g., when used as scaffold coatings).

Safety

All the components of the body are either dia-, para-, superpara-, ferri-, or ferromagnetic. The magnetic fields required to produce obvious effects in the body are quite large. Even red blood cells, which each contain micrograms of the Fe protein haemoglobin, show a relatively low response to large fields or steep field gradients, although this low value is enough to be used in functional MRI. Some other natural Fe-containing compounds in the body are ferritin, transferrin and the cytochromes.

In 1987, the US Food and Drug Administration (FDA); based on positive clinical and safety experience, classified magnets with field strength of less than 2T as nonsignificant risk devices. Additional positive experiences prompted the FDA to increase this threshold to 8T in 2003 (for adults). Experiments with strong static magnetic field (8T) reduce the flow rate of human blood by 30 per cent in *in vitro* tests (Haik et al., 2001). Conceivably, magnetic fields above 3T might affect the normal behaviour of erythrocytes. Recent studies evaluating human subjects for adverse effects in physiological or neurocognitive functions resulting from exposure to static magnetic fields (up to 8T) from MRI systems have not shown any clinically relevant effects (Duncan and Izzo, 2005).

Toxicity

The toxicity of NPs depends on many factors such as the dose, chemistry, method of administration, size, biodegradability, solubility, pharmacokinetics and biodistribution. The risk-benefit trade-off needs to be considered to judge whether the risks can be justified. In general, the size, surface area, shape, composition and coating of an NP are the most important characteristics regarding cytotoxicity and modifications of the NP surface are crucial to minimize toxicological effects (Park et al., 2006).

All nanosized particles can potentially prove harmful if they are inhaled and subsequently absorbed via the lung or swallowed and then absorbed across the gastrointestinal tract (Duncan and Izzo, 2005). In 20-100 mg/ml concentrations, large magnetic particles surprisingly show higher cytotoxicity than smaller ones even after normalizing for surface area (Yin et al., 2005), in spite of their lower surface-to-volume ratio.

For a magnetic carrier as a potential drug delivery vector, it is necessary, at the very least, to analyse its: (i) toxicity, teratogenicity and mutagenicity in cellular and animal models; (ii) hematocompatibility; (iii) biodegradation, (iv) immunogenicity; and (v) pharmacokinetics (body distribution, metabolism, bioavailability, elimination, organ-specific toxicity) before the start of preclinical testing. The contrast agents based on magnetic NPs currently on the market, either involving superparamagnetic Fe oxides or paramagnetic metals encapsulated in a chelating agent satisfy current regulations regarding use in patients. The same applies to the magnetic drug delivery systems that have already been commercialized, MagNaGel®[32], FluidMAG® and TargetMAG® (Table 12.2).

Future Challenges

Magnetic NPs are being used as drug delivery vectors and as tools for hyperthermia/thermal ablation. Magnetic drug delivery is a promising technology to treat cancer, with many products already on the market. The difficulties in the use of external magnetic fields can sometimes be avoided by using internal magnets placed near the target by minimally invasive surgery (Rosengart et al., 2005). Magnetic fluid hyperthermia/thermal ablation is being applied but is limited by the fact that the tumour needs to be localized. This route makes this unsuitable for preventive medicine, or for treating early-stage tumours.

The greatest therapeutic potential appears to be associated with applications involving 'intelligent' particles with a magnetic core (to direct the particles to the vicinity of the target and also for hyperthermia or for temperature-enhanced release of the drug), a recognition layer (to which suitable receptors are attached) and a therapeutic load (adsorbed inside the pores or hosted within internal cavities of the particles (Arruebo et al., 2007).

The major challenge is related to the development of suitable recognition layers. Here useful recognition moieties need to be identified and attached to the particles; they must also be loaded to a high density while maintaining their desired characteristics.

The biomedical uses of magnetic NPs are by no means restricted to drug delivery. Novel applications are also likely in MRI, where contrast agents could be tagged with a recognition moiety, cell sorting/targeting, bioseparation, sensing, enzyme immobilization, immunoassays and gene transfection/detection systems (Arruebo et al., 2007).

Nanomagnetism and its *in vivo* Potential

Magnetic nanoparticles seem to offer great potential for *in vivo* use in delivering personalized medicine. Biocompatible nanoparticles that can be drawn toward a magnet are being explored as site-specific drug delivery agents (Gould, 2006). Transfection of cells

Table 12.2 Selected companies engaged in the development and production of magnetic micro- and nanoparticles (after Arruebo et al., 2007).

Company/Website*	Applications
Bangs Laboratories (bangslabs.com)	Cell separation, DNA and RNA purification, immunoassays
Micromod Partikeltechnologie (micromod.de)	Drug delivery, biomagnetic separation, nucleic acid purification
Guerbet (guerbet.com)	X-ray and MRI contrast agents
Ademtech (ademtech.com)	Cell sorting, biomagnetic separation
Invitrogen Corp. (invitrogen.com)	Immunoassay and nucleic acid *in vitro* diagnostics, DNA and RNA isolation, protein purification, cell separation and expansion
MagForce Nanotechnologies (magforce.com)	Hyperthermia
Spherotech (spherotech.com)	Cell separation, enzyme immunoassay
Alnis Biosciences (alnis.com)	Drug delivery for anti-cancer and infective treatments MagNaGel® 105 and smart contrast agents
Sirtex Medical (sirtex.com)	Radiation therapy
Biophan Technologies (sirtex.com)	Drug delivery
Magnamedics (magnamedics.com)	Drug delivery, *in vitro* diagnostics
Chemicell (chemicell.com)	Drug delivery (FluidMAG®), gene transfection and detection

*(Note: All websites are preceded by www.).

with nanoparticles observable by magnetic resonance imaging (MRI) facilitates monitoring of experimental cell therapies, but one size does not necessarily fit all.

Most interest in the clinical use of magnetic nanoparticles has focused on iron oxide because of the chemical stability, biological compatibility and ease of manufacture of magnetite (Fe_3O_4) and maghemite (γ-Fe_2O_3) nanoparticles.

Mixtures of both these compounds can be synthesized in a single step by alkaline co-precipitation of Fe^{2+} salts. Synthesis is generally done in an aqueous solution of an appropriate macromolecule which limits the growth of the magnetic core, while also forming a coating that helps control particle dispersion and aggregation. The iron oxide component of such mixtures is gradually recycled, naturally. The human body contains around 3–4 g Fe in the proteins ferritin, haemosiderin, transferritin and haemoglobin. As the magnetic nanoparticles break down, any soluble Fe becomes part of this normal Fe pool, which is then regulated by the body (Mornet et al., 2004). But since a clinical dose usually includes only few milligrams of Fe per kilogram body weight, the chances of Fe overload are slim.

In nanoparticulate form, both Fe_2O_4 and γ-Fe_2O_3 show superparamagnetic behaviour at room temperature, i.e., they magnetize strongly under an applied magnetic field but retain no permanent magnetism after the field is removed (Gould, 2004, 2006). This behaviour raises hopes that iron oxide nanoparticles could improve the accuracy of drug delivery by dragging attached therapeutic agents to specific areas in the body through an applied magnetic field. The on/off switching means that particles are unlikely to clump together during manufacture or after an applied magnetic field is removed, leading to easy dispersal.

Fe_3O_4/γ-Fe_2O_3 combinations have already been approved for clinical use as MRI contrast agents that work by changing the relaxation rates of water protons trying to realign with a static magnetic field following the application of radiofrequency (RF) pulses. Iron oxide-based contrast agents affect transverse relaxation times (termed T2 decay). This leads to 'negative contrast', or dark spots, on T2-weighted MR images. They do not affect longitudinal relaxation, or T1 decay. The agents are termed superparamagnetic iron oxides (SPIO) if individual particles are larger than 50 nm, or ultra-small superparamagnetic iron oxides (USPIO) if less than 50 nm in diameter. SPIO contrast agents find special use for imaging liver and spleen where they tend to amass shortly after intravenous administration. The USPIO agents are better for MR-based lymphography in view of their tendency to accumulate in the lymph nodes.

Maximizing Magnetism

But iron oxide nanoparticles may not necessarily be the best material for MR-guided cell tracking. Negative contrast from the iron oxide particles sometimes extends far beyond its immediate surroundings, leading to distortions in the background image, or large 'blooming artifacts' that obscure adjacent anatomy. This is a drawback to the utilization of SPIO-based contrast for tracking stem cells or transplanted cells, where the exact location and extent of the cells are crucial.

Some doubts have also been expressed about the suitability of Fe_3O_4 and γ-Fe_2O_3 in magnetically targeted drug delivery. There is some doubt whether iron oxide NPs could really be moved around the human body by magnetic force—the saturation magnetization and hence the magnetic moment per unit volume of SPIO nanoparticles is too low.

Another option is to use transition metal nanoparticles, such as pure Fe and Co, or metallic alloys or compounds, such as FeCo. These metallic nanoparticles, especially FeCo, have a larger magnetic moment than their iron oxide counterparts. Or, smaller concentrations of magnetic material, or smaller particles, could be used to produce the same magnetic effect; this allows using ultra-small (less than 10 nm) nanoparticles, which are critical for the delivery of small molecules and pieces of DNA. However, this class of nanomaterials also has disadvantages. Synthesis of stable, monodisperse transition metal nanoparticles suitable for use in aqueous environments is not easy. These pure metal nanoparticles are also ferromagnetic at room temperature, rather than superparamagnetic; this means that once magnetized, they continue to remain so regardless of whether an external magnetic field is withdrawn; they are also prone to clumping. Researchers are seeking suitable coatings that would prevent particulate aggregation and ensure chemical stability. Options being considered include inert metals, such as Au and Ag, peptide capping ligands and silica (Bai and Wang, 2005).

Carbon could be a possible coating for transition metal nanoparticles. Simultaneous evaporation of Fe and graphite in argon plasma yields a mixture of carbon-coated Fe and iron oxide nanoparticles with an average size of 200 nm. Preliminary haematological *in vitro* tests on rabbit and human blood samples have indicated good biocompatibility (Gould, 2006).

The carbon-coated particles are being studied in preclinical trials as possible vehicles for magnetically targeted chemotherapy delivery. The porosity and large specific area of the inorganic shell allows rapid adsorption of therapeutic agents. The drug molecules are then desorbed from the nanoparticles very slowly. The delivery agents can be loaded with their therapeutic armoury quickly and early release of the payload into the bloodstream is minimized.

Carbon might, in principle, be used to coat Co nanoparticles too, but many researchers hesitate of trying these elements for *in vivo* applications, since unlike Fe, they are not already present in the body in significant quantities. The toxicity of elements such as Co is not known.

Effective Delivery

Whatever the pros and cons of using nanoscale iron oxide for *in vivo* applications, (U)SPIOs are the only magnetic nanoparticles that are yet approved for clinical use. And the drawbacks may probably be surmounted to some extent. The nanoparticles' weak magnetic responsiveness may be strengthened by maximizing the magnetic field at the target site. Some have suggested to do this by implanting an Au-plated permanent magnet within the organ to be treated—a strategy that might enable nanoscale magnetic carriers to deliver chemotherapy agents to tumours deep within the body (Gould, 2006).

Another option is to optimize the shape and strength of externally placed magnets. Researchers are looking into using magnetically responsive nanoparticles to treat patients with stage III or IV ovarian cancer whose malignancy has spread to the peritoneum. Although intraperitoneal administration of taxane- and Pt-containing regimens has been beneficial, many patients dislike the temporary insertion of the catheter used for drug delivery. An alternative is to administer the chemotherapy agents via 20 nm silica-coated, magnetite-based nanoparticles under the influence of an external magnet.

This approach also enables the targeting of these drugs to the tumour or peri-tumoural environment, as well as less toxicity as compared to the free drugs.

In these approaches the critical variables are the design and selection of the vectoring device and the particle and coating chemistry. It is important, therefore, to deal with both these issues carefully.

According to C. Plank of the Institute of Experimental Oncology, Technical University of Munich and his co-workers from the Ludwigs-Maximilians University Munich, gas-filled microbubbles tend to increase the magnetic responsiveness of SPIO-based drug delivery agents by concentrating the particles together, but without causing clumping or blocking blood vessels. Flexible 2–5 μm diameter microbubbles can do this work. In fact, microbubbles are already used clinically to enhance ultrasound images. But demonstrating delivery by using magnetically responsive microbubbles is novel. Plank et al. use 100–200 nm particles containing a high proportion of Fe_3O_4, which are incorporated into the lipid shell of C_3F_8-filled bubbles along with a therapeutic agent by vigorous shaking. Some of these magnetic nanoparticles are coated with a detergent; these can be easily incorporated into the lipid bubble shell.

The magnetic retention of bubbles is much greater than retention of an equivalent dose of 'free' magnetic nanoparticles. 1MHz ultrasound pulses burst the bubbles and release their cargo. Animal studies will confirm whether or not the delivered therapeutic agents remain functional following their ultrasound-induced delivery.

Researchers at the University of Chicago and Argonne National Laboratory, Illinois, have adopted a different approach—coating the magnetic nanoparticles with oleic acid, to promote hydrophobicity. These coated particles are then embedded with a therapeutic agent in a polymer matrix. Enough of magnetite can be incorporated into the carrier that the magnetization value is much higher than any other carriers. The carrier is much easier to direct and to hold in target positions against strong, arterial blood flow according to Axel Rosengart (University of Chicago). Application of ultrasound of an appropriate intensity causes the polymer beads to resonate and then break, releasing the therapeutic agent. But there is an additional benefit from using ultrasound; Rosengart wishes to use the magnetic beads to deliver the 'clot-busting' thrombolysis agent rt-PA to stroke and heart attack patients. The porosity of blood clots increases when exposed to ultrasound, which speeds up lysis. Possibly, therefore, using ultrasound-triggered delivery will further increase the efficacy of targeted rt-PA delivery (Gould, 2006).

The important lesson is that one size—and one composition—does not fit all when it comes to *in vivo* applications for magnetic nanoparticles. An example: an agent that hunts down widely dispersed metastatic cancer cells by using MRI may not prove very effective for dragging chemotherapy molecules toward a well-defined tumour site. The correct nanoparticles must be found for each specific job.

Polymer Nanoconjugates

Two distinct current approaches to the search for improved anti-cancer treatments are: (a) genomics and proteomics research which assists in the identification of unique targets that will aid the synthesis of the 'perfect fit' drug molecule with exquisite therapeutic activity and no side effects (Atkins and Gershell, 2002); and (b) the design of systems for drug targeting that can better guide drugs precisely to the tumour cells, at increased concentrations and away from sites of dose-limiting toxicity (see Torchilin, 2005; Duncan, 2003, 2003a). The approach (a) has proved difficult to realize in practice. Poorly predictive preclinical models, lack of tumour target specificity, lack of effective cellular and intracellular delivery and emergence of drug resistance have hindered progress. As regards the second approach, first generation technologies include liposomes, antibody-drug conjugates and also several polymer-conjugates carrying either low-molecular-weight drugs or proteins. Willis (2004) expressed considerable optimism that application of nanotechnology to medicine will significantly advance the diagnosis and treatment of cancer; in fact these hybrid multi-component polymer-containing systems may be viewed as the first-generation of 'nanomedicines' for cancer treatment.

During the past decade, the importance of synthetic and natural polymeric drug-delivery systems in oncology has increased with the advent of biodegradable polymeric implants (Anderson, 2001). In this form, they are used as a subcutaneous depot that slowly releases luteinising hormone-releasing hormone (LHRH) analogues for treatment of prostate and other hormone-dependent cancers. When implanted post-surgically, they provide local delivery of chemotherapy for treating brain cancer (Bolla et al., 2002; Guerin et al., 2004).

The term 'polymer therapeutics' covers several different families of polymer-based drugs, polymeric pro-drugs and polymer-based delivery systems; it includes the water-soluble polymer conjugates of several drugs and proteins. Unlike polymeric implants designed for sustained or local drug release, these water soluble therapeutic polymer-based conjugates are meant for parenteral administration, often in the treatment of disseminated metastatic disease (see Vicent and Duncan, 2006).

A combination of polymer chemistry and biomedical sciences has led to production of the first polymer-based nanomedicines for the diagnosis and treatment of cancer (see Vicent and Duncan, 2006). These water-soluble hybrid constructs are administered intravenously. They fall into two main categories: polymer-protein conjugates or polymer-drug conjugates. Polymer conjugation to proteins lowers immunogenicity, prolongs plasma half-life and enhances protein stability. Polymer-drug conjugation promotes tumour targeting through the enhanced permeability and retention (EPR) effect and, at the cellular level following endocytic capture, allows lysosomotropic drug delivery. The successful clinical application of polymer-protein conjugates (PEGylated enzymes and cytokines) and promising results emerging from clinical trials with polymer-bound chemotherapy (e.g., doxorubicin, paclitaxel, camptothecins) have laid a strong foundation for more sophisticated second-generation constructs that deliver the novel target-directed anti-cancer agents (e.g., modulators of the cell cycle, signal transduction inhibitors and antiangiogenic drugs) in addition to polymer-drug combinations (e.g., endocrine- and chemotherapy) (Vicent and Duncan, 2006).

Both, polymer-drug and polymer-protein conjugates must be carefully designed for their specific use, duly considering the nature of the individual drug payload (protein, low-molecular-mass drug) and the location of each molecular pharmacological target. Both families of polymer conjugates can be tailor-made by using a basic tripartite structure containing a water-soluble polymer, a linker and the bioactive agent (Table 12.3). The molecular mass and physico-chemical properties of the polymer govern biodistribution, elimination and metabolism of the conjugate as a whole; this makes the choice of a suitable polymer vital. The water-soluble polymeric carrier must be non-toxic, non-immunogenic and suitable for repeated administration. Poly(ethylene glycol) (PEG), N-

Table 12.3 Chemical characteristics of selected polymer anti-cancer conjugates (after Vicent and Duncan, 2006).

Compound	Polymer characteristics		Linker	Drug (loading)	Cleavage conditions
	Polymer	M mass (g/mol)			
Polymer-protein conjugates					
SMANCS	Styrene-maleic anhydride (SMA) copolymer	15,000	Amine	Neocarzinostatin	Non-biodegradable
Oncaspar®	m-PEG	5,000	Amide	L-asparaginase	Non-biodegradable
PEG-Asys®	Branched m-PEG	40,000	Amide	IFNα-2a	Non-biodegradable
PEG-intron™	m-PEG	12,000	Carbamate	IFNα-2b	β-lactamase or basic hydrolysis
Polymer-drug conjugates					
PK1, PK2	HPMA copolymer	30,000, 25,000	Amide	Doxorubicin (8.5 wt%; 7.5 wt%) and galactosamine (1.5–2.5 mol%)	Thiol protease cathepsin B
PROTHECAN™	PEG	40,000	Ester	Camptothecin (1.7 wt%)	Esterases or acid hydrolysis

Mw: Molecular weight; SMANCS: poly(styrene-co-maleic anhydride)-neocarzinostatin; HPMA: N-(2-hyroxypropyl) methacrylamide; m-PEG: monomethoxy poly(ethylene glycol); IFN-α: interferon-α

(2-hydroxypropyl-methacrylamide) (HPMA) copolymers and poly(glutamic acid) (PGA) are the most commonly tested in a clinical setting. Of these, only PGA is biodegradable; so the molecular masses of PEG and HPMA copolymers have been limited to <40kDa to ensure eventual renal elimination. For non-degradable polymers, the polymer-drug or protein linker is important (Table 12.3). Although polymer-protein and polymer-drug conjugates show many similarities, the biological rationales behind their respective designs differ.

A selection of polymer-protein conjugates that have entered into routine clinical use in oncology is shown in Table 12.4.

Although polymer anti-cancer conjugates are rapidly being added to the anti-cancer armoury, several challenges are yet to be addressed to develop this technology further. Better polymeric carriers are being developed. There is a strong need to develop high-molecular-mass; biodegradable polymeric carriers that can better exploit EPR-mediated tumour targeting. PEG-polyacetals that show pH-dependent degradation (Tomlinson et al., 2002) and dextrins (Hreczuk-Hirst et al., 2001) which are degraded by amylase are potential options for such carriers. Researchers should move away from heterogeneous, random-coiled, polymeric carriers towards better defined polymer structures. As dendrimers and dendronized polymers integrate the features of a mono-disperse nanoscale

Table 12.4 Ten selected polymer-protein and polymer-drug conjugates (after Vicent and Duncan, 2006).

S.No.	Compound	Name	Comment
Polymer-protein conjugates			
1.	SMANCS	Zinostatin Stimalmer®	Hepatocellular carcinoma
2.	PEG-L-asparaginase	Oncaspar®	Acute lymphoblastic leukaemia
3.	PEG-GCSF	Neulasta™	Prevention of neutropenia associated with cancer and AIDS chemotherapy
4.	PEG-interferon α-2a	PEG-Asys®	Hepatitis B and C
5.	PEG-arginine deiminase	ADI-PEG20	Hepatocellular carcinoma
Polymer-drug conjugates			
6.	Polyglutamate-paclitaxel	CT-2103; XYOTAXTM	Non-small cell lung cancer; ovarian cancer
7.	HPMA copolymer-doxorubicin	PK1; FCE28068	Lung and breast cancer
8.	HPMA copolymer-carboplatin platinate	AP5280	Various
9.	HPMA copolymer-DACH-platinate	AP5346	Various
10.	PEG-camptothecin	PROTHECAN™	Various

Notes: SMANCS: poly(styrene-co-maleic anhydride)-neocarzinostatin; G-CSF: granulocyte colony-stimulating factor; HPMA: N-(2-hydroxypropyl) methacrylamide; PEG: poly(ethylene glycol); Status: (1-4, marketed; 5. undergoing Phase I trials; 6-10, Phase I-III trials).

geometry with high end-group density at their surface, they are attractive options for immobilization of anti-cancer drugs (Malik et al., 1999) and/or as targeting moieties (Shukla et al., 2003). However, their dendrimer safety and chemical characteristics need to be established.

There is also a need to improve the existing therapeutic strategies. For example, one possible mechanism of resistance that affects polymer conjugates requiring endocytic uptake and lysosomal enzyme activation might be reduced internalization or a decrease in the levels of an activating enzyme; this is prompting development of polymer-based strategies for extracellular drug delivery. Polymer-directed enzyme pro-drug therapy (PDEPT) is a two-step approach that utilizes a polymer-bound enzyme to activate a polymer-drug conjugate, present in the tumour interstitium, where the linker is a substrate for the activating enzyme (Satchi-Fainaro et al., 2003).

Another welcome development is the recent emergence of polymer conjugates containing drugs directed against novel anti-cancer targets (Rowinsky, 2003; Steeg, 2003; Alam, 2003; Cao, 2004 and Ranson, 2004). The first polymeric anti-angiogenic conjugate, HPMA copolymer-TNP-470 has been described (Satchi-Fainaro et al., 2004). Attempts are being made to develop therapies that target the apoptotic signalling cascade at the molecular level: promising *in vivo* results have been observed for a targeted proapoptotic anti-cancer drug delivery system for the treatment of ovarian cancer (Dharap et al., 2003).

Use of polymer-drug conjugates in combination therapy also offers an important opportunity to enhance tumour response rates (see Vicent and Duncan, 2006). The polymeric carrier is a good platform for the delivery of a cocktail of drugs simultaneously. It may soon become possible to design polymer-drug combinations for improved treatment of breast and prostate cancers.

Similar novel nanomedicines based on polymer-protein conjugates are also being used to successfully treat diseases other than cancer (e.g., PEG-interferon-α can be used to cure hepatitis C).

Ferrofluids

Certain novel forms of therapy for combating cancer use magnetic fields to apply forces to ferrofluids. Ferrofluids are suspensions of extremely fine magnetic particles in a carrier fluid. They have become important in various fields of application. These fluids contain magnetic nanoparticles (diameter approx 10 nm). These nanoparticles (NPs) can be coated with long-chain molecules that prevent agglomeration. This enables the particles to remain homogeneously distributed for many years. A striking property of ferrofluids is that magnetic fields, generated with standard electromagnets are used to apply forces to the NPs thus allowing the fluid or other properties of a ferrofluid to be modified. This possibility has attracted biomedical applications that require physiologically compatible (biocompatible) ferrofluids. This has inspired the development of ferrofluids with water as the carrier fluid and iron oxide particles coated with starch molecules, for example, as the magnetic component (Odenbach, 2007). One major goal of biomedical research based on the use of ferrofluids is the development of novel forms of therapy for cancer patients. Two approaches are available. In magnetic 'drug targeting', a chemotherapeutic agent is bound to the surface coating of the particles. After injecting the suspension prepared in this way into the artery supplying the tumour, magnetic force is applied to concentrate these particles in the tumour. Only small amounts of a chemotherapeutic agent can achieve a high concentration of the active substance in the tumour and at the same time, only a small amount, if any, of the drug reaches other parts of the body. This minimizes any adverse effects while improving the therapeutic effects.

The second strategy is to heat the tumour tissue. The higher temperature damages the tissue and makes it more susceptible to other forms of therapy. To do this locally, at the tumour site, magnetic NPs are localized in the tumour tissue. Alternating magnetic fields continuously remagnetize the particles, while the associated release of energy heats the tissue. This technique is termed magnetic hyperthermy. In contrast to approaches in which the magnetic suspension is injected directly into the tumour, current research focus is on incorporating specific markers on the particles which can then lodge onto the tumour tissue, allowing those tumours to be reached which cannot be injected directly. It also avoids damaging the tumour and so minimizes any detachment or the release of cancerous cells (Odenbach, 2007).

Direct injection localizes the NPs within the region of the tumour, while new magnetic and chemical drug targeting techniques facilitate study of the efficiency of particle storage in the tumour tissue and of how the particles are distributed within the tumour.

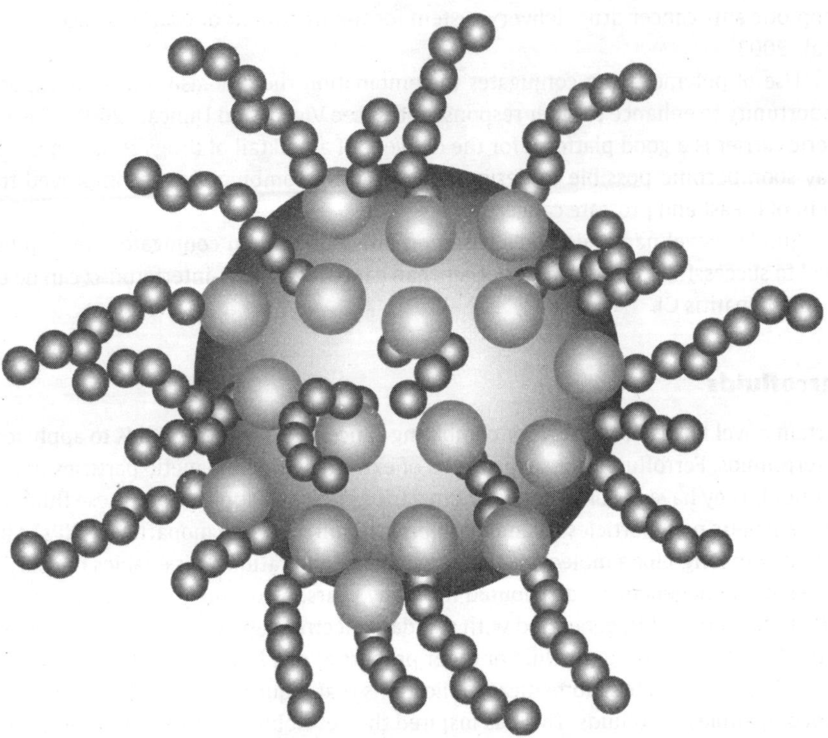

Fig. 12.6 Ferrofluids containing magnetic nanoparticles coated with long-chain molecules. For clarity, the surface coating is not shown to scale in the modelled particles (after Odenbach, 2007).

Research is underway to examine the NP distribution by means of X-ray microtomography. Since the X-ray absorption depends on the density of the object being examined, its radiography gives a two-dimensional 'projection' of the object's inner structure. Unlike X-rays, tomography gives information on the three dimensional distribution of the material and is achieved by recording radiographic images from various different angles. When these images are combined mathematically, the 3-D information can be back-calculated. Although tomographic techniques are standard medical procedures, their spatial resolution is limited to a few millimeters. Modern tomography cameras, which use synchrotron radiation, produce 3-D datasets with a spatial resolution of a few microns. In fact, X-ray microtomography can be an ideal method to localize magnetic particles in treated tumours.

A new synchrotron tomography camera is being designed that may allow 3-D investigations with a high temporal and spatial resolution. Such a camera could be used in future projects to study the time-dependent particle distribution in test animals after dosing and will significantly reduce the number of experiments required (Odenbach, 2007).

References

Achen, M.G., McColl, B.K., Stacker, S.A. Focus on lymphangiogenesis in tumour metastasis. Cancer Cell 7:121-127 (2005).

ACS. Cancer Facts and Figures 2007. American Cancer Society, Atlanta (2007).

Acuff, R. Vitamin E:Bioavailability and function of natural and synthetic forms. Am J. Nat. Med. 5 (1998).

Adams, E.J., Chien, Y.H., Garcia, K.C. Science 308:227-231 (2005).

Adams, G.P., Weiner, L.M. Monoclonal antibody therapy of cancer. Nature Biotechnol. 23:1147-1157 (2005).

Akashi, K., Traver, D., Miyamoto, T., Weissman, I.L. Nature 404:193-197 (2000).

Akerman, M.E. et al. PNAS (USA) 99:12617-12621 (2002).

Alam, J.J. Apoptosis:target for novel drugs. TIBTECH 21:479-483 (2003).

Alberts, B. et al. Essential Cell Biology. Garland Publishing, New York (1998).

Alexiou, C. et al. Cancer Res. 60:6641 (2000).

Al-Hajj, M. et al. Prospective identification of tumourigenic breast cancer cells. PNAS (USA) 100:3983-3988 (2003).

Al-Tassan, N. et al. Inherited variants of MYH associated with somatic G:C to T:A mutations in colorectal tumours. Nature Genet. 30:227-232 (2002).

Anderson, J.M. Biological responses to materials. Ann. Rev. Mat. Res. 31:81-110 (2001).

Anderson, R. et al. Teenage girls and elderly women living in northern Europe have low winter vitamin D status. Eur. J. Clin. Nutr. 59:533-541 (2005).

Antoniou, A. et al. Average risks of breast and ovarian cancer associated with mutations in BRCA1 or BRCA2 detected in case series unselected for family history:A combined analysis of 22 studies. Am. J. Hum. Genet. 72:1117-1130 (2003).

Antony, A.C. Blood 79:2807 (1992).

Aoki, Y. et al. RNA interference may be more potent than antisense RNA in human cancer cell lines. Clin. Exp. Pharmacol. Physiol. 30:96-102 (2003).

Armanios, M.Y. et al. Telomerase mutations in families with idiopathic pulmonary fibrosis. N. Engl. J. Med. 356:1317-1326 (2007).

Arruebo, M. et al. Magnetic nanoparticles for drug delivery. Nanotoday 2 (3):22-32 (2007).

Ast, G. How did alternative splicing evolve? Nature Rev. Genetics. 5:773-782 (2004).

Ast, G. The alternative genome. Scientific Amer. 292:60-65 (2005).

Atanasijevic, T. et al. Calcium sensitive MRI contrast agents based on superparamagnetic iron oxide nanoparticles and calmodulin. PNAS (USA) 103:14707-14712 (2006).

Atkins, J.H., Gershell, L.J. Selective anticancer drugs. Nature Rev. Drug Discov. 1:491-492 (2002).

Azarova, A. et al. Roles of DNA topoisomerase II isozymes in chemotherapy and secondary malignancies. PNAS (USA) 104:11014-11019 (2007).

Bae, J.M., Jung, K.W., Won, Y.J. Estimation of cancer deaths in Korea for the upcoming years. J. Korean Med. Sci. 17:611-615 (2002).

Bae, Y. et al. Bioconjug. Chem. 16:122-130 (2005).

Bagwe, R.P. et al. Langmuir 22:4357 (2006).

Bahar, R. et al. Increased cell-to-cell variation in gene expression in ageing mouse heart. Nature 441:1011-1014 (2006).

Bai, J., Wang, J.P. Appl. Phys. Lett. 87:152502 (2005).

Baker, D.J. et al. BubR1 insufficiency causes early onset of aging-associated phenotypes and infertility in mice. Nature Genet. 36:744-749 (2004).

Baker, D.J. et al. Early aging-associated phenotypes in Bub3/Rae1 haploinsufficient mice. J. Cell Biol. 172:529-540 (2006).

Baker, M. In biomarkers we trust? Nature Biotechnol. 23:297-304 (2005).

Baker, M. New-wave diagnostics. Nature Biotechnol. 24:931-938 (2006).

Balkwill, F., Coussens, L.M. Cancer:an inflammatory link. Nature 431:405-406 (2004).

Balkwill, F., Mantovani, A. Lancet 357:539-545 (2001).

Balkwill, F. et al. Smoldering and polarized inflammation in the initiation and promotion of malignant disease. Cancer Cell 7:211-217 (Mar. 2005).

Balzarini, J. Inhibition of HIV entry by carbohydrate-binding proteins. Antiviral Res. 71:237-247 (2006).

Balzarini, J. et al. Carbohydrate-binding agents efficiently prevent dendritic cell-specific intercellular adhesion molecule-3-grabbing nonintegrin (DC-SIGN)-directed HIV-1 transmission to T lymphocytes. Mol. Pharmacol. 71:3-11 (2007).

Banchereau, J., Palucka, A.K. Dendritic cells as therapeutic vaccines against cancer. Nature Rev. Immunol. 5:296-306 (2005).

Bao, S. et al. Glioma stem cells promote radioresistance by preferential activation of the DNA damage response. Nature 444:756-760 (2006).

Barber, T.D. et al. Somatic mutations of EGFR in colorectal cancers and glioblastomas. N. Engl. J. Med. 351:2883 (2004).

Bardeesy, N., DePinho, R.A. Nature Rev. Cancer 2:897-909 (2002).

Baricault, L. et al. Use of HT-29, a cultured human colon cancer cell line, to study the effect of fermented milks on colon cancer cell growth and differentiation. Carcinogenesis 16:245-252 (1995).

Barone, W. et al. Nature Mater. 4(1):86 (2005).

Bartosch, B., Cosset, F.L. Strategies for retargeted gene delivery using vectors derived from lentiviruses. Curr. Gene Ther. 4:427-443 (2004).

Bazell, R. HER2:The Making of Herceptin, a Revolutionary Treatment for Breast Cancer. Random House (1998).

BDWG (Biomarkers Definitions Working Group). Biomarkers and surrogate endpoints :preferred definitions and conceptual framework. Clin. Pharmacol. Ther.69, 89-95 (2001).

Beckman, E.M. et al. Recognition of a lipid antigen by CD1-restricted [illegible]+T cells. Nature 372:691-694 (1994).

Bensaad, K. et al. TIGAR, a p53-inducible regulator of glycolysis and apoptosis. Cell 126:107-120 (2006).

Benson, J.D. et al. Validating cancer drug targets. Nature 446:451-456 (2006).

Bergers, G., Benjamin, L.E. Tumourigenesis and the angiogenic switch. Nature Rev. Cancer 3:401-410 (2003).

Bernal, A. et al. Emerging opportunities in functional informatics. Pharma Geonomics 9:38-44 (2003).

Bernard, O., Hozumi, N., Tonegawa, S. Sequences of mouse immunoglobulin light chain genes before and after somatic changes. Cell 15:1133-1144 (1978).

Bernstein, B.E. et al. A bivalent chromatin structure marks key developmental genes in embryonic stem cells. Cell 125:315-326 (2006).

Besaratinia, A. et al. DNA lesions induced by UVA1 and B radiation in human cells:comparative analyses in the overall genome and in the p53 tumour- suppressor gene. PNAS (USA) 102:10058-10063 (2005).

Bestor, T. et al. Cancer Cell 8:479-484 (2005).

Bielas, J.H., Loeb, L.A. Quantification of random genomic mutations. Nature Methods 2:285-290 (2005).

Bielas, J.H. et al. Human cancers express a mutator phenotype. PNAS (USA) 103:18238-18242 (2006).

Bielas, J.H., Venkatesan, R.N., Loeb, L.A. LOH-proficient embryonic stem cells:a model of cancer progenitor cells? Trends Genet. 23:154-157 (2007).

Biffi, A. et al. Antiproliferative effect of fermented milk on the growth of a human breast cancer cell line. Nutr. Cancer 28:93-99 (1997).

Bikle, D.D. What is new in vitamin D:2006-2007. Curr. Opin. Rheumatol. 19(4):383-388 (2007).

Bild, A.H. et al. Oncogenic pathway signatures in human cancers as a guide to targeted therapies. . Nature 439:353-355 (2006).

Billings, P.R. Three barriers to innovative diagnostics. Nature Biotech. 24:917-918 (2006).

Bilodeau, M.T. et al. Total synthesis of a human breast tumour associated antigen. J. Am. Chem. Soc. 117:7840-7841 (1995).

Bischoff-Ferrari et al. Estimation of optimal serum concentrations of 25-hydroxyvitamin D for multiple health outcomes. Am. J. Clin. Nutr. 84:18-28 (2006).

Bissell, M.J., Labarge, M.A. Context, tissue plasticity, and cancer:are tumour stem cells also regulated by the microenvironment? Cancer Cell 7:17-23 (2005).

Blanco, R. et al. Telomerase abrogation dramatically accelerates TRF2-induced epithelial carcinogenesis. Genes Dev. 21:206-220 (2007).

Blattman, J.N., Greenberg, P.D. Cancer immunotherapy:A treatment for the masses. Science 305:200-205 (2004).

Blazej, R.G., Kumaresan, P., Mathies, R.A. Microfabricated bioprocessor for integrated nanoliter-scale Sanger DNA sequencing. PNAS (USA) 103:7240-7245 (2006).

Blixt, O. et al. Printed covalent glycan array for ligand profiling of diverse glycan binding proteins. PNAS (USA) 101:17033-17038 (2004).

Blunt, J.W. et al. Natural Prod. Rep. 23:26-78 (2006).

Bodmer, W.F. J. Hum. Genet. 51:391-396 (2006).

Bogdanov Jr., A., Weissleder, R. The development of in vivo imaging systems to study gene expression. TIBTECH 16:5 (1998).

Boland, C.R., Goel, A. Somatic evolution of cancer cells. Semin. Cancer Biol. 15:436-450 (2005).

Bolla, M. et al. Long-term results with immediate androgen suppression and external irradiation in patients with locally advanced prostate cancer (an EORTC study):a phase III randomized trial. Lancet 360:103-108 (2002).

Bonjour, J.P., Chevalley, T., Fardellone, P. Calcium intake and vitamin D metabolism and action, in healthy conditions and in prostate cancer. Br. J. Nutr. 97(4):611-616 (2007).

Boons, G.-J., Demchenko, A.V. Recent advances in O-sialylation. Chem. Rev. 100:4539-4565 (2000).

Borg, N.A. et al. CD1d-lipid antigen recognition by the semi-invariant NKTT-cell receptor. Nature 448:44-49 (2007).

Boshoff, C. Understanding Cancer. Nature 444:549 (2006).

Bouillon, R. et al. Vitamin D and cancer. J. Steroid Biochem. Mol. Biol. 102:156-162 (2006).

Boveri, T. The Origin of Malignant Tumours. Williams and Wilkins, Baltimore (1914).

Boychyn, M. et al. Laboratory scaledown of protein purification processes involving fractional precipitation and centrifugal recovery. Biotechnol. Bioeng. 69:1-10 (2000).

Boyd, B.J. Technology Overviews, Colloidal Drug Delivery. Drug Delivery Report, Autumn/Winter, Oxford, p. 63 (2005).

Boyer, L.A. et al. Polycomb complexes repress development regulators in murine embryonic stem cells. Nature 441:349-353 (2006).

Brash, D.E. et al. A role for sunlight in skin cancer:UV-induced p53 mutations in squamous cell carcinoma. PNAS (USA) 88:10124-10128 (1991).

Brennan, F.R. et al. Mol. Biotechnol. 27:59 (2004).

Brenton, J.D., Aparicio, S.A., Caldas, C. Molecular profiling of breast cancer:portraits but not physiognomy. Breast Cancer Res. 3:77-80 (2001).

Brewster, D.H. et al. Recent trends in incidence of nonmelanoma skin cancers in the East of Scotland, 1992-2003. Br. J. Dermatol. 156:1295-1300 (2007).

Brock, K. et al. Associations with vitamin D deficiency in "at risk" Australians. J. Steroid Biochem. Mol. Biol. 89-90:581-588 (2004).

Brown, K.E. et al. Mol. Cell 3:207-217 (1999).

Brown, W.L. et al. RNA bacteriophage capsid-mediated drug delivery and epitope presentation. Intervirology 45:371-380 (2002).

Bruchez, M. et al. Semiconductor nanocrystals as fluorescent biological labels. Science 281:2013-2016 (1998).

Brulliard, M. et al. Nonrandom variations in human cancer ESTs indicate that mRNA heterogeneity increases during carcinogenesis. PNAS 104:7522-7527 (2007).

Brumby, A.M., Richardson, H.E. Using Drosophila melanogaster to map human cancer pathways. Nature Rev. Cancer 5:626-639 (2005).

Brummelkamp, T.R. et al. Stable suppression of tumourigenicity by virus-mediated RNA interference. Cancer Cell 2:243-247 (2002).

Buck, C.B. et al. Efficient intracellular assembly of papillomaviral vectors. J. Virol. 78:751-757 (2004).

Burke, K.E. et al. Effects of topical and oral vitamin E on pigmentation and skin cancer induced by ultraviolet radiation in Skh:2 hairless mice. Nutr. Cancer 38:87-97 (2000).

Burke, P.A. et al. Cancer Res. 62:4263 (2002).

Burnet, F.M. A modification of Jerne's theory of antibody production using the concept of clonal selection. Aust. J. Sci. 20:67-69 (1957).

Burns, A.J., Rowland, I.R. Antigenotoxicity of probiotics and prebiotics on faecal water-induced DNA damage in human colon adenocarcinoma cells. Mutat. Res. 551:233-243 (2004).

Cai, W. et al. Nano Lett. 6:669-676 (2006).

Calarese, D.A. et al. Antibody domain exchange is an immunological solution to carbohydrate cluster recognition. Science 300:2065-2071 (2003).

Callinan, P.A., Feinberg, A.P. The emerging science of epigenomics. Hum. Mol. Genet. 15:R95-R101 (2006).

Cantley, L.C. The phosphoinositide 3-kinase pathways. Science 296:1655 (2002).

Cao, Y. Antiangiogenic cancer therapy. Sem. Cancer Biol. 14:139-145 (2004).

Carmeleit, P., Jain, R.K. Angiogenesis in cancer and other diseases. Nature 407:249-257 (2000).

Carroll, N.M. et al. The effect of ganciclovir on herpes simplex virus-mediated oncolysis. J. Surg. Res. 69:413-417 (1997).

Cartwright, P. et al. LIF/STAT3 controls ES cell self-renewal and pluripotency by a Myc-dependent mechanism. Development 132:126-140 (2003).

Caruso, F. Nanoengineering of particle surfaces. Adv. Mater. 13:11-22 (2001).

Caruthers, M.H. Gene synthesis machines:DNA chemistry and its uses. Science 230:281-285 (1985).

Caussinus, E., Gonzalez, C. Induction of tumour growth by altered stem-cell asymmetric division in Drosophila melanogaster. Nature Genet. 37:1125-1129 (2005).

Cavallaro, U. et al. N-CAM modulates tumour-cell adhesion to matrix by inducing FGF-receptor signalling. Nature Cell Biol. 3:650-657 (2001).

Cawthon, R.M. et al. Association between telomere length in blood and mortality in people aged 60 years or older. Lancet 361:393-395 (2003).

CGHFBC (Collaborative Group on Hormonal Factors in Breast Cancer). Familial breast cancer:Collaborative reanalysis of individual data from 52 epidemiological studies including 58209 women with breast cancer and 101986 women without the disease. Lancet 358:1389-1399 (2001).

Chah, S. et al. Chem. Biol. 12:323 (2005).

Chakeres, D.W., de Vocht, F. Prog. Biophys. Molec. Biol. 87:255 (2005).

Chambers, A.F., Groom, A.C., MacDonald, I.C. Dissemination and growth of cancer cells in metastatic sites. Nature Rev. Cancer 2:562-572 (2002).

Chan, W.C., Nie, S. Quantum dot bioconjugates for ultrasensitive nanoisotopic detection. Science 281:2016-2019 (1998).

Chang, Y.S. et al. Mosaic blood vessels in tumours:frequency of cancer cells in contact with flowing blood. PNAS (USA) 97:14608-14613 (2000).

Cheadle, J.P., Sampson, J.R. MUTYH-associated polyposis – from defect in base excision repair to clinical genetic testing. DNA Repair (Amst.) 6:274-279 (2007).

Check, E. Human genome:patchwork people. Nature 437:1084-1086 (2005).

Chen, R.J. et al. Noncovalent functionalization of carbon nanotubes for highly specific electronic biosensors. PNAS (USA) 100(9):4984-4989 (2003).

Chen, Y. et al. Inhibition of hepatitis B virus replication by stably expressed shRNA. Biochem. Biophys. Res. Commun. 311:398-404 (2003).

Chen, Y. et al. Anal. Chem. 79:960 (2007).

Cheng, J. et al. Preparation of hybridization analysis of DNA/RNA from E. coli on microfabricated bioelectronic chips. Nature Biotechnol. 16:541-546 (1998).

Cheng, M.M.-C. et al. Curr. Opin. Chem. Biol. 10:11-19 (2006).

Cheong, I. + 6 others. A bacterial protein enhances the release and efficacy of liposomal cancer drugs. Science 314:1308-1311 (2006).

Cheshier, S., Morrison, S.J., Liao, X., Weissman, I.L. In vivo proliferation and cell cycle kinetics of long-term self-renewing haematopoietic stem cells. PNAS (USA) 96:3120-3125 (1999).

Chester, J. et al. Tumour antigen-specific induction of transcriptionally targeted retroviral vectors from chimeric immune receptor-modified T cell. Nature Biotechnol. 20:256-263 (2002).

Chiba, H. et al. Actinohivin, a novel anti-HIV protein from actinomycetes that inhibits syncytium formation:isolation, characterization, and biological activities. Biochem. Biophys. Res. Commun. 282:595-601 (2001).

Chin, L. et al. Essential role for oncogenic Ras in tumour maintenance. Nature 400:468-472 (1999).

Chiocca, E.A. Guided genes for tumour warfare. Nature Biotechnol. 20:235-236 (2002).

Christenson, L.J. et al. Incidence of basal cell and squamous cell carcinomas in a population younger than 40 years. JAMA 294:681-690 (2005).

Christofori, G. New signals from the invasive front. Nature 441:444-450 (2006).

Clark, G.F. et al. Viewing AIDS from a glycobiological perspective:potential linkages to the human fetoembryonic defence system hypothesis. Mol. Hum. Reprod. 3:5-13 (1997).

Clark, J.H. The effect of long ultraviolet radiation in the development of tumours induced by 20-methylcholanthrene. Cancer Res. 24:207-211 (1964).

Clarke, M.F., Becker, M.W. Stem cells:the real culprits in cancer? Sci. Amer., pp. 53-59 (Jul., 2006).

Clarke, M.F., Fuller, M. Stem cells and cancer:Two faces of eve. Cell 124:1111-1115 (Mar. 2006).

Cleaver, J.E., Kraemer, K.H. Xeroderma pigmentosum. Pp. 2949-2971. In:Scriver, C.R. et al. (eds.) The Metabolic Basis of Inherited Disease. McGraw-Hill, New York (1989).

Clevers, H. Stem cells, asymmetric division and cancer. Nature Genet. 37:1027-1028 (2005).

Cole, C., Conzen, S. Polyomaviridae:the viruses and their replication. Pp. 2141-2174. In:Knipe, D.M., Howley, P.M. (eds.). Fields Virology (4th ed.). Lippincott, Williams and Wilkins, Baltimore (2001).

Cole, K.S. et al. Removal of N-linked glycosylation sites in the V1 region of simian immunodeficiency virus gp120 results in redirection of B-cell responses to V3. Virol. 78:1525-1539 (2004).

Collado, M., Serrano, M. The power and the promise of oncogene-induced senescence markers. Nature Rev. Cancer 6:472-476 (2006).

Collins, M.K., Cerundolo, V. Gene therapy meets vaccine development. TIBTECH 22:623-626 (2004).

Conacci-Sorrell, M.E. et al. Nr-CAM is a target gene of the [illegible]-catenin/LEF-1 pathway in melanoma and colon cancer and its expression enhances motility and confers tumourigenesis. Genes Dev. 16:2058-2072 (2002).

Cooper, E.L. General Immunology. Pergamon Press, New York (1982).

Corso, S., Comoglio, P.M., Giordano, S. Cancer therapy:can the challenge be met? Trends Mol. Med. 11:284-292 (2005).

Cory, S., Adams, J.M. The Bcl1 family:regulators of the cellular life-or-death switch. Nature Rev. Cancer 2:647-656 (2002).

Coultas, L., Chawengsaksophak, K., Rossant, J. Endothelial cells and VEGF in vascular development. Nature 438:937-945 (2005).

Couvreur, P., Vauthier, C. Nanotechnology:intelligent design to treat complex disease. Pharm. Res. 23:1417-1450 (2006).

Couzin, J. T cells a boon for colon cancer prognosis. Science 313:1868-1869 (2006).

Cox, A.L. et al. Identification of a peptide recognized by five melanoma-specific human cytotoxic T cell lines. Science 264:716-719 (1994).

Crespi, B.J., Summers, K. Evolutionary biology of cancer. Trends in Ecology and Evolution 20:545-552 (2005).

Crespi, B.J., Summers, K. Positive selection in the evolution of cancer. Biol. Rev. 81:407-424 (2006).

Cristofanilli, M., Mendelsohn, J. Circulating tumour cells in breast cancer:Advanced tools for "tailored" therapy? PNAS (USA) 103:17073-17074 (2006).

Crnkovic-Mertens, I. et al. Induction of apoptosis in tumour cells by siRNA-mediated silencing of the livin/ML-IAP/KIAP gene. Oncogene 22:8330-8336 (2003).

Croft, J.A. et al. J. Cell. Biol. 145:1119-1131 (1999).

Croul, S. et al. Brain tumours and polyomaviruses. J. Neurovirol. 9:173-182 (2003).

Cui, J. et al. Requirement of V[illegible]14NKT cells in IL-12-mediated rejection of tumours. Science 278:1623-1626 (1997).

Cui, Y. et al. Nanowire nanosensors for highly sensitive and selective detection of biological and chemical species. Science 293:1289-1292 (2001).

Curtis, H.J. Biological mechanisms underlying the aging process. Science 141:686-694 (1963).

Dahan, M. et al. Diffusion dynamics of glycine receptors revealed by single quantum dot tracking. Science 302:442-445 (2003).

Dahl, F. et al. Multigene amplification and massively parallel sequencing for cancer mutation discovery. PNAS (USA) 104:9387-9392 (2007).

Dalla-Favera, R. et al. Mechanism of activation and biological role of the c-myc oncogene in B-cell lymphomagenesis. Ann. N.Y. Acad. Sci. 511:207-218 (1987).

Dalmay, T., Edwards, D.R. Oncogene 25:6170-6175 (2006).

Dalton, W.S., Friend, S.H. Cancer biomarkers – an invitation to the table. Science 312:1165-1168 (2006).

Damelin, M. et al. Decatenation checkpoint deficiency in stem and progenitor cells. Cancer Cell 8:479-484 (2005).

Damania, B. DNA tumour viruses and human cancer. Trends Microbiol. 15:38-44 (2006).

Daniel, M.C., Astruc, D. Gold nanoparticles:assembly, supramolecular chemistry, quantum-size-related properties, and applications toward biology, catalysis, and nanotechnology. Chem. Rev. 104:293-346 (2004).

Darrow, A.L. et al. Virus-based expression systems facilitate rapid target in vivo functionality validation and high-throughput screening. J. Biomol. Screen. 8, 65-71 (2003).

Daser, A., Rabbitts, T. Genes Dev. 18:965-974 (2004).

Davey, B. Immunology. Affil. East West Press, New Delhi (1994).

David, S.S., O'Shea, V.L., Kundu, S. Base-excision repair of oxidative DNA damage. Nature 447:941-950 (2007).

Davies, H. et al. Mutations of the BRAF gene in human cancer. Nature 417:949-954 (2002).

Davis, B.G. Recent developments in oligosaccharide synthesis. J. Chem. Soc. Perkin Trans. 1:2137-2160 (2000).

de Visser, K.E., Korets, L.V., Coussens, L.M. De novo carcinogenesis promoted by chronic inflammation is B lymphocyte dependent. Cancer Cell 7:411-423 (2005).

de Visser, K. et al. Paradoxical roles of the immune system during cancer development. Nature Rev. Cancer 6:24-37 (2006).

Dews, M. et al. Nature Genet. 38:1060-1065 (2006).

De Weerd-Kastelein, E.A., Keijzer, W., Bootsma, D. Genetic heterogeneity of xeroderma pigmentosum demonstrated by somatic cell hybridization. Nature New Biol. 238:80-83 (1972).

De Weese, T.L. et al. A phase I trial of CV706, a replication-competent, PSA selective oncolytic adenovirus, for the treatment of locally recurrent prostate cancer following radiation therapy. Cancer Res. 61:7464-7472 (2001).

DeBaun, M.R. et al. Epigenetic alternations of H19 and L9T1 distinguish patients with Beckwith-Wiedemann syndrome with cancer and birth defects. Am J. Hum. Genet. 70:604-611 (2002).

DeMello, A.J. Control and detection of chemical reactions in microfluidic systems. Nature 442:394 (2006).

DeMello, J., DeMello, A. Lab-on-a-Chip 4:316 (2004).

Dharap, S.S. et al. Molecular targeting of drug delivery systems to ovarian cancer by BH3 and LHRH peptides. J. Control. Release 91:61-73 (2003).

Di Bussolo, V., Kim, Y.-J., Gin, D.Y. Direct oxidative glycosylations with glycal donors. J. Am. Chem. Soc. 120:13515-13516 (1998).

Di Micco, R. et al. Oncogene-induced senescence is a DNA damage response triggered by DNA hyper-replication. Nature 444:638-642 (2006).

Diffey, B.L. Solar ultraviolet radiation effects on biological systems. Phys. Med. Biol. 36:299-328 (1991).

Dingli, D., Nowak, M.A. Infectious tumour cells. Nature 443:35-36 (2006).

Dirks, P.B. Stem cells and brain tumours. Nature 444:687-688 (2006).

Dittrich, P.S., Manz, A. Anal. Bioanal. Chem. 382:1771-1782 (2005).

Doe, C.Q., Bowerman, B. Asymmetric cell division:fly neuroblast meets worm zygote. Curr. Opin. Cell Biol. 13:68-75 (2001).

Doherty, J.K. et al. The HER-2/Neu receptor tyrosine kinase gene encodes a secreted autoinhibitor. PNAS (USA) 96:10869-10874 (1999).

Dokland, T. Scaffolding proteins and their role in viral assembly. Cell Mol. Life Sci. 56:580-603 (1999).

Donahue, S.L. et al. Carcinogens induce genome-wide loss of heterozygosity in normal stem cells without persistent chromosomal instability. PNAS (USA) 103:11642-11646 (2006).

Donnelly, I.J. et al. DNA vaccines. Annu. Rev. Immunol. 15:617-648 (1997).

Douglas, J.T. et al. Targeted gene delivery by tropism-modified adenoviral vectors. Nature Biotechnol. 14:1574-1578 (1996).

Douma, S. et al. Suppression of anoikis and induction of metastasis by the neurotrophic receptor TrkB. Nature 430:1034-1039 (2004).

Dranoff, G. Cytokines in cancer pathogenesis and cancer therapy. Nature Rev. Cancer 4:11-22 (2004).

Dreyer, W.J., Bennett, J.C. The molecular basis of antibody formation:a paradox. PNAS (USA) 54:864-869 (1965).

Druker, B.J. et al. N. Engl. J. Med. 344:1031-1037 (2001).

Dulbecco, R. Reactivation of ultra-violet-inactivated bacteriophage by visible light. Nature 162:949-950 (1949).

Duncan, R. The dawning era of polymer therapeutics. Nature Rev. Drug Discov. 2:347-360 (2003).

Duncan, R. Polymer-drug conjugates. pp. 239-260. In:Budman, D. et al. (eds.) Handbook of Anticancer Drug Development. Lippincott Williams and Wilkins (2003a).

Duncan, R., Izzo, L. Adv. Drug Delivery Rev. 57:2215 (2005).

Duncan, R. Nature Rev. Cancer 6:688-701 (2006).

Easton, D.F. et al. Genome-wide association study identifies novel breast cancer susceptibility loci. Nature 447:1087-1092 (2007).

Ein-Dor, L. et al. Thousands of samples are needed to generate a robust gene list for predicting outcome in cancer. PNAS (USA) 103:5923-5928 (2006).

Elghanian, R. et al. Selective colorimetric detection of polynucleotides based on the distance-dependent optical properties of gold nanoparticles. Science 277:1078-1081 (1997).

Ellington, A.D., Szostak, J.W. Nature 355:85 (1992).

El-Nezami, H.S. + 9 others. Probiotic supplementation reduces a biomarker for increased risk of liver cancer in young men from Southern China. Am. J. Clin. Nutr. 83:1199-1203 (2006).

Emens, L.A. Trastuzumab:targeted therapy for the management of HER-2/neu-overexpressing metastatic breast cancer. Am. J. Ther. 12:243-253 (2005).

Engelman, J.A., Luo, J., Cantley, L.C. Nature Rev. Genet. 7:606 (2006).

Ernst, B., Hart, G.W., Sinay, P. Carbohydrates in Chemistry and Biology Pt. 1. Chemistry of Saccharides. Wiley-VCH, Weinheim (2000).

Ernst, P. et al. Curr. Biol. 14:2063-2069 (2004).

Eshhar, Z. et al. Subunits of the immunoglobulin and T-cell receptors. PNAS (USA) 90:720-724 (1993).

Esquela-Kerscher, A., Slack, F.J. Oncomirs – microRNAs with a role in cancer. Nature Rev. Cancer 6:259-269 (2006).

Esser, M.T. et al. Cyanovirin-N binds to gp120 to interfere with CD4-dependent human immunodeficiency virus type 1 virion binding, fusion, and infectivity but does not affect the CD4 binding site on gp120 or soluble CD4-induced conformational changes in gp120. J. Virol. 73:4360-4371 (1999).

Etienne-Mannevile, S., Hall, A. Rho GTPases in cell biology. Nature 420:629-635 (2002).

Evans, G. et al. Construction of HSC-2D PAGE:a two-dimensional gel electrophoresis database of heart proteins. Electrophoresis 18:471-479 (1997).

Fang, J. et al. Cancer Res. 63:3567-3574 (2003).

Farmer, H. et al. Targeting the DNA repair defect in BRCA mutant cells as a therapeutic strategy. Nature 434:917-921 (2005).

Farokhzad, O.C. et al. Nanoparticle-aptamer bioconjugates result in significant tumour reduction in vivo. PNAS (USA) 103:6315-6320 (2006).

Fearnhead, N.S., Britton, M.P., Bodmer, W.F. The ABC of APC. Hum. Mol. Genet. 10:721-733 (2001).

Feinberg, A.P. Phenotypic plasticity and the epigenetics of human disease. Nature 447:433-440 (2007).

Feinberg, A.P., Vogelstein, B. Hypomethylation distinguishes genes of some human cancers from their normal counterparts. Nature 301:89-92 (1983).

Feinberg, A.P., Tycko, B. The history of cancer epigenetics. Nature Rev. Cancer 4:143-153 (2004).

Feinberg, A.P., Ohlsson, R., Henikoff, S. The epigenetic progenitor origin of human cancer. Nature Rev. Genet. 7:21-33 (2006).

Feling, R.H. et al. Angew. Chem. Int. Edn. 42:355-357 (2003).

Felley, C., Michetti, P. Probiotics and Helicobacter pylori. Best Pract. Res. Clin. Gastroenterol. 17:785-791 (2003).

Ferrara, N., Kerbel, R.S. Angiogenesis as a therapeutic target. Nature 438:967-974 (2005).

Ferrari, M. Cancer nanotechnology:opportunities and challenges. Nature Rev. Cancer 5:161-171 (2005).

Ferrari, M. Curr. Opin. Chem. Biol. 9:343 (2005).

Finkel, T., Serrano, M., Blasco, M.A. The common biology of cancer and ageing. Nature 448:767-774 (2007).

Fisher, K.D. et al. Polymer-coated adenovirus permits efficient retargeting and evades neutralizing antibodies. Gene Ther. 8:341-348 (2001).

Fisher, P.B. Cancer Res. 65:10128-10138 (2005).

Fleming, T.R., DeMets, D.L. Surrogate endpoints in clinical trials:are we being misled? Ann. Intern. Med. 125:605-613 (1996).

Fliss, M.S. et al. Facile detection of mitochondrial DNA mutations in tumours and bodily fluids. Science 287:2017-2019 (2000).

Fok, S.Y. et al. BMC Cancer 6:151 (2006).

Folkman, J. Role of angiogenesis in tumour growth and metastasis. Semin. Oncol. 29:15-18 (2002).

Forsberg, E.C. et al. PloS Genet. 1:e28 (2005).

Fortina, P. et al. TIBTECH 23:168-173 (2005).

Fortina, P. et al. Applications of nanoparticles to diagnostics and therapeutics in colorectal cancer. TIBETCH 25:145-151 (2007).

Fraga, M.F. et al. Loss of acetylation at Lys16 and trimethylation at Lys20 of histone H4 is a common hallmark of human cancer. Nature Genet. 37:391-400 (2005).

Frangioni, J.V. Translating in vivo diagnostics into clinical reality. Nature Biotech. 24:909-913 (2006).

Frangioni, J.V., Hajjar, R.J. Circulation 110:3378-3383 (2004).

Frank, R., Hargreaves, R. Clinical biomarkers in drug discovery and development. Nature Rev. Drug Discov. 2, 566-580 (2003).

Fraser, D.R. Exploration of possible mechanisms linking vitamin D status and dietary calcium to prostate cancer. Br. J. Nutr. 97:596-597 (2007).

Freeman, M.W. et al. J. Appl. Phys. 31:S404 (1960).

Freeman, W.M., Gioia, L. The maturation of nucleic acid technologies. TIBTECH 17:44-45 (1999).

Freire, T. et al. Carbohydrate antigens:synthesis aspects and immunological applications in cancer. Mini Rev. Med. Chem. 6:1357-1373 (2006).

Frick, G.S. et al. Guanylyl cyclase C:a molecular marker for staging and postoperative surveillance of patients with colorectal cancer. Expert Rev. Mol. Diagn. 5:701-713 (2005).

Friedberg, E.C., Walker, G.C., Siede, W. DNA Repair and Mutagenesis. Amer. Soc. Microbiol. Press, Washington, D.C. (1995).

Friedberg, E.C. The intersection between the birth of molecular biology and the DNA repair and mutagenesis field. DNA Repair 1:855-867 (2002).

Friedberg, E.C. DNA damage and repair. Nature 421:436-440 (2003).

Fuerer, C., Iggo, R. Adenoviruses with Tcf binding sites in multiple early promoters show enhanced selectivity for tumour cells with constitutive activation of the wnt signalling pathway. Gene Ther. 9:270-281 (2002).

Gale, N.W. et al. Haploinsufficiency of delta-like legand results in embryonic lethality due to major defects in arterial and vascular development. PNAS (USA) 101:15949-15954 (2004).

Galonic, D.P., Gin, D.Y. Chemical glycosylation in the synthesis of glycoconjugate antitumour vaccines. Nature 446:1000-1006 (2007).

Gangopadhyay, R., De, A. Chem. Mater. 12(3):608 (2000).

Gao, C.F. et al. Proliferation and invasion:plasticity in tumour cells. PNAS (USA) 102:10528-10533 (2005).

Gao, C.F. et al. Chromosome instability, chromosome transcriptome, and clonal evolution of tumour cell populations. PNAS (USA) 104:8995-9000 (2007).

Garber, K. Energy deregulation:licensing tumours to grow. Science 312:1158-1159 (2006).

Garcia-Echeverria, C. et al. In vivo antitumour activity of NVP-AEW541 – A novel, potent, and selective inhibitor of the IGF-IR kinase. Cancer Cell 5:231-239 (2004).

Garland, C.F. et al. The role of vitamin D in cancer prevention. Am. J. Public Health 96:252-261 (2006).

Garrod, A.E. Inborn Errors of Metabolism. Oxford Univ. Press, Oxford (1909).

Gavert, N. et al. L1, a novel target of β-catenin signalling transforms cells and is expressed at the invasive front of colon cancers. J. Cell Biol. 168:633-642 (2005).

Geng, X. et al. In pursuit of carbohydrate-based HIV vaccines, part 2:the total synthesis of high-mannose-type gp120 fragments – evaluation of strategies directed to maximal convergence. Angew. Chem. Int. Ed. Engl. 43:2562-2565 (2004).

Gensler, H.L., Welch, K. Prevalence of tumour prevention rather than tumour enhancement when repetitive UV radiation treatments precede initiation and promotion. Carcinogenesis 13:9-13 (1992).

George, S.K. et al. Chemoenzymatic synthesis of sialylated glycopeptides derived from mucins and T-cell stimulating peptides. J. Am. Chem. Soc. 123:11117-11125 (2001).

Gibbs, J.B. Mechanism-based target identification and drug discovery. Science 287:1969-1973 (2000).

Gilbert, P.B. et al. Correlation between immunologic responses to a recombinant glycoprotein 120 vaccine and incidence of HIV-1 infection in a phase 3 HIV-1 preventive vaccine trial. J. Infect. Dis. 191:666-677 (2005).

Gillock, E.T. et al. Polyomavirus major capsid protein VP1 is capable of packaging cellular DNA when expressed in the baculovirus system. J. Virol. 71:2857-2865 (1997).

Gilroy, D.W. et al. Inflammatory resolution:new opportunities for drug discovery. Nature Rev. Drug Discov. 3:401-416 (2004).

Glaser, S.L. et al. Epstein-Barr virus-associated Hodgkin's disease:epidemiologic characteristics in international data. Int. J. Cancer 70:375-382 (1997).

Gloeckler Ries, L.A. et al. Cancer survival and incidence, from the surveillance, epidemiology, and end results (SEER) program. Oncologist 8:541-552 (2003).

Glomm, W.R. Functionalized gold nanoparticles for application in biotechnology. J. Disp. Sci. Tech. 26:389-414 (2005).

Godar, D.E. Methods Enzymol. 319:309-330 (2000).

Goedert, J.J. (Ed.). Infectious Causes of Cancer:Targets for Intervention. Humana Press, Totowa, New Jersey (2000).

Gold, L. J. Biol. Chem. 270:13581 (1995).

Golub, T.R. et al. Molecular classification of cancer:class discovery and class prediction by gene expression monitoring. Science 286:531 (1999).

Gonzalez, E. et al. The influence of CCL3L1 gene-containing segmental duplications on HIV-1 AIDS susceptibility. Science 307:1434-1440 (2005).

Gorelik, L., Flavell, R.A. Nature Med. 7:1118 (2001).

Gotteland, M., Cruchet, S. Suppressive effect of frequent ingestion of Lactobacillus johnsonii La1 on Helicobacter pylori colonization in asymptomatic volunteers. J. Antimicrob. Chemother. 51:1317-1319 (2003).

Gould, P. Materials Today 7(2):36 (2004).

Gould, P. Nanomagnetism shows in vivo potential. Nanotoday 1(4):34-39 (2006).

Gowher, H., Leismann, U., Jeltsch, A. DNA methylation in Drosophila melanogaster. EMBO J. 19:6918-6923 (2000).

Gozuacik, D., Kimchi, A. Oncogene 23:2891-2906 (2004).

Graewal, H. Antioxidants in oral cancer prevention. Amer. J. Clin. Nutr. 62(Suppl. 6):1410S-1416S (1995).

Grant, G.A., Crankshaw, M.W., Gorka, J. Edman sequencing as tool for characterization of synthetic peptides. Methods Enzymol. 289:395-419 (1997).

Grant, W.B., Holick, M.F. Benefits and requirements of vitamin D for optimal health:a review. Altern. Med. Rev. 10:94 111 (2005).

Grant, W.B., Garland, C.F., Gorham, E.D. An estimate of cancer mortality rate reductions in Europe and the U.S. with 1000 I.U. of oral vitamin D per day. Rec. Results Cancer Res. 174:225-234 (2007).

Greenman, C. et al. Patterns of somatic mutation in human cancer genome. Nature 446:153-158 (2007).

Gref, R. et al. Biodegradable long-circulating polymeric nanospheres. Science 263:1600-1603 (1994).

Greger, V., Passarge, E., Hopping, W., Messmer, E., Horsthemke, B. Epigenetic changes may contribute to the formation and spontaneous regression of retinoblastoma. Human Genet. 83:155-158 (1989).

Gridley, T. Vessel guidance. Nature 445:722-723 (2007).

Griffith, T.S., Broghammer, E.L. Suppression of tumour growth following intralesional therapy with TRAIL recombinant adenovirus. Mol. Ther. 4:257-266 (2001).

Grimm, E.A., Wei, Q. Genetic variants of the ADPRT, XRCC1, and APE1 genes and risk of cutaneous melanoma. Carcinogenesis 7:1894-1901 (2006).

Grimm, J. et al. Use of gene expression profiling to direct in vivo molecular imaging of lung cancer. PNAS (USA) 102:14404-14409 (2005).

Grossarth-Maticek, R. et al. Use of Iscardor, an extract of European mistletoe (Viscum album) in cancer treatment:prospective non-randomized and randomized match-pair studies nested within a cohort study. Alternative Therapies 7:57-66 68-72, 74-76 (2001).

Gu, F. et al. Targeted nanoparticles for cancer therapy. Nanotoday 2:14-21 (2007).

Guerin, C. et al. Recent advances in brain tumour therapy:local intracerebral drug delivery by polymers. Invest. New Drugs 22:27-37 (2004).

Gupta, P.K. et al. J. Pharmacol. Sci. 78:290 (1989).

Haber, D.A., Settleman, J. Drivers and passengers. Nature 446:145-146 (2007).

Häder, D.P., Kumar, H.D., Smith, R.C., Worrest, R.C. Effects of solar UV radiation on aquatic ecosystems and interactions with climate change. Photochem. Photobiol. Sci. 6:267-285 (2007).

Häfeli, U.O. et al. J. Biomed. Mater. Res. 28:901 (1994).

Häfeli, U.O. et al. Nucl. Med. Biol. 22:147 (1995).

Haik, Y. et al. J. Magn. Matr. 225:180 (2001).

Hakomori, S. Tumour malignancy defined by aberrant glycosylation and sphingo (glycol) lipid metabolism. Cancer Res. 56:5309-5318 (1996).

Hakomori, S., Zhang, Y. Glycosphingolipid antigens and cancer therapy. Chem. Biol. 4:97-104 (1997).

Hamaguchi, T. et al. Br. J. Cancer 92:1240-1246 (2005).

Hammond, S.M. MicroRNA therapeutics:a new niche for antisense nucleic acids. Trends Mol. Med. 12:99-101 (2006).

Han, J. et al. Genetic variation in XRCC1, sun exposure, and risk of skin cancer. Br. J. Cancer 91:1604-1609 (2004).

Han, S.Y. et al. Hepatoprotective effect of lactic acid bacteria, inhibitors of beta-glucuronidase production against intestinal microflora. Arch. Pharm. Res. 28:325-329 (2005).

Hanash, S. Disease proteomics. Nature 422:226-232 (2003).

Hanash, S., Harnessing immunity for cancer marker discovery. Nature Biotechnol. 21:37-38 (2003a).

Hanash, S.M. et al. Integrating cancer genomics and proteomics in the post-genome era. Proteomics 2, 69-75 (2002).

Hanawalt, P.C., Haynes, R.H. The repair of DNA. Sci. Am. 216:36-43 (1967).

Handley, S., Page, M., Northcote, P. Anti-cancer sponge:the race is on for aquaculture supply. Water & Atmosphere 14(3), p. 14-15 (Sept. 2006).

Harley, C.B., Futcher, A.B., Greider, C.W. Telomeres shorten during ageing of human fibroblasts. Nature 345:458-460 (1990).

Harris, S., Foord, S.M. Transgenic gene knock-outs:functional genomics and therapeutic target selection. Pharmacogenomics 1:433-443 (2000).

Hartwell, L. et al. Cancer biomarkers:a systems approach. Nature Biotech. 24:905-908 (2006).

Hashizume, H. et al. Am. J. Pathol. 156:1363 (2000).

Hassan, M. et al. Technol. Cancer Res. Treat. 3:451-457 (2004).

Hayashi, I. et al. Effects of oral administration of Echinacea purpurea (American herb) on incidence of spontaneous leukaemia viruses in AKR/J mice. Nihon Rinsho Meneki Gakkai Kaishi 24:10-20 (2001).

Hayward, S.W. et al. Malignant transformation in a nontumourigenic human prostatic epithelial cell line. Cancer Res. 61:8135-8142 (2001).

He, X. et al. J. Nanosci. Nanotechnol. 4:585 (2004).

Helenius, A., Aebi, M. Roles of N-linked glycans in the endoplasmic reticulum. Annu. Rev. Biochem. 72:1019-1049 (2004).

Helling, F. et al. GD3 vaccines for melanoma:superior immunogenicity of keyhole limpet hemocyanin conjugate vaccines. Cancer Res. 54:197-203 (1994).

Hellström, M. et al. Dll4 signalling through Notch1 regulates formation of tip cells during angiogenesis. Nature 445:776-780 (2007).

Hengartner, M.O., Horvitz, H.R. C. elegans cell survival gene ced-9 encodes a functional homolog of the mammalian proto-oncogene bcl-2. Cell 76:665-676 (1994).

Herbig, U. et al. Science 311:1257 (2006).

Hernandez, L.M. Implications of Genomics for Public Health:Workshop Summary. Committee on Genomics and the Public's Health in the 21st Century, National Academies Press, Washington, D.C. (2005).

Herr, J.K. et al. Anal. Chem. 78:2918 (2006).

Hicks, D.G., Tubbs, R.R. Assessment of the HER2 status in breast cancer by fluorescence in situ hybridization:a technical review with interpretive guidelines. Hum. Pathol. 36:250-261 (2005).

Hicks, J.F. et al. J. Am. Chem. Soc. 124(44):13322 (2002).

Hieronymus, H. et al. Cancer Cell 10:321-330 (2006).

Hilario, M. et al. Processing and classification of protein mass spectra. Mass Spectrom. Rev. 25:409-449 (2006).

Hildemann, W.H. Essentials of Immunology. Elsevier, New York (1984).

Hileman, E.O. et al. Cancer Chemother. Pharmacol. 53:209-219 (2004).

Hippert, M., O'Toole, P.S., Thorburn, A. Cancer Res. 66:9349-9351 (2006).

Hirsch, L.R. et al. Ann. Biomed. Eng. 34:15 (2006).

Hochedlinger, K. et al. Reprogramming of a melanoma genome by nuclear transplantation. Genes Dev. 18:1875-1885 (2004).

Holick, M.F. Sunlight and vitamin D for bone health and prevention of autoimmune diseases, cancers, and cardiovascular disease. Am. J. Clin. Nutr. 80:1678S-1688S (2004).

Holliday, R. A new theory of carcinogenesis. Brit. J. Cancer 40:513-522 (1979).

Holliday, R. The significance of DNA methylation in cellular aging. Pp. 269-283. In:Woodhead, A.D. et al. (eds.) Molecular Biology of Aging. Plenum, New York (1984).

Holliday, R. The inheritance of epigenetic defects. Science 238:163-170 (1987).

Holliday, R. Epigenetics:an overview. Dev. Genet. 15:453-457 (1994).

Holliday, R. Epigenetics comes of age in the twentyfirst century. J. Genet. 81:1-4 (2002).

Hollingsworth, M.A., Swanson, B.J. Mucins in cancer:protection and control of the cell surface. Nature Rev. Cancer 4:45-60 (2004).

Homey, B., Muller, A., Zlotnik, A. Nature Rev. Immunol. 2:175 (2002).

Hong, S. et al. Chem. Biol. 14:107 (2007).

Hood, L., Weissman, I., Wood, W. Immunology. 2 ed. Benjamin/Cummings, Menlo Park (1983).

Hope, K.J., Jin, L., Dick, J.E. Nature Immunol. 5:738 (2004).

Howley, P., Lowy, D. Papillomaviruses and their replication. Pp. 2197-2229. In:Knipe, D.M., Howley, P.M. (eds.) vide infra (2001).

Hozumi, N., Tonegawa, S. Evidence for somatic rearrangement of immunologlobulin genes coding for variable and constant regions. PNAS (USA) 73:3628-3632 (1976).

Hreczuk-Hirst, D. et al. Dextrins as potential carriers for drug targeting:tailored rates of dextrin degradation by introduction of pendant groups. Int. J. Pharm. 230:57-66 (2001).

Hu, M. et al. Distinct epigenetic changes in the stromal cells of breast cancers. Nature Genet. 37:899-905 (2005).

Huang, N., Banavali, N.K., MacKerell Jr., A.D. Protein-facilitated base flipping in DNA by cytosine-5-methyltransferase. PNAS (USA) 100:68-73 (2003).

Huang, P. et al. Cancer Cell 10:241-252 (2006).

Huang, X. et al. Science 275:547-550 (1997).

Huber, M.A., Kraut, N., Beug, H. Molecular requirements for epithelial-mesenchymal transition during tumour progression. Curr. Opin. Cell Biol. 17:548-558 (2005).

Huhtinen, P. et al. In:Pandalai, S.G. (Ed.). Recent Research and Developments in Bioconjugate Chemistry. Research Signpost, Kerala 2:85 (2005).

Hulka, B.S. Cancer screening. Degrees of proof and practical application. Cancer 62 Suppl. 9:1776-1780 (1988).

Hunkapiller, T. et al. Large-scale and automated DNA sequence determination. Science 354:59-67 (1991).

Huntly, B.J.P., Gilliland, D.G. Leukaemia stem cells and the evolution of cancer-stem-cell research. Nature Rev. Cancer 5:311-321 (2005).

IARC. IARC Monographs on the Evaluation of Carcinogenic Risks to Humans. Vol. 56. Solar and Ultraviolet Radiation. Intl. Agency Res. Cancer, Lyon (France) (1992).

IARC. Evaluation of Carcinogenic Risks to Humans. Monograph (vol. no. 60). Internat. Agency for Research on Cancer. WHO, Geneva (Feb. 1994).

Ilyin, S.E. et al. Emerging paradigms in applied bioinformatics. BioSilico 3, 86-88 (2003).

Ilyin, S.E., Belkowski, S.M., Plata-Salaman, C.R. Biomarker discovery and validation:technologies and integrative approaches. TIBTECH. 22(8):411-416 (2004).

Immonen, A. et al. AdvHSV-tk gene therapy with intravenous ganciclovir improves survival in human malignant glioma:a randomized, controlled study. Mol. Ther. 10:967-972 (2004).

Inoue, A. Loss-of-function screening by randomized intracellular antibodies:Identification of hnRNP-K as a potential target for metastasis. PNAS (USA) 104:8983-8988 (2007).

Inoue, M. et al. Regular consumption of green tea and the risk of breast cancer recurrence:follow-up study from the hospital-based Epidemiol. Res. Prog., Aichi Cancer Center (HERPACC) Japan 167:175-182 (2001).

Interlandi, J. Drugs target epigenetic changes in cancer cells. Sci. Amer. 296:24 (Apr. 2007).

Ishikawa, H. et al. Randomized trial of dietary fibre and Lactobacillus casei administration for prevention of colorectal tumours. Int. J. Cancer 116:762-767 (2005).

Ito, M. The photodynamic effect of acridine orange and ultraviolet on the mouse skin carcinogenesis by 20-methylcholanthrene. Nagoya Med. J. 12:247-259 (1966).

Jablonka, E., Lamb, J.M. Epigenetic Inheritance and Evolution. Oxford University Press, Oxford (1995).

Jager, E. et al. Simultaneous humoral and cellular immune response against cancer-testis antigen NY-ESO-1:definition of human histocompatibility leukocyte antigen (HLA)-A2-binding peptide epitopes. J. Exp. Med. 187:265-270 (1998).

Jänne, P. et al. Science doi:10.1126/science.1141478 (2007).

Jänne, P.A., Engelman, J.A., Johnson, B.E. Epidermal growth factor receptor mutations in non-small cell lung cancer:implications for treatment and tumour biology. J. Clin. Oncol. 23:3227-3234 (2005).

Jemal, A. et al. CA Cancer J. Clin. 54:8-29 (2004); 57:43-66 (2007).

Jensen, E.V., Jordan, V.C. The oestrogen receptor:a model for molecular medicine. Clin. Cancer Res. 9:1980-1989 (2003).

Jenster, G. The role of the androgen receptor in the development and progression of prostate cancer. Semin. Oncol. 26:407-421 (1999).

Jerne, N.K. The natural selection theory of antibody formation. PNAS (USA) 412:849-857 (1955).

Jiang, L.I., Nadeau, J.H. 129/Sv mice:a model system for studying germ cell biology and testicular cancer. Mammal. Genome 12:89-94 (2001).

Jimenez-Lara, A.M. Colorectal cancer:Potential therapeutic benefits of vitamin D. Int. J. Biochem. Cell Biol. 39:672-677 (2007).

Jo, W.S., Chung, D.C. Genetics of hereditary colorectal cancer. Semin. Oncol. 32:11-23 (2005).

John, E.M., Koo, J., Schwartz, G.G. Sun exposure and prostate cancer risk:evidence for a protective effect of early-life exposure. Cancer Epidemiol. Biomarkers Prev. 16:1283-1286 (2007).

Jones, P.A., Baylin, S.B. The fundamental role of epigenetic events in cancer. Nature Rev. Genet. 3:415-428 (2002).

Joyce, J.A. Therapeutic targeting of the tumour microenvironment. Cancer Cell 7:513-520 (2005).

Kaelin, W.J. Jr. The concept of synthetic lethality in the context of anticancer therapy. Nature Rev. Cancer 5:689-698 (2005).

Kagan, E. et al. Comparison of antigen constructs and carrier molecules for augmenting the immunogenicity of the monosaccharide epithelial cancer antigen Tn. Cancer Immunol. Immunother. 54:424-430 (2005).

Kain, S.R. Green fluorescent protein (GFP):applications in cell-based assays for drug discovery. Drug. Discov. Today 4:304-312 (1999).

Kaiser, J. First pass at cancer genome reveals complex landscape. Science 313:1370 (2006).

Kang, Y. et al. A multigenic program mediating breast cancer metastasis to bone cancer. Cell 3:537-549 (2003).

Kano, M.R. et al. Improvement of cancer-targeting therapy using nanocarriers for intractable solid-tumours by inhibition of TGF-β signalling. PNAS (USA) 104:3460-3465 (2007).

Kantarjian, H. et al. N. Engl. J. Med. 346:645-652 (2002).

Kaplan, R.N. et al. VEGFR1-positive haematopoietic bone marrow progenitors initiate the pre-metastatic niche. Nature 438:820-827 (2005).

Karhadkar, S.S. et al. Hedgehog signalling in prostate regeneration, neoplasia and metastasis. Nature 431:707-712 (2004).

Karin, M. et al. Innate immunity gone awry:linking microbial infections to chronic inflammation and cancer. Cell 124:823-835 (2006).

Kauffman, H.M. et al. Transplantation 74:358-362 (2002).

Kay, N.E. et al. Blood 104:100a (2004); 109:405 (2007).

Keith, D.R. Herbal tonics. Health'N Vitality (Magazine) Issue No. 42, pp. 10-12 (April/May 2006).

Kelly, P.N., Dakic, A., Adams, J.M., Nutt, S.L., Strasser, A. Tumour growth need not be driven by rare cancer stem cells. Science 317:337 (2007).

Kelner, A. Effect of visible light on the recovery of Streptomyces griseus conidia from ultraviolet irradiation injury. PNAS (USA) 45:73-79 (1949).

Kensil, C.R., Patel, U., Lennick, M., Marciani, D. Separation and characterization of saponins with adjuvant activity from Quillaja saponaria Molina cortex. J. Immunol. 146:431-437(1991).

Kensil, C.R., Saponins as vaccine adjuvants. Crit. Rev. Ther. Drug Carr. Syst. 13:1-55 (1996).

Kerbel, R., Folkman, J. Nature Rev. Cancer 2:727 (2002).

Kerbel, R.S. Antiangiogenic therapy:A universal chemosensitization strategy for cancer? Science 312:1171-1174 (2006).

Keren, K. et al. DNA templated carbon nanotube field-effect transistor. Science 302:1380-1382 (2003).

Khaled, A. et al. Nano Lett. 5:1797 (2005).

Kidd, P.M. The use of mushroom glucans and proteoglycans in cancer. Altern. Med. Rev. 5:4-27 (2000).

Kim, H., Chen, J., Yu, X. Ubiquitin-binding protein RAP80 mediates BRCA1-dependent DNA damage response. Science 316:1202-1203 (2007).

Kim, J.E., Jeong, D.W., Lee, H.J. Expression, purification, and characterization of arginine deiminase from Lactococcus lactis spp. lactis ATCC 7962 in Escherichia coli BL21. Protein Expr. Purif. 53:9-15 (2007).

Kim, J.-E. et al. Cancer chemopreventive effects of lactic acid bacteria. J. Microbiol. Biotechnol. 17:1227-1235 (2007).

Kim, J.J., Wright, T.C., Goldie, S.J. J. Am. Med. Assoc. 287:2382-2390 (2002).

Kim, N.W. et al. Specific association of human telomerase activity with immortal cells and cancer. Science 266:2011-2015 (1994).

Kim, S. et al. E. coli moves into the plastic age. Nature Biotechnol. 22(1):93-99 (2004).

Kim, S.Y. et al. Cytoplasmic fraction of Lactococcus lactis ssp. Lactis induces apoptosis in SNU-1 stomach adenocarcinoma cells. Biofactors 22:119-122 (2004).

Kim, Y.J. et al. Synthetic studies of complex immunostimulants from Quillaja saponaria:synthesis of the potent clinical immunoadjuvant QS-21Aapi. J. Am. Chem. Soc. 128:11906-11915 (2006).

Kinzler, K.W. et al. Identification of FAP locus genes from chromosome 5q21. Science 253:661-665 (1991).

Kinzler, K.W., Vogelstein, B. The Genetic Basis of Human Cancer. McGraw-Hill, New York (1998).

Knight, J.A. et al. Vitamin D and reduced risk of breast cancer:A population-based case-control study. Cancer Epidemiol. Biomarker Prev. 16:422-429 (2007).

Knipe, D.M., Howley, P.M. (eds.) Fields Virology (4th edn.). Lippincott Williams and Wilkins, Baltimore (2001).

Knox, P.G. et al. Inhibition of metalloproteinase cleavage enhances the cytotoxicity of Fas ligand. J. Immunol. 170:677-685 (2003).

Kobinger, G.P. et al. Filovirus-pseudotyped lentiviral vector can efficiently and stably transduce airway epithelia in vivo. Nature Biotechnol. 19:225-230 (2001).

Kocks, C., Rajewsky, K. Stable expression and somatic hypermutation of antibody V regions in B-cell developmental pathways. Annu. Rev. Immunol. 7:537-559 (1989).

Kola, I., Landis, J. Nature Rev. Drug Discov. 3:711-715 (2004).

Komarova, N.L., Wodarz, D. Drug resistance in cancer:principles of emergence and prevention. PNAS (USA) 102:9714-9719 (2005).

Kong, J. et al. Nanotube molecular wires as chemical sensors. Science 287:622-625 (2000).

Kops, G.J., Weaver, B.A., Cleveland, D.W. Nature Rev. Cancer 5:773-785 (2005).

Kowalski, K. et al. Dalton Trans., 743 (2007).

Kramata, P. et al. Patches of mutant p53-immunoreactive epidermal cells induced by chronic UVB irradiation harbour the same p53 mutations as squamous cell carcinomas in the skin of hairless SKH-1 mice. Cancer Res. 65:3577-3585 (2005).

Kramberger, P. et al. Concentration of plant viruses using monolithic chromatographic supports. J. Virol. Methods 120:51-57 (2004).

Kremer, A. et al. A bioinformatics perspective on proteomics:data storage, analysis and integration. Biosci. Rep. 25:95-106 (2005).

Krieg, A.M. CpG motifs in bacterial DNA and their immune effects. Annu. Rev. Immunol. 20:709-760 (2002).

Krishnamurthy, J. et al. p16INK4a induces an age-dependent decline in islet regenerative potential. Nature 443:453-457 (2006).

Krivtsov, A.V. et al. Transformation from committed progenitor to leukaemia stem cell initiated by MLL-F9. Nature 442:818-822 (2006).

Krynska, B. et al. Detection of human neurotropic JC virus DNA sequence and expression of the viral oncogenic protein in pediatric medulloblastomas. PNAS (USA) 96:11519-11524 (1999).

Kubota, Y. Faecal intestinal flora in patients with colon adenoma and colon cancer. Nippon Shokakibyo Gakkai Zasshi 87:771-779 (1990).

Kumar, H.D. Modern Concepts of Biotechnology. Vikas Publishing House, New Delhi (1998).

Kumar, H.D. Genomics and Cloning:Technology and Applications. East-West Press, New Delhi (2004).

Kumar, H.D. Management of nutritional and health needs of malnourished and vegetarian people in India. Pp. 311-321. In:Cooper, E.L., Yamaguchi, N. (eds.). Complementary and Alternative Approaches to Biomedicine. Kluwer/Plenum, New York, Dordrecht (2004).

Kumar, H.D., Häder, D.P. Global Aquatic and Atmospheric Environment. Springer, Heidelberg (1999).

Kurashige, S. et al. Effects of astragali radix extract on carcinogenesis, cytokine production, and cytotoxicity in mice treated with a carcinogen, N-butyl-N'-butanolnitrosamine. Cancer Invest. 17:30-35 (1999).

Kwon, H.C. et al. J. Am. Chem. Soc. 128:1622-1632 (2006).

Kwong, P.D. et al. Oligomeric modelling and electrostatic analysis of the gp120 envelope glycoprotein of human immunodeficiency virus. J. Virol. 74:1961-1972 (2000).

Laghi, L. et al. JC virus DNA is present in the mucosa of the human colon and in colorectal cancers. PNAS (USA) 96:7484-7489 (1999).

Lai, W.B., Middleberg, A.P.J. The production of human papillomavirus type 16 L1 vaccine product from Escherichia coli inclusion bodies. Bioprocess Biosyst. Eng. 25:121-128 (2002).

Lamb, J. et al. The connectivity map:using gene expression signatures to connect small molecules, genes and disease. Science 313:1929-1935 (2006).

Lanciotti, J. et al. Targeting adenoviral vectors using heterofunctional polyethylene glycol FGF2 conjugates. Mol. Ther. 8:99-107 (2003).

Lander, E.S. et al. Initial sequencing and analysis of the human genome. Nature 409:860-921 (2001).

Lange, J.R. et al. Melanoma in children and teenagers:an analysis of patients from the National Cancer Data Base. J. Clin. Oncol. 25:1363-1368 (2007).

Langer, R. Drug delivery and targeting. Nature 392:5-10 (1998).

Langer, R., Tirrell, D.A. Designing materials for biology and medicine. Nature 428:487 (2004).

Lappe, J.M., Travers-Gustafson, D., Davies, K.M., Recker, R.R., Heaney, R.P. Vitamin D and calcium supplementation reduces cancer risk:results of a randomized trial. Am. J. Clin. Nutr. 85:1586-1591 (2007).

Laroy, W., Contreas, R., Callewaert, N. Glycome mapping on DNA sequencing equipment. Nature Protocols 1:397-405 (2006).

Lawrence, T. Inflammation and cancer:a failure of resolution? TIBTECH 28(4):162-165 (2007).

Lawrence, T. et al. Anti-inflammatory lipid mediators and insights into the resolution of inflammation. Nature Rev. Immunol. 2:787-795 (2002).

Le Naour, F. Contribution of proteomics to tumour immunology. Proteomics 1:1295-1302 (2001).

Lebedeva, I.V. + 8 others. Strategy for reversing resistance to a single anticancer agent in human prostate and pancreatic carcinomas. PNAS (USA) 104:3484-3489 (2007).

Lee, C.-Y., Robinson, K.J., Doe, C.Q. Lgl, Pins and aPKC regulate neuroblast self-renewal versus differentiation. Nature 439:594-598 (2006).

Lee, H.-W. et al. Essential role of mouse telomerase in highly proliferative organs. Nature 392:569-574 (1998).

Lee, J.Y., Engelman, J.A., Cantley, L.C. PI3K charges ahead. Science 317:207-208 (2007).

Lee, K.W., Lee, H.J. The roles of polyphenols in cancer chemoprevention. Biofactors 26:105-121 (2006).

Lee, S.-Y., Jeoung, D. The reverse proteomics for identification of tumour antigens. J. Microbiol. Biotechnol. 17:879-890 (2007).

Lehtinen, M., Paavonen, J. Int. J. STD AIDS 14:787-792 (2003).

Lengauer, C., Kinzler, K.W., Vogelstein, B. Genetic instabilities in human cancers. Nature 396:643-649 (1998).

Levine, B. Autophagy 2:65-66 (2006).

Levine, B. Autophagy and cancer. Nature 446:745-747 (2007).

Lewis, C.E., Pollard, J.W. Distinct role of macrophages in different tumour microenvironments. Cancer Res. 66:605-612 (2006).

Lewis, T.S. et al. Identification of novel MAP kinase pathway signalling targets by functional proteomics and mass spectrometry. Mol. Cell 6:1343-1354 (2000).

Li, K. et al. Use of RNA interference to target cyclin E-overexpressing hepatocellular carcinoma. Cancer Res. 63:3593-3597 (2003).

Li, R. et al. Identification of putative oncogenes in lung adenocarcinoma by a comprehensive functional genomic approach. Oncogene 25:2628-2635 (2006).

Li, Y. et al. Nature Mater. 3:38 (2004).

Li, Y. et al. Murine embryonic stem cell differentiation is promoted by SOCS-3 and inhibited by the zinc finger transcription factor Klf4. Blood 105:635-637 (2005).

Liang, X.H. et al. Induction of autophagy and inhibition of tumourigenesis by beclin 1. Nature 402:672-676 (1999).

Lidke, D.S. et al. Quantum dot ligands provide new insights into erbB/HER receptor-mediated signal transduction. Nature Biotechnol. 22(2):198-203 (2004).

Liebe, B., Kunz, H. Solid-phase synthesis of a tumour-associated sialyl-TN antigen glycopeptide with a partial sequence of the 'tandem repeat' of the MUC-1 mucin. Angew Chem. Int. Ed. 36:618-621 (1997).

Liede, K.E. et al. Beta carotene concentration in buccal mucosal cells with and without dysplastic oral leukoplakia after long term beta carotene supplementation in male smokers. Eur. J. Clin. Nutr. 52:872-876 (1998).

Lieu, R. et al. Cell 106:309-318 (2001).

Lin, E.Y. et al. Colony-stimulating factor 1 promotes progression of mammary tumours to malignancy. J. Exp. Med. 193:727-740 (2001).

Lin, E.Y., Pollard, J.W. Br. J. Cancer 90:2053-2058 (2004).

Lin, J. et al. Intakes of calcium and vitamin D and breast cancer risk in women. Arch. Intern. Med. 167:1050-1059 (2007).

Lips, P. Vitamin D status and nutrition in Europe and Asia. J. Steroid Biochem. Mol. Biol. 103(3-5):620-625 (2007).

Liu, G. et al. Omega 3 but not omega 6 fatty acids inhibit AP-1 activity transformation in JB6 cells. PNAS (USA) 98:7510-7515 (1998).

Liu, J. et al. Fabrication of hollow metal 'nano-caps' and their red-shifted optical absorption spectra. Adv. Mater. 17:1276-1281 (2005).

Livingston, P.O. Approaches to augmenting the immunogenicity of melanoma gangliosides:from whole melanoma cells to ganglioside-KLH conjugate vaccines. Immunol. Rev. 145:147-166 (1995).

Livingston, P.O., Ragupathi, G. Cancer vaccines targeting carbohydrate antigens. Hum. Vaccin. 2:137-143 (2006).

Loo, C. et al. Nanoshell-enabled photonics-based imaging and therapy of cancer. Technol. Cancer Res. Treat. 3:33-40 (2004).

Lopez, T., Hanahan, D. Elevated levels of IGF-1 receptor convey invasive and metastatic capability in a mouse model of pancreatic islet tumourigenesis. Cancer Cell 1:339-353 (2002).

Lorinez, T., Toth, J., Badalian, G., Timar, J., Szendroi, M. Pathol. Oncol. Res. 12:149-152 (2006).

Lovatt, T. et al. Polymorphism in the nuclear excision repair gene. ERCC2/XPD:association between an exon 6-exon 10 haplotype and susceptibility to cutaneous basal cell carcinoma. Hum. Mutat. 25:353-359 (2005).

Lowe, J.B., Marth, J.D. A genetic approach to mammalian glycan function. Annu. Rev. Biochem. 72:643-691 (2003).

Lowy, D., Howley, P. Papillomaviruses. Pp. 2231-2264. In:Knipe, D.M., Howley, P.M. (eds.). Vide supra (2001).

Lübbe, A.S. et al. Cancer Res. 56:, 4686, 4694 (1996).

Lupold, S.E. et al. Cancer Res. 62:4029 (2002).

Lynch, W.P., Sharpe, A.H., Snyder, E.Y. J. Virol. 73:6841-6851 (1999).

Lynch, T.J. et al. N. Engl. J. Med. 350:2129-2139 (2004).

Ma, L., Teruya-Feldstein, J., Weinberg, R.A. Tumour invasion and metastasis initiated by microRNA-10b in breast cancer. Nature 449:682-688 (2007).

MacFarlane, G.D. et al. Hypovitaminosis D in a normal, apparently healthy urban European population. J. Steroid Biochem. Mol. Biol. 89-90:621-622 (2004).

Mack, G.S. Epigenetic cancer therapy makes headway. J. Natl. Cancer Inst. 98:1443-1444 (2006).

Macleod, K. Tumour-suppressor genes. Curr. Opin. Genet. Dev. 10:81-93 (2000).

Madoz-Gurpide, J. et al. Protein based micro-arrays:a tool for probing the proteome of cancer cells and tissues. Proteomics 1:1279-1287 (2001).

Maeda, H., Matsumura, Y. Crit. Rev. Ther. Drug Carrier Syst. 6:193-210 (1989).

Maher, E.A. et al. Genes Dev. 15:1311-1333 (2001).

Maherali, N. et al. Cell Stem Cell 1:55-60 (2007).

Major, M.B. et al. Wilms tumour suppressor WTX negatively regulates WNT/β-catenin signalling. Science 316:1043-1045 (2007).

Malik, N. et al. Dendrimer-platinate:a novel approach to cancer chemotherapy. Anticancer Drugs 10:767-776 (1999).

Mankoff, D.A., Krohn, K.A. pp. 105-122. In:Teicher, B. (Ed.). Drug Resistance in Cancer. Humana Press, Totowa, NJ (2006).

Mantovani, A. An infernal triangle. Nature 448:547-548 (2007).

Margulies, M. et al. Genome sequencing in microfabricated high-density picolitre reactors. Nature 437:376-380 (2005).

Marris, E. Drugs from the deep. Nature 443:904-905 (2006).

Martienssen, R.A., Colot, V. DNA methylation and epigenetic inheritance in plants and fungi. Science 293:1070-1074 (2001).

Martin, F. et al. Retrovirus targeting by tropism restriction to melanoma cells. J. Virol. 73:6923-6929 (1999).

Martinez-Cruz, L.A. et al. GARBAN :genomic analysis and rapid biological annotation of cDNA microarray and proteomic data. Bioinformatics 19, 2158-2160 (2003).

Martins, C.P., Brown-Swigart, L., Evan, G.I. Cell 127:1323-1334 (2006).

Marx, J. Encouraging results for second generation anti-angiogenic drugs. Science 308:1248-1249 (2005).

Marx, J. Autophagy:Is it cancer's friend or foe? Science 1160-1161 (2006).

Marx, J. Recruiting the cell's own guardian for cancer therapy. Science 315:1211-1213 (2007).

Marx, J. Cancer's perpetual source? Science 317:1029-1031 (2007).

Maser, R.S., DePinho, R.A. Science 297:565-569 (2002).

Mathieu, C. et al. Vitamin D and 1,25-dihydroxyvitamin D3 as modulators in the immune system. J. Steroid Biochem. Mol. Biol. 89-90:449-452 (2004).

Matoba, S. et al. p53 regulates mitochondrial respiration. Science 312:1650-1653 (2006).

Matteucci, E., Locati, M., Desiderio, M.A. Hepatocyte growth factor enhances CXCR4 expression favouring breast cancer cell invasiveness. Exp. Cell. Res. 310:176-185 (2005).

Mattner, J. et al. Exogenous and endogenous glycolipid antigens activate NKT cells during microbial infections. Nature 434:525-529 (2005).

Mazurier, F., Doedens, M., Gan, O.I., Dick, J.E. Rapid myeloerythroid repopulation after intrafemoral transplantation of NOD-SCID mice reveals a new class of human stem cells. Nature Med. 9:959-963 (2003).

McKelvey, W. et al. A second look at the relation between colorectal adenomas and consumption of foods containing partially hydrogenated oil. Epidemiology 11:469-473 (2000).

McKenzie, R.L. et al. Changes in biologically-active ultraviolet radiation reaching the Earth's surface. Photochem. Photobiol. Sci. 6:218-231 (2007).

McKerrow, J.H. et al. A functional proteomics screen of proteases in colorectal carcinoma. Mol. Med. 6:450-460 (2000).

McNeil, S.E. Nanotechnology for the biologist. J. Leukoc. Biol. 78:585-594 (2005).

Medintz, I.L. et al. J. Am. Chem. Soc. 126(1):30 (2004).

Meindl, S. et al. Vitamin D receptor ablation alters skin architecture and homeostasis of dendritic epidermal T cells. Br. J. Dermatol. 152:231-241 (2005).

Melzer, D. et al. A common variant of the p16(INK4a) genetic region is associated with physical function in older people. Mech. Ageing Dev. Published online, doi:10.1016/j.mad.2007.03.005 (27 March 2007).

Meng, S. et al. uPAR and HER-2 gene status in individual breast cancer cells from blood and tissues. PNAS (USA) 103:17361-17365 (2006).

Merrifield, B. Concept and early development of solid-phase peptide synthesis. Methods Enzymol. 289:3-13 (1997).

Meyerhardt, J.A., Mayer, R.J. Systemic therapy for colorectal cancer. N. Engl. J. Med. 352:476-487 (2005).

Meyerson, M. Broken genes in solid tumours. Nature 448:545-546 (2007).

Michaloglou, C. et al. BRAFE600-associated senescence-like cell cycle arrest of human naevi. Nature 436:720-724 (2005).

Miki, Y. et al. A strong candidate for the breast and ovarian-cancer susceptibility gene BRCA1. Science 266:66-71 (1994).

Miled, N. et al. Mechanism of two classes of cancer mutations in the phosphor-inositide 3-kinase catalytic subunit. Science 317:239-242 (2007).

Miller, N., Whelan, J. Progress in transcriptionally targeted and regulatable vectors for genetic therapy. Hum. Gene Ther. 8:803-815 (1997).

Mills, G.P., Lu, Y., Kohn, E.C. Linking molecular therapeutics to molecular diagnostics:inhibition of the FRAP/RAFT/TOR component of the PI3K pathway preferentially blocks PTEN mutant cells in vitro and in vivo. PNAS (USA) 98:10031-10033 (2001).

Milner, J.A. Mechanisms by which garlic and allyl sulfur compounds suppress carcinogen bioactivation. Adv. Exp. Med. Biol. 492:69-81 (2001).

Mincer, T.J. et al. Appl. Environ. Microbiol. 68:5005-5011 (2002).

Minn, A.J. et al. Genes that mediate breast cancer metastasis to lung. Nature 436:518-524 (2005).

Misteli, T. et al. Nature 408:877-881 (2000).

Moghimi, S.M. et al. Nanomedicine:current status and future prospects. FASEB J. 19:311-330 (2005).

Mohandas, K.M. Genetic predisposition to cancer. Curr. Sci. 81:482-489 (2001).

Moody, D.B. How a T cell sees sugar. Nature 448:36-37 (2007).

Moolten, F.L. Cancer Res. 46:5276-5768 (1986).

Moon, R. et al. Science 316:1043-1046 (2007).

Moore, G.L. et al. Predicting crossover generation in DNA shuffling. PNAS (USA) 98:3226-3231 (2001).

Moore, P.S., Chang, Y. Kaposi's sarcoma-assciated herpesvirus immunoevasion and tumourigenesis: two sides of the same coin? Annu. Rev. Microbiol. 57:609-639 (2003).

Mornet, S. et al. J. Mater. Chem. 14:2161 (2004).

Morreale, G. et al. Bioprocess-centered molecular design (BMD) for the efficient production of an interfacially active peptide. Biotechnol. Bioeng. 87:912-923 (2004).

Morrison, S.J., Kimble, J. Asymmetric and symmetric stem-cell divisions in development and cancer. Nature 441:1068-1074 (2006).

Mrozek, E. et al. Ann. Oncol. 16:1087 (2005).

Mueller, K., Zieris, K. Arch. Pharm. (Weinheim) 325:219-223 (1992).

Muggia, F.M. Curr. Oncol. Rep. 3:156-162 (2001).

Muller, H.J. Artificial transmutation of the gene. Science 66:84-87 (1927).

Müller, S., Hanisch, F.G. Recombinant MUC1 probe authentically reflects cell-specific O-glycosylation profiles of endogenous breast cancer mucin. High density and prevalent core 2-based glycosylation. J. Biol. Chem. 277:26103-26112 (2002).

Mullin, G.E., Dobs, A. Vitamin D and its role in cancer and immunity:a prescription for sunlight. Nutr. Clin. Pract. 22:305-322 (2007).

Murby, M. et al. Hydrophobicity engineering to increase solubility and stability of a recombinant protein from respiratory syncytial virus. Eur. J. Biochem. 230:38-14 (1995).

Murgia, C. et al. Cell 126:477-487 (2007).

Nador, R.G. et al. Primary effusion lymphoma:a distinct clinicopathologic entity associated with the Kaposi's sarcoma-associated herpes virus. Blood 88:645-656 (1996).

Narita, M., Lowe, S.W. Nature Med. 11:920-922 (2005).

Naugler, W.E. et al. Gender disparity in liver cancer due to sex differences in MyD88-dependent IL-6 production. Science 317:121-124 (2007).

Neuberger, T. et al. J. Magn. Mater. 293:483 (2005).

Newton, J.R. et al. Neoplasia 8:772 (2006).

Nichkova, M. et al. Anal. Chem. 77:6864 (2005).

Nicklin, S.A. et al. In vitro and in vivo characterization of endothelial cell selective adenoviral vectors. J. Gen. Med. 6:300-308 (2004).

Nicolaou, K.C., Mitchell, H.J. Adventures in carbohydrate chemistry:new synthetic technologies, chemical synthesis, molecular design, and chemical biology. Angew. Chem. Int. Ed. 40:1576-1624 (2001).

Nicolaou, K.C., Snyder, S.A. The essence of total synthesis. PNAS (USA) 101:11929-11936 (2004).

Niemeyer, C.M. Bioconjugation Protocols:Strategies and Methods. Humana Press, Totowa, New Jersey (2004).

Nieth, C. et al. Modulation of the classical multidrug resistance (MDR) phenotype by RNA interference (RNAi). FEBS Lett. 545:144-150 (2003).

NIH. Near-Term Technology Development for Genome Sequencing. Natl. Inst. of Health, Bethesda, RFA-HG-04-002 (Feb. 2004).

Nilsson, C.L. Bacterial proteomics and vaccine development. Am. J. Pharmacogenomics 2:49-65 (2002).

Nobile, C. et al. Covert human immunodeficiency virus replication in dendritic cells and in DC-SIGN-expressing cells promotes long-term transmission to lymphocytes. J. Virol. 79:5386-5399 (2005).

Noguera-Troise, I. et al. Blockade of DII4 inhibits tumour growth by promoting non-productive angiogenesis. Nature 444:1032-1037 (2006).

Nord, K. et al. Nature Biotechnol. 15:772 (1997).

Norval, M. et al. The effects on human health from stratospheric ozone depletion and its interactions with climate change. Photochem. Photobiol. Sci. 6:232-251 (2007).

Norval, M. et al. Health effects (Unpublished work – UNEP Panel, Malaysia, Aug. 2007).

Nossal, G.J.V., Lederberg, J. Antibody production by single cells. Nature 181:1419-1420 (1958).

Nossal, G.J.V. The double helix and immunology. Nature 421:440-444 (2003).

Nurse, R. Converging on ▯-catenin in Wilms tumour. Science 316:988-989 (2007).

O'Brien, C.A. et al. A human colon cancer cell capable of initiating tumour growth in immunodeficient mice. Nature 445:106-110 (2007).

O'Neal, D.P. et al. Photo-thermal tumour ablation in mice using near infrared-absorbing nanoparticles. Cancer Lett. 209:171-176 (2004).

O'Neill, J. et al. Promises and challenges of targeting Bcl-2 anti-apoptotic proteins for cancer therapy. Biochim. Biophys. Acta 1705:43-51 (2004).

O'Brien, S.G. et al. N. Engl. J. Med. 348:994-1004 (2003).

O'Connell, J.B. et al. Colon cancer survival rates with the new American Joint Committee on Cancer sixth edition staging. J. Natl. Cancer Inst. 96:1420-1425 (2005).

Odenbach, S. Great benefits from the smallest particles. German Res 1:18-21 (2007).

Oh, J.S. et al. Clin. Vaccine. Immunol. 13:520 (2006).

Ohashi, Y. & 15 others. Habitual intake of lactic acid bacteria and risk reduction of bladder cancer. Urol. Int. 68:273-280 (2002).

Ohsumi, Y., Molecular dissection of autophagy:two ubiquitin-like systems. Nature Rev. Mol. Cell Biol. 2:211-216 (2001).

Okita, K., Ichisaka, T., Yamanaka, S. Generation of germline-competent induced pluripotent stem cells. Nature 448:313-317 (2007).

Okuhata, Y. Adv. Drug Delivery Rev. 37:121 (1999).

Old, L.J., Chen, Y.T. New paths in human cancer serology. J. Exp. Med. 187:1163-1167 (1998).

Orimo, A. et al. Stromal fibroblasts present in invasive human breast carcinomas promote tumour growth and angiogenesis through elevated SDF-1/CXCL12 secretion. Cell 121:335-348 (2005).

Ouerfelli, O. et al. Synthetic carbohydrate-based antitumour vaccines:challenges and opportunities. Expert Rev. Vaccines 4:677-685 (2005).

Overwijk, W.W., Restifo, N.P. Autoimmunity and the immunotherapy of cancer:targeting the "self" to destroy the "other". Crit. Rev. Immunol. 20:433-450 (2000).

Paciotti, G.F. et al. Colloidal gold:a novel nanoparticle vector for tumour directed drug delivery. Drug Deliv. 11:169-183 (2004).

Padilla, De Jesus, O.L. et al. Bioconjug. Chem. 13:453 (2002).

Paegel, B.M. et al. High throughput DNA sequencing with a microfabricated 96-lane capillary array electrophoresis bioprocessor. PNAS (USA) 99:574-579 (2002).

Paegel, B.M., Blazej, R.G., Mathies, R.A. Curr. Opin. Biotechnol. 14:42-50 (2003).

Paez, J.G. et al. EGFR mutations in lung cancer:Corelation with clinical response to Gefitinib therapy. Science 304:1497-1500 (2004).

Pagliaro, L.C. et al. Repeated intravesical instillations of an adenoviral vector in patients with locally advanced bladder cancer:a phase I study of p53 gene therapy. J. Clin. Oncol. 21:2247-2253 (2003).

Paik, S. et al. A multigene assay to predict recurrence of tamoxifen-treated, node-negative breast cancer. N. Engl. J. Med. 351:2817-2826 (2004).

Pal, S.K. Use of alternative cancer medicines in India. Lancet Oncol. 3:394-395 (2002).

Pal, S.K. Complementary and alternative medicine:overview. Curr. Sci. 82:518-524 (2002a).

Pal, S.K. Cancer treatment with traditional herbal medicines. Curr. R&D Highlights, 26-31 (April-June, 2006).

Pal, S.K., Fatima, S.H., Mehrotra, R. Oral cancer treatment with an alternative poly-herbal therapy 'HUMA' in two patients with advanced disease. Elements 4:12-16 (2006).

Palmer, D.H., Young, L.S., Mautner, V. Cancer gene-therapy:clinical trials. TIBTECH 24:76-82 (2006).

Pankhurst, Q.A. et al. J. Phys. D. Appl. Phys. 36:R167 (2003).

Pantophlet, R., Burton, D.R. gp120:target for neutralizing HIV-1 antibodies. Annu. Rev. Immunol. 24:739-769 (2006).

Papadopoulos, N., Kinzler, K.W., Vogelstein, B. The role of companion diagnostics in the development and use of mutation-targeted cancer therapies. Nature Biotechnol. 24:985-995 (2006).

Parada, L.A. et al. Curr. Biol. 12:1692-1697 (2002).

Park, S.I. et al. J. Magn. Magn. Mater. 304:e406 (2006).

Park, T.K. et al. Total synthesis and proof of structure of a human breast tumour (globo-H) antigen. J. Am. Chem. Soc. 118:11488-11500 (1996).

Park, Y.G. et al. Sipa1 is a candidate for the metastasis efficiency modifier locus Mtes1. Nature Genet. 37(10):1055-1062 (2005).

Parkinson, G.N., Lee, M.P.H., Neidle, S. Crystal structure of parallel quadruplexes from human telomeric DNA. Nature 417:876-880 (2002).

Paroo, Z., Corey, D.R. Challenges for RNAi in vivo. TIBTECH 22:390-394 (2004).

Parson, A.B. The Proteus Effect:Stem Cells and Their Promise for Medicine. Joseph Henry Press (2004).

Pashov, A. et al. Antigenic properties of peptide mimotopes of HIV-1-associated carbohydrate antigens. J. Biol. Chem. 280:28959-28965 (2005).

Passegue, E. A game of subversion. Nature 442:754-755 (2006).

Patolsky, F. et al. J. Am. Chem. Soc. 125(46):13918 (2003).

Patolsky, F. et al. Electrical detection of single viruses. PNAS (USA) 101(39):14017-14022 (2004).

Pattenden, L.K. et al. Towards the preparative and large-scale precision manufacture of virus-like particles. TIBTECH 23:523-529 (2005).

Patton, W.F. Detection technologies in proteome analysis. J. Chromatogr. B771:3-31 (2002).

Paweletz, C.P. et al. Reverse phase protein micro-arrays which capture disease progression show activation of pro-survival pathways at the cancer invasion front. Oncogene 20:1981-1989 (2001).

Peabody, D.S., Al-Bitar, L. Isolation of viral coat protein mutants with altered assembly and aggregation properties. Nucleic Acids Res. 29:E113 (2001).

Pearce, M.S. et al. Skin cancer in children and young adults:28 years experience from the Northern Region Young Person's Malignant Disease Registry, UK. Melanoma Res. 13:421-426 (2003).

Pearse, A.M., Swift, K. Transmission of devil facial-tumour disease. Nature 439:549 (2006).

Pearson, H. Beyond the double helix. Nature 421:310-312 (2003).

Peek, R.M. Jr., Blaser, M.J. Helicobacter pylori and gastrointestinal tract adenocarcinomas. Nature Rev. Cancer 2:28-37 (2002).

Pegram, M.D., Konecny, G., Slamon, D.J. The molecular and cellular biology of HER2/neu gene amplification/overexpression and the clinical development of Herceptin (trastuzumab) therapy for breast cancer. Cancer Treat. Res. 103:57-75 (2000).

Pelham, R.J. et al. Identification of alterations in DNA copy number in host stromal cells during tumour progression. PNAS (USA) 103:19848-19853 (2006).

Pellieux, C., Dewilde, A., Pierlot, C., Aubry, J.M. Methods Enzymol. 319:197-207 (2000).

Pellman, D. Aneuploidy and cancer. Nature 446:38-39 (2007).

Pellois, J.P. et al. Individually addressable parallel peptide synthesis on microchips. Nature Biotechnol. 20:922-926 (2002).

Pennisi, E. DNA's molecular gymnastics. Science 312:1467-1468 (2006).

Perl, A.K. et al. Reduced expression of neural cell adhesion molecule induces metastatic dissemination of pancreatic □ tumour cells. Nature Med. 5:286-291 (1999).

Peto, R. et al. Can dietary beta carotene materially reduce human cancer rates? Nature 290:201-207 (1981).

Petricoin, E.F. et al. Clinical proteomics:translating benchside promise into bedside reality. Nature Rev. Drug Discov. 1:683-695 (2002).

Petros, J.A. et al. mtDNA mutation increase tumourigenicity in prostate cancer. PNAS (USA) 102:719-724 (2005).

Phair, R.D., Misteli, T. High mobility of protein in mammalian cell nucleus. Nature 404:604-609 (2000).

Pharoah, P.D.P. et al. Polygenic susceptibility to breast cancer and implications for prevention. Nature Genet. 31:33-36 (2002).

Phiel, C.J. et al. Histone deacetylase is a direct target of valproic acid, a potent anticonvulsant, mood stabilizer, and teratogen. J. Biol. Chem. 276:36734-36741 (2001).

Piccart-Gebhart, M.J. et al. N. Engl. J. Med. 353:1659-1672 (2005).

Piccirillo, S.G.M. et al. Bone morphogenetic proteins inhibit the tumourigenic potential of human brain tumour-initiating cells. Nature 444:761-765 (2006).

Pierceall, W.E. et al. Mutations in the p53 tumour-suppressor gene in human cutaneous squamous cell carcinomas. Mol. Carcinog. 4:445-449 (1991).

Pinaud, F. et al. Biomaterials 27:1679 (2006).

Pinhasov, A. et al. Gene expression analysis for high throughput screening applications. Comb. Chem. High Throughput Screen. 7, 133-140 (2004).

Pipas, J.M. Common and unique features of T antigens encoded by the polyomavirus group. J. Virol. 66:3979-3985 (1992).

Pissuwan, D., Valenzuela, S.M., Cortie, M.B. Therapeutic possibilities of plasmonically heated gold nanoparticles. TIBTECH 24:62-67 (2006).

Pollard, J.W. Tumour-educated macrophages promote tumour progression and metastasis. Nature Rev. Cancer 4:71-78 (2004).

Ponsonby, A.L., Lucas, R.M., van der Mei, I.A. UVR, vitamin D and three autoimmune diseases – multiple sclerosis, type 1 diabetes, rheumatoid arthritis. Photochem. Photobiol. 81:1267-1275 (2005).

Pontecorvo, G. Trends in Genetic Analysis. Columbia Univ. Press, New York (1958).

Portakal, O. et al. Coenzyme Q10 concentrations and antioxidant status in tissue of breast cancer patients. Clin. Biochem. 33:279-284 (2000).

Qu, X. et al. Promotion of tumourigenesis by heterozygous disruption of the beclin 1 autophagy gene. J. Clin. Invest. 112:1809-1820 (2003).

Quaranta, V. et al. Clin. Chim. Acta 24:173-179 (2005).

Quillin, P. Beating Cancer With Nutrition. Nutrition Times Press, Tulsa (2001).

Radisky, D.C. et al. Rac1b and reactive oxygen species mediate MMP-3 induced EMT and genomic instability. Nature 436:123-127 (2005).

Ragupathi, G. Carbohydrate antigens as targets for active specific immunotherapy. Cancer Immunol. Immunother. 43:152-157 (1996).

Ragupathi, G., Gathuru, J., Livingston, P. Antibody inducing polyvalent cancer vaccines. Cancer Treat. Res. 123:157-180 (2005).

Rainov, N.G. A phase III clinical evaluation of herpes simplex virus type 1 thymidine kinase and ganciclovir gene therapy as an adjuvant to surgical resection and radiation in adults with previously untreated glioblastoma multiforme. Hum. Gene Ther. 11:2389-2401 (2000).

Rajagopalan, H. et al. Nature Rev. Cancer 3:695-701 (2003).

Rajendran, J.G., Krohn, K.A. pp. 689-696. In:Bailey, D.L. et al. (eds.). Positron Emission Tomography: Principles and Practice. Springer, London (2002).

Rakoff-Nahoum, S., Medzhitov, R. Regulation of spontaneous intestinal tumourigenesis through the adaptor protein MyD88. Science 317:124-127 (2007).

Ranson, M. Epidermal growth factor receptor tyrosine kinase inhibitors. Br. J. Cancer 90:2250-2255 (2004).

Reimer, A.B. et al. Induction of IgG antibodies against the GD2 carbohydrate tumour antigen by vaccination with peptide mimotopes. Eur. J. Immunol. 36:1267-1274 (2006).

Rickinson, A., Kieff, E. Epstein-Barr virus. Pp. 2575-2627. In:Knipe, D.M., Howley, P.M. (eds.). vide supra (2001).

Ridgway, J. et al. Inhibition of Dll4 signalling inhibits tumour growth deregulating angiogenesis. Nature 444:1083-1087 (2006).

Rivera, M.N., Haber, D.A. Nature Rev. Cancer 5:699 (2005).

Rivera, M.N. et al. An X chromosome gene, WTX, is commonly inactivated in Wilms tumour. Science 315:642-646 (2007).

Robbins, R.J. et al. J. Clin. Endocrinol. Metab. 91:498-505 (2006).

Roberts, A.B., Wakefield, L.M. The two faces of transforming growth factor (beta) in carcinogenesis. PNAS (USA) 100:8621-8623 (2003).

Roberts, L.K., Daynes, R.A. Modification of the immunogenic properties of chemically induced tumours arising in hosts treated concomitantly with ultraviolet light. J. Immunol. 125:438-447 (1980).

Roberts, R.J., Cheng, X. Annu. Rev. Biochem. 67:181-198 (1998).

Robinson, W.H. et al. Autoantigen micro-arrays for multiplex characterization of autoantibody responses. Nature Med. 8:295-301 (2002).

Robosky, L.C. et al. In vivo toxicity screening programs using metabonomics. Comb. Chem. High Throughput Screen 5:651-662 (2002)

Rogulski, K.R. et al. Double suicide gene therapy augments the antitumour activity of a replication-competent lytic adenovirus through enhanced cytotoxicity and radiosensitization. Hum. Gene Ther. 11:67-76 (2000).

Rolan, P. et al. Use of biomarkers from drug discovery through clinical practice:Report, 9th Europ. Fed. Pharma. Sci. Conf. on Optimizing Drug Development. Clin. Pharmacol. Ther. 73:284-291 (2003).

Romond, E.H. et al. N. Engl. J. Med. 353:1673-1684 (2005).

Rosengart, A.J. et al. J. Magn. Magn. Mater. 293:633 (2005).

Rossant, J. The magic brew. Nature 448:260-262 (2007).

Roth, J.A. et al. p53 tumour-suppressor gene therapy for cancer. Oncology (Williston Park) 13 (Suppl. 5):148-154 (1999).

Rountree, M.R. et al. DNA methylation, chromatin inheritance, and cancer. Oncogene 20:3156-3165 (2001).

Rowinsky, E.K. Signal events:cell signal transduction and its inhibition in cancer. Oncologist 8 (Suppl. 3):5-17 (2003).

Rozkov, A., Enfors, S.O. Analysis and control of proteolysis of recombinant proteins in Escherichia coli. Adv. Biochem. Eng. Biotechnol. 89:163-195 (2004).

Rubenwolf, S. et al. Functional proteomics using chromophore-assisted laser inactivation. Proteomics 2:241-246 (2002).

Rudin, M., Weissleder, R. Molecular imaging in drug discovery and development. Nature Rev. Drug Discov. 2, 123-131 (2003).

Rueda, P. et al. Effect of different baculovirus inactivation procedures on the integrity and immunogenicity of porcine parvovirus-like particles. Vaccine 19:726-734 (2000).

Ruffner, H. et al. PNAS (USA) 98:5134 (2001).

Ryan, R.M., Green, J., Lewis, C.E. Bioessays 28:84 (2006).

Saal, L.H. et al. Poor prognosis in carcinoma is associated with a gene expression signature of aberrant PTEN tumour suppressor pathway activity. PNAS (USA) 104:7564-7569 (2007).

Sabatini, D.M. mTOR and cancer:insights into a complex relationship. Nature Rev. Cancer 6:729-734 (2006).

Saebo, K.B. (Ed.). Comprehensive Summaries of Uppsala Dissertations from the Faculty of Medicine. Uppsala University, Sweden (2004).

Sagata, N. Untangling checkpoints. Science 298:1905-1906 (2002).

Sahin, U. et al. Human neoplasms elicit multiple specific immune responses in the autologous host. PNAS (USA) 92:11810-11813 (1995).

Sakakura, C. et al. Inhibition of colon cancer cell proliferation by antisense oligonucleotides targeting the messenger RNA of the Ki-ras gene. Anticancer Drugs 6:553-561 (1995).

Salata, O.V. Applications of nanoparticles in biology and medicine. J. Nanobiotech. 2:3 (2004).

Sala-Tora, O. et al. Biol. Blood Marrow Transplant. 12:511-517 (2006).

Saluz, H.P., Jiricny, J., Jost, J.P. Genomic sequencing reveals a positive correlation between the kinetics of strand specific DNA demethylation of the overlapping estradiol/glucocorticoid receptor binding site and the rate of avian vitellogenin mRNA synthesis. PNAS (USA) 83:7167-7171 (1986).

Sampson, J.R. et al. MutYH (MYH) and colorectal cancer. Biochem. Soc. Trans. 33:679-683 (2005).

Samuels, Y. et al. High frequency of mutations of the PIK3CA gene in human cancers. Science 304:554-555 (2004).

Sasongko, L. et al. Clin. Pharmacol. Ther. 77:503-514 (2005).

Satchi-Fainaro, R. et al. PDEPT:polymer-directed enzyme prodrug therapy. 2. HPMA copolymer-beta-lactamase and HPMA copolymer C-Dox as a model combination. Bioconjug. Chem. 14:797-804 (2003).

Satchi-Fainaro, R. et al. Targeting angiogenesis with a conjugate of HPMA copolymer and TNP-470. Nature Med. 10:255-261 (2004).

Satyakumar, S., Babu, R.S. Nanotechnology:A new approach in cancer therapy. Pharma Times 38(4) (April 2006).

Satyanarayana, L., Asthana, S. Uterine cervical cancer – prevention and control. Curr. Sci. 93:447-448 (2007).

Sawyer, J.S. et al. J. Med. Chem. 46:3953-3956 (2003).

Sawyers, C. Targeted cancer therapy. Nature 432:294-297 (2004).

Scanlan, C.N. et al. The broadly neutralizing anti-human immunodeficiency virus type 1 antibody 2G12 recognizes a cluster of a1□2 mannose residues on the outer face of gp120. J. Virol. 76:7306-7321 (2002).

Scanlan, C.N. et al. Exploiting the defensive sugars of HIV-1 for drug and vaccine design. Nature 446:1038-1045 (2007).

Scanlan, M.J. et al. Characterization of human colon cancer antigens recognized by autologous antibodies. Int. J. Cancer 76:652-658 (1998).

Scanlan, M.J. et al. Antigens recognized by autologous antibody in patients with renal-cell carcinoma. Int. J. Cancer 83:456-464 (1999).

Scanlan, M.J. et al. Humoral immunity to human breast cancer:Antigen definition and quantitative analysis of mRNA expression. Cancer Immunity 1:4 (2001).

Schiedlmeier, B. et al. Multidrug resistance 1 gene transfer can confer chemoprotection to human peripheral blood progenitor cells engrafted in immunodeficient mice. Hum. Gene Ther. 13:233-242 (2002).

Schieke, S.M. et al. The mammalian target of rapamycin (mTOR) pathway regulates mitochondrial oxygen consumption and oxidative capacity. J. Biol. Chem. 281:27643-27652 (2006).

Schmitz, V. et al. Treatment of colorectal and hepatocellular carcinomas by adenoviral mediated gene transfer of endostatin and angiostatin-like molecule in mice. Gut 53:561-567 (2004).

Schneider, D. et al. J. Mol. Biol. 228:862 (1992).

Schneider, R.M. et al. Directed evolution of retroviruses activable by tumour-associated matrix metalloproteases. Gene Ther. 10:1370-1380 (2003).

Schulze, R. Global radiation climate (German). Wiss. Forschungsber. 72:1-220 (1970).

Schwartz, G.G., Skinner, H.G. Vitamin D status and cancer:new insights. Curr. Opin. Clin. Nutr. Metab. Care 10:6-11 (2007).

Schweitzer, B. et al. Micro-arrays to characterize protein interactions on a whole-proteome scale. Proteomics 3, 2190-2199 (2003).

Schweitzer, C., Schmidt, R. Chem. Rev. 103:1685-1757 (2003).

Sebolt-Leopold, J.S., English, J.M. Mechanisms of drug inhibition of signalling molecules. Nature 441:457-462 (2006).

Seeberger, P.H., Werz, D.B. Synthesis and medical applications of oligosaccharides. Nature 446:1046-1051 (2007).

Seeman, N.C. TIBS 30:119-125 (2005).

Seitz, O., Kunz, H. A novel allylic anchor for solid-phase synthesis – synthesis of protected and unprotected O-glycosylated mucin-type glycopeptides. Angew. Chem. Int. Ed. 34:803-805 (1995).

Sellers, T.A. et al. Dietary folate intake, alcohol, and risk of breast cancer in prospective study of postmenopausal women. Epidemiology 12:420-428 (2001).

Service, R.F. New probes. Open windows on gene expression, and more. Science 280:1010-1011 (1998).

Service, R.F. Protein chips map yeast kinase network. Science 307:1854-1855 (2005).

Service, R.F. Nanotechnology takes aim at cancer. Science 310:1132-1134 (2005).

Seymour, R.M. et al. Evolution of the human ABO polymorphism by two complementary selective pressures. Proc. R. Soc. Lond. B271:1065-1072 (2004).

Shangguan, D. et al. Aptamers evolved from live cells as effective molecular probes for cancer study. PNAS (USA) 103:11838-11843 (2006).

Shankaran, V. et al. IFNγ and lymphocytes prevent primary tumour development and shape tumour immunogenicity. Nature 410:1107 (2001).

Sharma, S.V. et al. Nature Rev. Cancer 7:169-181 (2007).

Sharpless, N.E., DePinho, R.A. Gone but not forgotten. Nature 445:606-607 (2007).

Shaw, C.F., III. Gold-based therapeutic agents. Chem. Rev. 99:2589-2600 (1999).

Shaw, R.J., Cantley, L.C. Ras, PI(3)K and mTOR signalling controls tumour cell growth. Nature 441:424-430 (2006).

Shendure, J. et al. Accurate multiplex polony sequencing of an evolved bacterial genome. Science 309:1728-1732 (2005).

Shestopalov, I. et al. Lab-on-a-Chip 4:316 (2004).

Shih, C., Weinberg, R.A. Isolation of a transforming sequence from a human bladder carcinoma cell line. Cell 29:161-169 (1982).

Shin, H., Markey, M.K. A machine learning perspective on the development of clinical decision support systems utilizing mass spectra of blood samples. J. Biomed. Inform. 39:227-248 (2006).

Shipitsin et al. Cancer 11:259 (2007).

Shukla, S. et al. Synthesis and biological evaluation of folate receptor-targeted boronated PAMAM dendrimers as potential agents for neutron capture therapy. Bioconjug. Chem. 14:158-167 (2003).

Shukla, Y., Pal, S.K. Complementary and alternative cancer therapies:past, present and the future scenario. Asian Pac. J. Cancer Prev. 5:3-14 (2004).

Shum, P. Phototriggering of liposomal drug delivery systems. Adv. Drug Deliv. Rev. 53:273-284 (2001).

Siddiqui-Jain, A. et al. Direct evidence for a G-quadruplex in a promoter region and its targeting with a small molecule to repress c-MYC transcription. PNAS (USA) 99:11593-11598 (2002).

Siekmann, A.F., Lawson, N.D. Notch signalling limits angiogenic cell behaviour in developing zebrafish arteries. Nature 445:781-784 (2007).

Silva, J. et al. RNA-interference-based functional genomics in mammalian cells:reverse genetics coming of age. Oncogene 23:8401-8409 (2004).

Silver, L.M. Stalking life's second secret. Nature 431:905-906 (2004).

Silverman, J. et al. Multivalent avimer proteins evolved by exon shuffling of a family of human receptor domains. Nature Biotechnol. 23:1556 (2005).

Simberg, D. et al. Biomimetic amplification of nanoparticle homing to tumours. PNAS (USA) 932-936 (2007).

Simon, R., Wang, S.-J. Pharmacogenomics J., published online (17 Jan. 2006).

Simoneau, A.R. Rev. Urol. 2 (Suppl. 8):S56-S67 (2006).

Singh, S.K. et al. Identification of human brain tumour initiating cells. Nature 432:396-400 (2004).

Sjöblom, T. et al. The consensus coding sequences of human breast and colorectal cancers. Science 314:268-274 (2006).

Slamon, D.J. et al. N. Engl. J. Med. 344:783-792 (2001).

Slepushkin, V. et al. Methods Enzymol. 387:134 (2004).

Sliney, D.H. Physical factors in cataractogenesis:ambient ultraviolet radiation and temperature. Invest. Ophthalmol. Visual Sci. 27:781-790 (1986).

Slovin, S.F. et al. Carbohydrate vaccines in cancer:immunogenicity of a fully synthetic globo H hexasaccharide conjugates in man. PNAS (USA) 96:5710-5715 (1999).

Slovin, S.F., Keding, S.J., Ragupathi, G. Carbohydrate vaccines as immunotherapy for cancer. Immunol. Cell Biol. 83:418-428 (2005).

Smith, J.E. et al. Trends Anal. Chem. 25:848 (2006).

Smith-Warner, S.A. et al. Alcohol and breast cancer in women:a pooled analysis of cohort studies. JAMA 279:535-540 (1998).

So, E. et al. Cancer Cell 3:161-171 (2003).

Sobhian, B. et al. RAP80 targets BRCA1 to specific ubiquitin structure at DNA damage sites. Science 316:1198-1199 (2007).

Soda, M. et al. Identification of the transforming EML4-ALK fusion gene in non-small cell lung cancer. Nature 448:561-566 (2007).

Sofuni, A. et al. J. Gastroenterol. 40:518-525 (2005).

Sotiriou, C., et al. Breast cancer classification and prognosis based on gene expression profile from a population based study. PNAS (USA) 100:10393-10398 (2003).

Soussi, T. The humoral response to the tumour-supressor gene product p53 in human cancer:implications for diagnosis and therapy. Immunol. Today 17:354-356 (1996).

Sova, P. et al. A tumour-targeted and conditionally replicating oncolytic adenovirus vector expressing TRAIL for treatment of liver metastases. Mol. Ther. 9:496-509 (2004).

Speicher, M.R., Carter, N.P. Nature Rev. Genet. 6:782-792 (2005).

Stallings, R.L. Are chromosomal imbalances important in cancer? Trends Genet. 23:278-283 (2007).

Steeg, P.S. Metastasis suppressors alter the signal transduction of cancer cells. Nature Rev. Cancer 3:55-53 (2003).

Steeg, P.S. Micromanagement of metastasis. Nature 449:671-673 (2007).

Steinman, R.M., Mellman, I. Immunotherapy:Bewitched, bothered, and bewildered no more. Science 305:197-200 (2004).

Steitz, J. et al. Evaluation of genetic melanoma vaccines in cdk4-mutant mice provides evidence for immunological tolerance against authochthonous melanomas in the skin. Int. J. Cancer 118:373-380 (2006).

Stemmer, W.P. Rapid evolution of a protein in vitro by DNA shuffling. Nature 370:389-391 (1994).

Stenbäck, F. Studies on the modifying effect of ultraviolet radiation on chemical skin carcinogenesis. J. Invest. Dermatol. 64:253-257 (1975).

Stephens, P. et al. Intragenic ERBB2 kinase mutations in tumours. Nature 431:525-526 (2004).

Stephens, P. et al. Nature Genet. 37:590-592 (2005).

Stewart, G.S. et al. Nature 421:961 (2003).

Stiles, M.E., Holzapfel, W.H. Lactic acid bacteria of foods and their current taxonomy. Int. J. Food Microbiol. 36:1-29 (1997).

Stix, G. Blockbuster dreams. Sci. Amer. 295:60-63 (May 2006).

Stix, G. A malignant flame. Sci. Amer. 297:60-67 (Jul. 2007).

Stoeckli, M. et al. Imaging mass spectrometry:a new technology for the analysis of protein expression in mammalian tissues. Nature Med. 7:493-496 (2001).

Strate, L.L., Syngal, S. Hereditary colorectal cancer syndromes. Cancer Causes Control 16:201-213 (2005).

Streit, M. et al. Thrombospondin-2:a potent endogenous inhibitor of tumour growth and angiogenesis. PNAS (USA) 96:14888-14893 (1999).

Sturm, R.A. Skin colour and skin cancer – MC1R, the genetic link. Melanoma Res. 12:405-416 (2002).

Stylianou, S., Clarke, R.B., Brennan, K. Aberrant activation of notch signalling in human breast cancer. Cancer Res. 66:1517-1525 (2006).

Su, Z. et al. A combinatorial approach for selectively including programmed cell death in human pancreatic cancer cell. PNAS (USA) 98:10332-10337 (2001).

Surh, Y.J. Cancer chemoprevention with dietary phytochemicals. Nature Rev. Cancer 3:768-780 (2003).

Takahashi, K., Yamanaka, S. Induction of pluripotent stem cells from mouse embryonic and adult fibroblast cultures by defined factors. Cell 126:663-676 (2006).

Takamura, S. et al. DNA vaccine-encapsulated virus-like particles derived from an orally transmissible virus stimulate mucosal and systemic immune responses by oral administration. Gene Ther. 11:628-635 (2004).

Takeda, K., Kaisho, T., Akira, S. Annu. Rev. Immunol. 21:335 (2003).

Tanabe, H. et al. Evolutionary conservation of chromosome territory arrangements in cell nuclei from higher primates. PNAS (USA) 99:4424-4429 (2002).

Tang, Z. et al. Spontaneous organization of single CdTe nanoparticles into luminescent nanowires. Science 297:237 (2002).

Tansil, N.C., Gao, Z. Nanoparticles in biomolecular detection. Nanotoday 1(1):28-37 (2006).

Tenesa, A. et al. Association of MutYH and colorectal cancer. Br. J. Cancer 95:239-242 (2006).

Terranova, R. et al. Histone and DNA methylation defects at Hox genes in mice expressing a SET domain-truncated form of Mll. PNAS (USA) 103:6629-6634 (2006).

Texter, J., Tirrell, M. Chemical processing by self-assembly. AIChE J. 47:1706-1710 (2001).

Thannickal, V.J., Fanburg, B.L. Am. J. Physiol. 279:L1005-L1028 (2000).

Theobald, M. et al. Targeting p53 as a general tumour antigen. PNAS (USA) 92:11993-11997 (1995).

Thiery, J.P. Epithelial-mesenchymal transitions in tumour progression. Nature Rev. Cancer 2:442-454 (2002).

Thomas, K.G., Kamat, P.V. Chromophore-functionalized gold nanoparticles. Acc. Chem. Res. 36:888-898 (2003).

Thompson, I.M. et al. J. Am. Med. Assoc. 294:66-70 (2005).

Thune, I. et al. Physical activity and the risk of breast cancer. New England J. Med. 336:1269-1275 (1997).

Thurston, G. et al. J. Clin. Invest. 101:1401 (1998).

Timoféeff-Ressovsky, N.W., Zimmer, K.G., Delbrück, M. Über die Natur der Genmutation und der Genkostruktur. Nachr. Ges. Wiss. Gottingen FG VI Biol. N.F. 1:189-245 (1935).

Tolar, J., Neglia, J.P. J. Pediatr. Hematol. Oncol. 25:430-434 (2003).

Tolley, D.A. et al. The effect of intravesical mitomycin C on recurrence of newly diagnosed superficial bladder cancer:A further report with 7 years of followup. J. Urol. 155:1233-1238 (1996).

Tomalia, D.A. Prog. Polym. Sci. 30:294 (2005).

Tomlinson, C.C., Damania, B. The K1 protein of Kaposi's sarcoma-associated herpesvirus activates the Akt signalling pathway. J. Virol. 78:1918-1927 (2004).

Tomlinson, R. et al. Pendent chain functionalized polyacetals that display pH-dependent degradation:a platform for the development of novel polymer therapeutics. Macromolecules 35:473-480 (2002).

Torchilin, V.P. Recent advances with liposomes as pharmaceutical carriers. Nature Rev. Drug Discov. 4:145-160 (2005).

Torrance, C.J. et al. Use of isogenic cancer cells for high-throughput screening and drug discovery. Nature Biotechnol. 19:940-945 (2001).

Touze, A., Coursaget, P. In vitro gene transfer using human papillomavirus-like particles. Nucleic Acids Res. 26:1317-1323 (1998).

Tsai, C.C. et al. Cyanovirin-N inhibits AIDS virus infections in vaginal transmission models. AIDS Res. Hum. Retroviruses 20:11-18 (2003).

Tsao, M.S. et al. Erlotinib in lung cancer – molecular and clinical predictors of outcome. N. Engl. J. Med. 353:133-144 (2005).

Turro, N.J., Chow, M.F., Rigaudy, J. J. Am. Chem. Soc. 101:1300-1302 (1979).

Turro, N.J., Chow, M.F. J. Am. Chem. Soc. 103:7218-7224 (1981).

Ummat, A. et al. Tissue Engineering and Artificial Organs. Pp. 1-42. In:Yarmush, M.L. CRC Press, Boca Raton (2006).

USDA. Nutrition and Your Health:Dietary Guidelines for Americans. US Dept. of Agriculture, Washington, D.C. (2000).

Vainio, H., Wilbourn, J., Tomatis, L. Identification of environmental carcinogens:the first step in risk assessment. In Mehlman, M.A., Upton, A. (eds.) The Identification and Control of Environmental and Occupational Diseases. Princeton Sci. Publ. Co., Princeton (1994).

Valiathan, M.S. Towards Ayurvedic Biology. Ind. Acad. Sci., Bangalore (2006).

Valk-Lingbeek, M.E., Bruggeman, S.W., van Lohuizen, M. Stem cells and cancer:the polycomb connection. Cell 118:409-418 (2004).

van de Vijver, M.J. et al. A gene-expression signature as a predictor of survival in breast cancer. N. Engl. J. Med. 347:1999-2009 (2002).

Van den Eynde, B. et al. A new family of genes coding for an antigen recognized by autologous cytolytic T lymphocytes on a human melanoma. J. Exp. Med. 182:689-698 (1995).

Van der Bruggen, P. et al. A gene encoding an antigen recognized by cytolytic T lymphocytes on a human melanoma. Science 254:1643-1647 (1991).

Van der Leun, J.C., de Gruijl, F.R. Climate change and skin cancer. Photochem. Photobiol. Sci. 1:324-326 (2002).

Van der Rhee, H.J., de Vries, E., Coebergh, J.W. Does sunlight prevent cancer? A systematic review. Eur. J. Cancer 42:2222-2232 (2006).

van Der Velden, J. et al. Effects of calcium, inorganic phosphate, and pH on isometric force in single skinned cardiomyocytes from donor and failing human hearts. Circulation 104:1140-1146 (2001).

Van Eyk, J.E. Proteomics:unravelling the complexity of heart disease and striving to change cardiology. Curr. Opin. Mol. Therapeut. 3:546-553 (2001).

Van Schanke, A. et al. Single UVB overexposure stimulates melanocyte proliferation in murine skin, in contrast to fractionated or UVA-1 exposure. J. Invest. Dermatol. 124:241-247 (2005).

van't Veer, L.J. et al. Gene expression profiling predicts clinical outcome of breast cancer. Nature 415:530-536 (2002).

van't Veer, P. et al. Consumption of fermented milk products and breast cancer:A case-control study in The Netherlands. Cancer Res. 49:4020-4023 (1989).

Varambally, S. et al. The polycomb group protein EZH2 is involved in progression of prostate cancer. Nature 419:624-629 (2002).

Varki, A. et al. Essentials of Glycobiology. Cold Spring Harbor Laboratory Press (1999).

Varmus, H. The new era in cancer research. Science 312:1162-1165 (2006).

Vassilev, L.T. et al. In vivo activation of the p53 pathway by small-molecule antagonists of MDM2. Science 303:844-848 (2004).

Vayalil, P., Kuttan, G., Kuttan, R. Protective effects of Rasayanas on cyclophosphamide and radiation-induced damage. J. Alter. Compl. Med. 8:787-796 (2002).

Venkitaraman, A.R. Cell 108:171 (2002).

Ventura, A. et al. Restoration of p53 function leads to tumour regression in vivo. Nature 445:661-665 (2007).

Vicent, M.J., Duncan, R. Polymer conjugates:nanosized medicines for treating cancer. TIBTECH 24:39-47 (2006).

Villa, L.L. et al. Prophylactic quadrivalent human papillomavirus (types 6, 11, 16, and 18) L1 virus-like particle vaccine in young women:a randomized double-blind placebo-controlled multicentre phase II efficacy trial. Lancet Oncol. 6:271-278 (2005).

Vliegenthart, J.F. Carbohydrate based vaccines. FEBS Lett. 580:2945-2950 (2006).

Vogelstein, B., Kinzler, K.W. (eds.). The Genetic Basis of Human Cancer. McGraw-Hill, New York (1998).

Vogelstein, B., Kinzler, K.W. Nature Med. 10:789-799 (2004).

Vogt, P.K., Kang, S., Elsliger, M.A., Gymnopoulos, M. Trends Biochem. Sci. 10.1016/j.tibs.2007.05.005 (2007).

Volkin, D.B. et al. Human papilloma virus vaccine with disassembled and reassembled virus-like particles. US Patent Office 6:245, 568 (2001).

von Eschenbach, A., Collins, F. http://cancergenome.nih.gov/about/TCGA_ executive_summary.pdf (2005).

Vondriska, T.M., Ping, P. Functional proteomics to study protection of the ischaemic myocardium. Expert Opin. Therapeut. Targets 6:563-570 (2002).

Waddington, C.H. An Introduction to Modern Genetics. Allen and Unwin, London (1939).

Walker, F., Olson, M.F. Targeting Ras and Rho GTPases as opportunities for cancer therapies. Curr. Opin. Genet. Dev. 15:62-68 (2005).

Wallace, D.C. Mitochondrial diseases in man and mouse. Science 283:1482-1488 (1999).

Wang, A.H.-J. et al. Molecular structure of a left-handed double helical DNA fragment at atomic resolution. Nature 282:680-686 (1979).

Wang, B. et al. Abraxas and RAP80 form a BRCA1 protein complex required for the DNA damage response. Science 316:1194-1196 (2007).

Wang, L. et al. Silica nanoparticles as fluorescent probes for bioanalytical application. Anal. Chem. 78:646-654 (2006).

Wang, L. et al. The Kaposi's sarcoma-associated herpesvirus (KSHV/HHV8) K1 protein induces expression of angiogenic and invasion factors. Cancer Res. 64:2774-2781 (2004).

Wang, L., Dai, W., Lu, L. Ultraviolet radiation-induced K(+) channel activity involving p53 activation in corneal epithelial cells. Oncogene 24:3020-3027 (2005).

Wang, S. et al. Nano Lett. 2(8):817 (2002).

Wang, Y. et al. Nature Genet. 37:750 (2005).

Wang, Y., Tang, Z., Kotov, N.A. Bioapplication of nanosemiconductors. Nanotoday, 20-31 (2005).

Watanabe, N. et al. Pancreas 13:395-400 (1996).

Watson, J.D., Crick, F.H.C. A structure for deoxyribose nucleic acid. Nature 171:737-738 (1953).

Watson, J.D. The Double Helix. A Personal Account of the Discovery of the Structure of DNA. Atheneum, New York (1968).

WCRC (World Cancer Research Fund and American Institute for Cancer Research). Food, Nutrition, and the Prevention of Cancer:A Global Perspective. Amer. Inst. Cancer Res., Washington, D.C. (1997).

Weaver, B.A. et al. Cancer Cell 11:25-36 (2007).

Weber, W.A. J. Nucl. Med. 46:983-995 (2005).

Wei, G. et al. Cancer Cell 10:331-342 (2006).

Wei, X. et al. Antibody neutralization and escape by HIV-1. Nature 422:307-312 (2003).

Weinberg, R.A. The Biology of Cancer. Garland Science, New York (2006).

Weinstein, I.B. Cancer. Addiction to oncogenes – the Achilles heal of cancer. Science 297:63-64 (2002).

Weinstein, J.N. et al. An information-intensive approach to the molecular pharmacology of cancer. Science 275:343-349 (1997).

Weinstein, J.N., Pommier, Y. Connecting genes, drugs and diseases. Nature Biotech. 24:1365-1366 (2006).

Weissleder, R. Molecular imaging in cancer. Science 312:1168-1170 (2006).

Welm, A.L. et al. The macrophage-stimulating protein pathway promotes metastasis in a mouse model for breast cancer and predicts poor prognosis in humans. PNAS (USA) 104:7570-7575 (2007).

Wernig, M. et al. In vitro reprogramming of fibroblasts into a pluripotent ES-cell-like state. Nature 448:318-324 (2007).

West, J.L., Halas, N.J. Applications of nanotechnology to biotechnology. Curr. Opin. Biotechnol. 11:215-217 (2000).

West, J.L., Halas, N.J. Engineered nanomaterials for biophotonics applications:improving sensing, imaging, and therapeutics. Annu. Rev. Biomed. Eng. 5:285-292 (2003).

Westbrook, J.A. et al. Zooming-in on the proteome:very narrow-range immobilized pH gradients reveal more protein species and isoforms. Electrophoresis 22:2865-2871 (2001).

Widder, K.J. et al. Proc. Soc. Exp. Biol. Med. 158:141 (1978).

Willard, D.M. et al. Nano Lett. 1(9):469 (2001).

Williams, C.L. Importance of dietary fibre in childhood. J. Am. Diet. Assoc. 95:1140-1146, 1149 (1995).

Willis, R.C. Good things in small packages. Nanotech advances are producing mega-results in drug delivery. Modern Drug Discov. 7:30-36 (2004).

Willuda, J. et al. Cancer Res. 59:5758 (1999).

Wilson, A.S., Power, B.E., Molloy, P.L. DNA hypomethylation and human diseases. Biochim. Biophys. Acta 1775:138-162 (2007).

Winterfeld, G.A., Khodair, A.I., Schmidt, R.R. O-glycosyl amino acids by 2-nitrogalactal concatenation – synthesis of a mucin-type O-glycan. Eur. J. Org. Chem. 1009-1021 (2003).

Wittwer, C.T. et al. BioTechniques 22:130-138 (1997).

Wodarz, D., Komarova, N. Can Loss of apoptosis protect against cancer? Trends Genet. 23:232-236 (2007).

Wolpowitz, D., Gilchrest, B.A. The vitamin D questions:how much do you need and how should you get it? J. Am. Acad. Dermatol. 54:301-317 (2006).

Wong, E.L., Damania, B. Linking KSHV to human cancer. Curr. Oncol. Rep. 7:349-356 (2005).

Wood, R.D. DNA repair in eukaryotes. Annu. Rev. Biochem. 65:135-167 (1996).

Woodcock, J. A Framework for Biomarker and Surrogate Endpoint Use in Drug Development. US Food and Drug Administration, Rockville, MD (2004).

Wooster, R. et al. Identification of the breast cancer susceptibility gene BRCA2. Nature 378:789-792 (1995).

Wu, C.-t. and Morris, J.R. Genes, genetics and epigenetics:A correspondence. Science 293:1103-1105 (2001).

Wu, X. et al. Immunofluorescent labelling of cancer marker Her2 and other cellular targets with semiconductor quantum dots. Nature Biotechnol. 21(1):41-46 (2003).

Xi, L.F. et al. Human papillomavirus type 16 and 18 variants:Race-related distribution and persistence. J. Natl. Cancer Inst. 15:1045-1052 (2006).

Xiao, Y. et al. Science 299:1877 (2003).

Xin, H. et al. High throughput siRNA-based functional target validation J. Biomol. Screen. 9, 286-293 (2004).

Xu, L.H. et al. Chem. Biol. 10:91 (2003).

Xue, W. et al. Senescence and tumour clearance is triggered by p53 restoration in murine liver carcinomas. Nature 445:656-660 (2007).

Yachi, A. et al. Immuno-chemical analysis of human adenocarcinoma-associated antigen YH206 detected by a monoclonal antibody. Jap. J. Med. 25:127-134 (1986).

Yamada, M. et al. Aged human skin removes UVB-induced pyrimidine dimers from the epidermis more slowly than younger adult skin in vivo. Arch. Dermatol. Res. 297:294-302 (2006).

Yamamoto, A. et al. Detection of autoantibodies against L-myc oncogene products in sera from lung cancer patients. Int. J. Cancer 22:283-289 (1996).

Yamamoto, M., Curiel, D.T. Technol. Cancer Res. Treat. 4:315 (2005).

Yan, J. et al. Dye-doped nanoparticles for bioanalysis. Nanotoday 2:44-50 (2007).

Yang, Y.A. et al. Lifetime exposure to a soluble TGF-□ antagonist protects mice against metastasis without adverse side effects. J. Clin. Invest. 109:1607-1615 (2002).

Yang, J. et al. Diagnosis of liver cancer using HPLC-based metabonomics avoiding false-positive results from hepatitis and hepatocirrhosis diseases. J. Chromatogr. B:Analyt. Technol. Biomed. Life Sci. 813:59-65 (2004).

Yarden, Y., Sliwkowski, M. Nature Rev. Mol. Cell Biol. 2:127-137 (2001).

Yin, H. et al. Biomaterials 26:5818 (2005).

Yoon, S.S. et al. An oncolytic herpes simplex virus type 1 selectively destroys diffuse liver metastases from colon carcinoma. FASEB J. 14:301-311 (2000).

You, C.-C., Chompoosor, A, Rotello, V.M. The biomacromolecule-nanoparticle interface. Nanotoday 2:34-42 (2007).

Yu, X. et al. The BRCT domain is a phosphor-protein binding domain. Science 302:639-643 (2003).

Zeelenberg, I.S., Ruuls-Van Stalle, L., Roos, E. The chemokine receptor CXCR4 is required for outgrowth of colon carcinoma micrometastases. Cancer Res. 63:3833-3839 (2003).

Zhang, X.W. et al. Molecular diagnosis of human cancer type by gene expression profiles and independent component analysis. Eur. J. Hum. Genet. 13:1303-1311 (2005).

Zhang, X. et al. Moving cancer diagnostics from bench to bedside. TIBTECH 25:166-173 (2007).

Zhao, X. et al. J. Am. Chem. Soc. 125:11474 (2003).

Zhao, X. et al. A rapid bioassay for single bacterial cell quantitation using bioconjugated nanoparticles. PNAS (USA) 101:15027-15032 (2004).

Zhou, B.-B.S., Elledge, S.J. The DNA damage response:putting checkpoints in perspective. Nature 408:433-439 (2000).

Zhou, G. et al. 2D differential in-gel electrophoresis for the identification of oesophageal scans; cell cancer-specific protein markers. Mol. Cell. Proteomics 1:117-124 (2001).

Zhou, S. & 17 others. Frequency and phenotypic implications of mitochondrial DNA mutations in human squamous cell cancers of the head and neck. PNAS (USA) 104:7540-7545 (2007).

Zhu, P. et al. Cell 124:615-629 (2006).

Zhu, X. et al. Synthesis of the trisaccharide and tetrasaccharide moieties of the potent immunoadjuvant QS21. Eur. J. Org. Chem. 965-973 (2004).

Zika, E., Gurwitz, D., Ibaretta, D. Pharmacogenetics and pharmacogenomics:state-of-the-art and potential socio-economic impact in the EU, Inst. Prosp. Technol. Studies and Europ. Commission Joint Res. Council (2006).

Zimmer, C. Evolved for cancer. Sci. Amer. 296:69-75 (2007).

Zimmermann, U., Pilwat, G. J. Biosci. 31:732 (1976).

Zingde, S.M. Cancer genes. Curr. Sci. 81:508-514 (2001).

Zinkernagel, R.M., Hengartner, H. Regulation of the immune response by antigen. Science 293:251-252 (2001).

Zitzmann, N. et al. Imino sugars inhibit the formation and secretion of bovine viral diarrhoea virus, a pestivirus model of hepatitis C virus:implications for the development of broad spectrum anti-hepatitis virus agents. PNAS (USA) 96:11878-11882 (1999).

Zolla-Pazner, S. Identifying epitopes of HIV-1 that induce protective antibodies. Nature Rev. Immunol. 4:199-210 (2004).

Zuo, X., Speicher, D.W. Comprehensive analysis of complex proteomes using microscale solution isoelectrofocusing prior to narrow pH range two-dimensional electrophoresis. Proteomics 2:58-68 (2002).

zur Hausen, H. Viruses in human cancers. Eur. J. Cancer 35:1174-1181 (1999).

Index

D

E

F

G